Gastrointestinal Function
in Diabetes Mellitus

Other titles in the Wiley *Diabetes in Practice* Series

Diabetic Nephropathy   (0 471 48992 1)
Edited by Christoph Hasslacher

Diabetes in Pregnancy: An International Approach to Diagnosis and Management   (0 471 96204 X)
Edited by Anne Dornhorst and David R. Hadden

Diabetic Complications   (0 471 96678 9)
Edited by Ken Shaw

Childhood and Adolescent Diabetes   (0 471 97003 4)
Edited by Simon Court and Bill Lamb

Hypoglycaemia in Clinical Diabetes   (0 471 98264 4)
Brian M. Frier and B. Miles Fisher

Exercise and Sport in Diabetes   (0 471 98496 5)
Edited by Bill Burr and Dinesh Nagi

Psychology of Diabetes Care   (0 471 97703 9)
Edited by Frank Snoek and T. Chas Skinner

The Foot in Diabetes Third Edition   (0 471 48974 3)
Edited by Andrew J. M. Boulton, Henry Connor and Peter R. Cavanagh

Nutritional Management of Diabetes Mellitus   (0 471 49751 7)
Edited by Gary Frost, Anne Dornhorst and Robert Moses

Gastrointestinal Function in Diabetes Mellitus

Edited by

Michael Horowitz

*Department of Medicine, University of Adelaide
and Endocrine and Metabolic Unit, Royal Adelaide Hospital
Adelaide, Australia*

Melvin Samsom

*Department of Gastroenterology and Hepatology
University Medical Centre
Utrecht, The Netherlands*

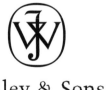

John Wiley & Sons, Ltd

This publication is designed to provide accurate and authoritative information in regard to the subject
matter covered. It is sold on the understanding that the Publisher is not engaged in rendering
professional services. If professional advice or other expert assistance is required, the services of a
competent professional should be sought.

Other Wiley Editorial Offices

John Wiley & Sons Inc., 111 River Street, Hoboken, NJ 07030, USA

Jossey-Bass, 989 Market Street, San Francisco, CA 94103-1741, USA

Wiley-VCH Verlag GmbH, Boschstr. 12, D-69469 Weinheim, Germany

John Wiley & Sons Australia Ltd, 33 Park Road, Milton, Queensland 4064, Australia

John Wiley & Sons (Asia) Pte Ltd, 2 Clementi Loop #02-01, Jin Xing Distripark, Singapore 129809

John Wiley & Sons Canada Ltd, 22 Worcester Road, Etobicoke, Ontario, Canada M9W 1L1

Wiley also publishes its books in a variety of electronic formats. Some content that appears
in print may not be available in electronic books.

Library of Congress Cataloging-in-Publication Data

Gastrointestinal function in diabetes mellitus / edited by Michael
Horowitz, Melvin Samsom.
      p. ; cm.—(Wiley diabetes in practice series)
Includes bibliographical references and index.
  ISBN 0-471-89916-X (cloth : alk. paper)
  1. Diabetes–Complications. 2. Gastrointestinal
system—Pathophysiology.
  [DNLM: 1. Diabetes Mellitus—complications. 2. Gastrointestinal
Motility. WK 840 G257 2004] I. Horowitz, Michael, 1953- II. Samsom,
Melvin. III. Diabetes in practice.
RC802.9 .G3625 2004
616.4'62—dc22
                                                        2003025309

British Library Cataloguing in Publication Data

A catalogue record for this book is available from the British Library

ISBN 0-471-89916-X

Typeset in 10.5/13pt Times by Laserwords Private Limited, Chennai, India
Printed and bound in Great Britain by TJ International, Padstow, Cornwall
This book is printed on acid-free paper responsibly manufactured from sustainable forestry
in which at least two trees are planted for each one used for paper production.

Contents

Gastrointestinal Function in Diabetes Mellitus.   Edited by Michael Horowitz and Melvin Samsom
© 2004 John Wiley & Sons, Ltd   ISBN: 0-471-89916-X

Preface

*'Would you tell me, please, which way I ought to go from here?' said Alice.
'That depends a good deal on where you want to get to', said the Cat. 'I don't
much care where', said Alice. 'Then it doesn't matter which way you go', said
the Cat. 'As long as I get somewhere', Alice added as an explanation. 'Oh,
you're sure to do that', said the Cat, 'if you only walk long enough'.*

Lewis Carroll, *Alice in Wonderland* (1856)

Progress might have been all right once, but it has gone on far too long.

Ogden Nash (1902–1971)

During the last 15–20 years, primarily as a result of the application of novel
investigative techniques, there has been a rapid expansion of knowledge relating
to the function of the gastrointestinal tract in diabetes mellitus. These insights
have been substantial and have led to the recognition that gastrointestinal function represents a hitherto inappropriately neglected, as well as important, aspect
of diabetes management. In particular, disordered gastrointestinal motor and
sensory function occur frequently in both type 1 and type 2 diabetes and may
be associated with significant clinical sequelae. Recent epidemiological studies
have established that there is a high prevalence of gastrointestinal symptoms in
the diabetic population and that these are associated with impaired quality of
life. Furthermore, upper gastrointestinal motility, even when normal, is central
to the regulation of postprandial blood glucose concentrations. Hence, diabetes
and the gastrointestinal tract are inextricably linked. The recent developments
in knowledge are not altogether surprising; although long recognised as a mul-
tisystem disorder, the history of diabetes since antiquity has been characterised
by periods of apparent neglect and rediscovery.

This book, which to our knowledge represents the first of its kind, was stimulated by the need to consolidate these advances, to illuminate an area that

Gastrointestinal Function in Diabetes Mellitus. Edited by Michael Horowitz and Melvin Samsom
© 2004 John Wiley & Sons, Ltd   ISBN: 0-471-89916-X

is perceived as increasingly important, but somewhat difficult to understand. Like Alice, the task we faced was somewhat daunting and has not proved easy. The book should also be viewed in context with the relatively recent, and fundamental, changes to the diagnosis and management of other aspects of diabetes—the latter relate particularly to recognition of the impact of chronic glycaemia and blood pressure control on both the development and progression of micro- and macro-vascular complications, and the effect of novel pharmaco-logical therapies. There have also been substantial changes to the processes of diabetes care and education, so that the challenges and demands made of the clinician/diabetologist have increased substantially—they should aim to achieve both euglycaemia and normal blood pressure in their patients. The primary rationale for our book is that a knowledge of gastroenterology, as it relates to diabetes, is also required.

The book aims to be comprehensive and to present the relevant information in context for both the clinician and clinical researcher. There are nine chapters: five are organ-specific, relating to oesophageal, gastric, intestinal, anorectal and hepatobiliary function; the four other chapters address epidemiological aspects of gastrointestinal function in diabetes, the effects of diabetes mellitus on gas-trointestinal function in animal models, the impact of gastrointestinal function on glycaemic control, and the evaluation of gastrointestinal autonomic function. All of the authors are recognised internationally for their expertise in the field and we wish to thank them most sincerely for their contributions. We also thank Layla Paggetti and Joan Marsh of John Wiley & Sons, Ltd, as well as Anouk de Vries and Sue Suter, for their unstinting support and encouragement. It should be recognised, as in any relatively new field of study, that there is a need for a constant reappraisal of concepts and ideas. As for Alice, it will be interesting to see where the journey takes us!

Michael Horowitz
Melvin Samsom
December 2003

List of Contributors

Thomas Abell

Professor of Medicine/Gastroenterology, The University of Mississipi Medical Center, Division of Digestive Diseases, 2500 N. State Street, Jackson, MS 39216–4505, USA

Louis M. A. Akkermans

Professor of Experimental Surgery, Gastrointestinal Research Unit, Department of Surgery, University Medical Center, PO Box 85500, 3508 GA, Utrecht, The Netherlands

Michael Camilleri

Professor of Medicine and Physiology, Mayo Clinic College of Medicine, Center for Enteric Neurosciences and Translational Epidemiological Research (C.E.N.T.E.R.) Charlton 8–110, 200 First St. S.W., Rochester, MN 55905, USA

Teresa F. Cutts

Director of Program Development, Church Health Center, Hope and Healing Facility, 1115 Union Avenue, Memphis, TN 38104, USA

Gaylen L. Edwards

Professor of Physiology, College of Veterinary Medicine, Department of Physiology and Pharmacology, University of Georgia, Athens, GA 30602, USA

Johann Hammer

Universitätsklinik für Innere Medizin IV, Abteilung für Gastroenterologie und Hepatologie, Währinger Gürtel 18–20, 1090 Vienna, Austria

Gastrointestinal Function in Diabetes Mellitus. Edited by Michael Horowitz and Melvin Samsom
© 2004 John Wiley & Sons, Ltd   ISBN: 0-471-89916-X

Bart van Hoek   Associate Professor of Hepatology, Department
of Gastroenterology and Hepatology, Leiden
University Medical Center, PO Box 9600,
2300 RC Leiden, The Netherlands

Michael Horowitz   Professor of Medicine, Department of Medicine,
University of Adelaide, and Director,
Endocrine and Metabolic Unit, Royal
Adelaide Hospital, North Terrace, Adelaide,
South Australia, Australia 5000

Karen L. Jones   NHMRC/Diabetes Australia, Senior Research
Fellow, Department of Medicine, University
of Adelaide, Royal Adelaide Hospital, North
Terrace, Adelaide, South Australia, Australia
5000

Marie-France Kong   Consultant Physician, Department of Diabetes
and Endocrinology, Leicester General
Hospital, Gwendolen Road, Leicester LE5
4PW, UK

Ian A. Macdonald   Professor of Metabolic Physiology, Institute of
Clinical Research and School of Biomedical
Sciences, University of Nottingham, Clifton
Boulevard, Nottingham NG7 2UH, UK

Ad A. M. Masclee   Associate Professor of Gastroenterology,
Department of Gastroenterology and
Hepatology, Leiden University Medical
Center, Building 1, C4-P, PO Box 9600, 2300
RC Leiden, The Netherlands

Michael A. Nauck   Professor of Medicine, Diabeteszentrum,
Kirchberg 21, 37431 Bad Lauterberg im Harz,
Germany

Nicholas W. Read   Professor of Medicine, Department of Medicine,
University of Sheffield, Sheffield S10 2TN,
UK

Melvin Samsom   Associate Professor of Gastroenterology,
Director, Department of Gastroenterology and
Hepatology, University Medical Center
Utrecht, PO Box 85500, 3508 GA Utrecht,
The Netherlands

André J. P. M. Smout   Professor of Gastroenterology, Department of Gastroenterology and Hepatology, University Medical Center Utrecht, PO Box 85500, 3508 GA Utrecht, The Netherlands

Wei Ming Sun   Director of Gastrointestinal Motility Laboratory, Division of Gastroenterology, Department of Internal Medicine, University of Michigan, 3912 Taubman Center, Ann Arbor, MI 48109, USA

Nicholas J. Talley   Professor of Medicine, Mayo Clinic College of Medicine, Center for Enteric Neurosciences and Translational Epidemiological Research (C.E.N.T.E.R.) Charlton 8–110, 200 First St. S.W., Rochester, MN 55905, USA

Miriam Thumshirn   Associate Professor of Medicine, Department of Gastroenterology, University Hospital, Raemistrasse 100, 8037 Zurich, Switzerland

Mark A. M. T. Verhagen   Department of Gastroenterology, Diaconessenhospital, Bosboomstraat 1, 3582 KE Utrecht, The Netherlands

Andrew A. Young   Vice President and Senior Research Fellow, Amylin Pharmaceuticals Inc., 9360 Towne Centre Drive, San Diego, CA 92121, USA

1

Epidemiology of Disordered Gastrointestinal Function and Impact of Chronic Gastrointestinal Symptoms on Quality of Life

Johann Hammer, Tom Abell, Teresa F. Cutts
and **Nicholas J. Talley**

Introduction

Patients with diabetes mellitus commonly complain of gastrointestinal symptoms, including chronic abdominal pain and bowel dysfunction, for which there is no structural cause [1–11]. It is now widely recognised, although only relatively recently, that complications involving the gastrointestinal tract represent an important cause of morbidity in patients with diabetes

Gastrointestinal Function in Diabetes Mellitus. Edited by Michael Horowitz and Melvin Samsom
© 2004 John Wiley & Sons, Ltd   ISBN: 0-471-89916-X

mellitus [12,13]. However, epidemiological studies of these problems remain sparse and the data are conflicting. In addition, aspects of quality of life have attracted increased interest in the past few years, as it has been shown that gastrointestinal problems can impair well-being and daily life in diabetes.

Epidemiology of gastrointestinal symptoms in diabetes

Prevalence of gastrointestinal symptoms in diabetes mellitus

Several studies have aimed to evaluate the frequency of gastrointestinal symptoms in patients with non-insulin-dependent and insulin-dependent diabetes, but at present no uniform picture can be drawn from these results. An enormous range in the prevalence of gastrointestinal symptoms has been identified in these studies. This probably relates in part to the methodology applied and the types of populations studied (Table 1.1). Although gastrointestinal symptoms were usually assessed by either interview or standard questionnaire, the criteria applied to identify relevant symptoms differed between the studies. Few studies compared symptoms in diabetic patients with adequately matched controls. Moreover potential confounders, such as the duration of disease, glycaemic control and the presence or absence of autonomic neuropathy or psychiatric disorders, were not corrected for in most of the studies.

An ideal study of the epidemiology of gastrointestinal symptoms needs to take into account a number of issues specific to patients with diabetes. An unselected sample of the diabetes population should be compared to an appropriately matched control population. The control group for population-based studies should be selected at random from the healthy population. However, for outpatient studies disease controls are usually more appropriate than healthy controls because the selection forces differ in the clinic [14]. The populations studied need to be carefully characterised, including by age and sex, type and duration of diabetes, type and success of therapy, the presence or absence of diabetic complications, and the type of complications. It is of particular importance that symptoms are assessed by adequately validated measures. However, although validated measures that evaluate gastrointestinal symptoms exist for a variety of diseases, no diabetes mellitus-specific questionnaire has been widely available. Recently, a disease-specific questionnaire, the Diabetes Bowel Symptom Questionnaire (DBSQ), has been developed for use in both epidemiological and clinical studies of patients with diabetes. The items included in this questionnaire assess both gastrointestinal symptoms in diabetes as well as diabetic disease status, and the instrument appears to be reliable and valid [11].

Outpatient studies of gastrointestinal symptoms in diabetes mellitus

The early literature emphasised the high prevalence of gastrointestinal symptoms in patients with diabetes complicated by neuropathy [15,16]. More than six

Table 1.1 Outpatient studies and population-based studies assessing gastrointestinal symptoms in diabetic patients

Reference	Population studied	Size of study population	Number of patients studied	Type of diabetes	Interview-based assessment	Questionnaire-based assessment	Control subjects studied	Patients with any gastrointestinal symptoms (%)
Dandona et al., 1983 [20]	Outpatients	N/A	285	NIDDM and IDDM (n = ?) (n = ?)	NO	Not validated questionnaire	YES	19%
Feldman and Schiller, 1983, [4]	Outpatients	N/A	136	NIDDM and IDDM (n = ?) (n = ?)	YES	N/A	NO	76%
Clouse and Lustmann, 1989 [17]	Outpatients	N/A	114	NIDDM and IDDM (n = 57) (n = 75)	YES	N/A	NO	68%
Maxton and Whorwell, 1991 [19]	Outpatients	N/A	200	NIDDM and IDDM (n = ?) (n = ?)	YES	N/A	YES	Not stated
Keshavarzian and Iber, 1987 [21]	Outpatients	N/A	75	IDDM (n = 75)	YES	N/A	NO	19%
Maser et al., 1990 [22]	Outpatients	N/A	168	IDDM (n = 168)	YES	N/A	NO	Not stated
Enck et al., 1994 [23]	Outpatients	N/A	190	NIDDM and IDDM (n = 68) (n = 75)	NO	Not validated questionnaire	YES	Not stated
Ko et al., 1999, [18]	Outpatients	N/A	149	NIDDM (n = 149)	NO	Not validated questionnaire	YES	71%
Dyck et al., 1993 [24]	General population	870	380	NIDDM and IDDM (n = 278) (n = 102)	YES	N/A	NO	Not stated
Schvarcz et al., 1995 [25]	General population	125	110	IDDM (n = 110)	NO	Validated questionnaire	YES	Not stated
Janatuinen et al., 1993 [26]	General population	624	538	NIDDM and IDDM (n = 451) (n = 87)	NO	Not validated questionnaire	YES	Not stated
Spångeus et al., 1999 [27]	General population	489	261	NIDDM and IDDM (n = 61) (n = 200)	NO	Validated questionnaire	YES	Not stated
Ricci et al., 2000 [28]	General population	?	483	NIDDM and IDDM (n = 61) (n = 200)	YES	N/A	YES	50%
Maleki et al., 2000 [29]	General population	?	?	NIDDM and IDDM (n = 217) (n = 138)	NO	Validated questionnaire	YES	Not stated
Hammer [30] Bytzer et al., 2000 [31]	General population	15 000	423	NIDDM and IDDM (n = 401) (n = 22)	NO	YES	YES	Not stated

N/A, not applicable

decades ago, Rundles reported that 'constipation, chronic diarrhoea, anorexia and nausea often accompany the development of diabetic neuropathy' [15]. He studied 125 patients with peripheral neuropathy selected from more than 3000 patients who were diagnosed with diabetes over a 7 year period. No information was given concerning age, gender or duration of disease. More than 60% of the patients reported gastrointestinal symptoms; 42% had constipation, this being the most frequent symptom, and 22% had chronic diarrhoea. However, it was also suggested, although not specifically quantified, that 'among an average group of diabetics receiving modern treatment, gastrointestinal disturbances' were 'probably no more frequent than among a similar group of non-diabetics'. In a follow-up study among 30 additional diabetic patients with neuropathy and gastrointestinal symptoms, abdominal pain was the most frequent symptom (in 70% of patients), followed by constipation, diarrhoea, vomiting and faecal incontinence [16].

Subsequently, a number of studies have evaluated gastrointestinal symptoms among outpatients with both type 2 (non-insulin) and type 1 (insulin-dependent) diabetes. In a sample of 136 outpatients attending a diabetes clinic, Feldman and Schiller [4] reported that 76% had one or more gastrointestinal symptoms which were, in most patients, chronic or frequently recurrent; nausea and vomiting occurred in 29%, dysphagia in 27%, abdominal pain in 34%, constipation in 60%, diarrhoea in 22% and faecal incontinence in 20% of the patients (Table 1). However, no control group was evaluated and the interview methodology applied was not well standardised, neither was the type of diabetes documented.

Clouse and Lustman [17] interviewed 114 outpatients with type 1 and type 2 diabetes; 68% reported at least one gastrointestinal symptom. Nausea was experienced by 21% of patients, abdominal pain by 32%, constipation by 12%, diarrhoea by 21% and bloating by 20%. However, no control group was evaluated.

Ko et al. [18] interviewed 149 patients with type 2 diabetes, using standard questions from a gastrointestinal symptom questionnaire, and 65 control subjects. They also found a high prevalence of gastrointestinal symptoms in Chinese outpatients with diabetes. Epigastric fullness was experienced by 17% of patients, abdominal pain by 16%, diarrhoea by 35% and constipation by 28% of patients; all of these symptoms were significantly more frequent than in the control group.

In contrast, Maxton and Whorwell [19] interviewed 200 patients with type 1 and type 2 diabetes attending a diabetic clinic, of whom 59 had signs of autonomic neuropathy, and 200 age- and sex-matched control subjects. They found that constipation was more common in patients with autonomic neuropathy (22% of patients) compared with patients without neuropathy (9%) and controls (7–14%). Diarrhoea was found in only 5% of patients with neuropathy and in 11% of patients without, and this was not significantly different from controls (3–6%). The prevalence of abdominal pain was also similar in patients with (19%) and without (21%) autonomic neuropathy and controls (20%).

Similarly, in 285 consecutive outpatients with type 1 and type 2 diabetes from a diabetic clinic in England, Dandona et al. [20] found a prevalence of 8% for diarrhoea and 5% for constipation, which was not significantly different from the prevalence in a control group of outpatients from other medical clinics. While the group of patients with diabetes who received biguanides had a higher prevalence of diarrhoea [20%], the prevalence of diarrhoea in patients who were on insulin or other oral hypoglycaemics was low (6%).

Other studies have evaluated gastrointestinal symptoms in outpatients who had type 1 diabetes. Keshavarzian and Iber [21] assessed gastrointestinal symptoms in 75 consecutive male patients with type 1 diabetes who had been on insulin for at least 5 years. Only 19% of the patients reported gastrointestinal symptoms, the most frequent being diarrhoea and constipation, with a prevalence of 5% each. Similarly, Maser et al. [22] evaluated gastrointestinal symptoms in a group of 168 patients with type 1 diabetes with a mean disease duration of 20.5 years; signs of autonomic neuropathy were present in 63 patients (37%). The prevalence of gastrointestinal symptoms was found to be low, with vomiting being the most frequent with a prevalence of 7%. Constipation was reported by only 3% of patients and none had diarrhoea. Enck and associates [23] evaluated 190 consecutive patients with type 1 and type 2 diabetes recruited from a diabetes research centre, and 180 age- and sex-matched controls. Symptoms arising from the upper gut were reported by 70% of patients with insulin-dependent diabetes and 44% of patients with non-insulin-dependent diabetes; 31% type 1 and 43% type 2, patients respectively, had symptoms from the lower gastrointestinal tract. However, the prevalence of gastrointestinal symptoms in diabetic patients did not differ from the prevalence in the control subjects.

In another survey using a validated questionnaire, Bytzer et al. [24] studied 892 randomly selected patients from a diabetes support group and 209 outpatients. To obtain information on recent glycaemic control, the authors measured glycated haemoglobin. Glycaemic control was predictive of upper, but not lower, gastrointestinal symptoms. Patients with diabetic complications had a higher frequency of most symptom groups and a higher symptom complexity.

Thus, although a number of outpatient studies have suggested that gastrointestinal symptoms are frequent, these results have not been confirmed by all investigators. Depending on the population studied, the prevalence of symptoms has varied considerably in patients with both type 1 and type 2 diabetes mellitus.

Population-based studies of gastrointestinal symptoms in diabetes mellitus

Population-based studies of gastrointestinal symptoms in diabetic patients have been relatively few and the results conflicting (Table 1.1). To date, a total of nine population-based studies have been undertaken evaluating gastrointestinal symptoms in subjects with diabetes mellitus [24–33]. Dyck *et al.* [24] studied 102 patients with type 1 and 278 patients with type 2 diabetes by interview. They were selected randomly from a cohort of individuals who were diagnosed with diabetes mellitus (1.3% of the total population) in the community of Rochester, Minnesota, USA ($n = 870$, 23% with type 1 and 77% with type 2 diabetes). This represents an underestimate because of the relatively high frequency of undiagnosed type 2 diabetes. Symptoms of "gastroparesis" were reported by none of the subjects with type 1 diabetes and by only 1% of subjects with type 2 diabetes. Nocturnal diarrhoea was reported by just 1% of these with type 1 diabetes and 0.5% with type 2 diabetes. The diagnostic criteria for gastroparesis and nocturnal diarrhoea were not stated and no control group was included.

Among a population of 125 subjects who were first diagnosed as having type 1 diabetes between 1960 and 1969 in the Swedish county of Örebro, Schvarcz *et al.* [25] surveyed 110 eligible subjects using a questionnaire that was previously validated for use in the general population. The prevalence of gastrointestinal symptoms was significantly higher among diabetic patients than among age- and sex-matched controls who were selected from a taxation register. In particular, anorexia (17.8% vs. 3.6%), vomiting (12.2% vs. 3.0%) and abdominal distension (42.3% vs. 24.4%) were more frequent amongst subjects with diabetes. However, the population studied was small, and only middle-aged patients who had long-standing type 1 diabetes were enrolled.

In a survey of 624 subjects with diabetes who were on a drug reimbursement register and 648 controls from the population register of Kuopio, a Finnish community, Janatuinen *et al.* [26] studied both subjects with type 1 ($n = 87$; mean age: men, 53 years; women, 56 years) and type 2 diabetes ($n = 451$; mean age: men, 56 years; women, 58 years). Subjects with type 1 diabetes had a mean disease duration of 17 years, while for those with type 2 diabetes the mean disease duration was 9 years. No differences were observed with respect to the prevalence of dysphagia, nausea, vomiting, abdominal pain, diarrhoea or constipation, and overall the prevalence of gastrointestinal symptoms was low (Figure 1.1). Frequent vomiting (once a week or more often) was experienced by 5% of patients, frequent abdominal pain ($\geq$ once a week) by 26%, constipation 'usually or always' by 16% and frequent diarrhoea ($\geq$ once a week] by 5% (Figure 1.1). However, the questionnaire used had not been validated, and patients with non-insulin-dependent diabetes mellitus who were on diet therapy only were not studied.

In another Scandinavian study, Spångéus *et al.* investigated subjects with diabetes aged 24–59 years and sex- and age-matched controls living in the Swedish county of Umeå [27]. Patients were identified by checking the registration forms

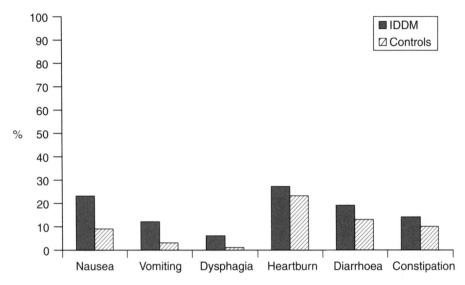

Figure 1.1 Prevalence of gastrointestinal symptoms in 110 type 1 patients compared to controls. $^*p < 0.05$ type 1 vs. control. From Schvarcz *et al.* [25], with permission

of 14 primary care centres within the county. The healthy controls were medical students and hospital staff. All were mailed a validated questionnaire that was previously used by Schvarcz *et al.* [25]. The response rate among the diabetics was 59% and among the controls was 53%. Half of the patients were female and most of the responders were identified as type 1 diabetics (200 vs. 61 type 2 diabetics). The medical records of the responders were checked for glucose control, body mass index, medications and diabetes-specific complications. Patients with both type 1 and type 2 diabetes reported gastrointestinal symptoms more often than the control group. Patients with type 1 diabetes had an increased frequency of constipation (19.5% vs. 6.5% in controls); nocturnal urgency, feelings of incomplete rectal evacuation and straining were also more frequent compared to controls. In contrast, patients with type 2 diabetes had a higher frequency of abdominal pain (28.3% vs. 14.3%) and faecal incontinence (4.9% vs. 0%); they also had a higher prevalence of a nocturnal urgency, feelings of incomplete evacuation at defecation and a need to strain at defecation. Diarrhoea was not more frequent in patients with diabetes compared to controls. Patients with signs of neuropathy had a higher frequency of gastrointestinal symptoms compared to patients who had no signs of neuropathy. Other diabetic complications, such as retinopathy and nephropathy, were not associated with a higher frequency of gastrointestinal symptoms. However, the results of this study are hard to interpret, since an inadequate response rate was achieved, the patients and control subjects were not randomly selected, the proportion with type 1 diabetes was inappropriately high and the methodology to identify diabetes complications was not standardised.

Ricci *et al.* reported on the frequency of upper gastrointestinal symptoms in a US national sample of patients with diabetes mellitus and controls who were identified by a telephone survey [28]. Of the 874 patients who identified themselves as diabetes sufferers, 483 completed a structured interview evaluating the presence of gastrointestinal symptoms within the past month. Two-thirds of the participants were women and the age range was 18–70+ years. The type of diabetes was not determined. Among the patients with diabetes, 50% reported an upper gastrointestinal symptom in the past month compared with 38% in the control group. Bloating and early satiety were more frequent in diabetics than in controls (Figure 1.4). The frequently of abdominal pain and nausea and vomiting, however, were similar in both of the groups.

A small population-based study from Olmsted County, Minnesota, evaluating the prevalence of gastrointestinal symptoms, was performed by Maleki *et al.* [29]. The authors detected no differences in the prevalence of most gastrointestinal symptoms between type 1 and type 2 diabetes and controls [30]. A slightly increased prevalence of constipation and laxative use in type 1 patients (27% vs. 19% in controls) was related to calcium channel blocker use, but not to autonomic neuropathy.

Another study was performed in Western Sydney, Australia [30]. These investigators assessed the frequency of gastrointestinal symptoms in 113 diabetics from an outpatient clinic, 400 diabetics that were selected at random from a diabetes support group, and a random sample of the general population ($n = 1000$) using a validated questionnaire; the response rates were 100%, 71% and 63%, respectively. After adjusting the results for age, sex and body mass index, none of the gastrointestinal symptoms reported was more frequent in the random diabetes population than in the control population. However, dysphagia, bloating, abdominal pain, constipation and diarrhoea were more frequent in outpatients with diabetes compared to the random diabetes population and controls. The authors also concluded that gastrointestinal symptoms may be related to glycaemic control, since the prevalence of nausea and dysphagia was greater in outpatients with glycated haemoglobin levels $\geq$ 10 mg%. Other data support this conclusion [31].

In a large study from Australia, Bytzer *et al.* [32] mailed a short questionnaire containing questions on the frequency of troublesome gastrointestinal symptoms and diabetic status to a random sample of 15 000 randomly chosen adults; 60% responded. Overall, 4.9% of the responders reported diabetes (95% of whom were type 2), who were generally older than controls. The authors evaluated the frequency of five symptom complexes, i.e. oesophageal (heartburn and/or dysphagia), upper gut dysmotility, any bowel symptom, diarrhoea and constipation. After adjusting for age and gender, all symptom complexes were more

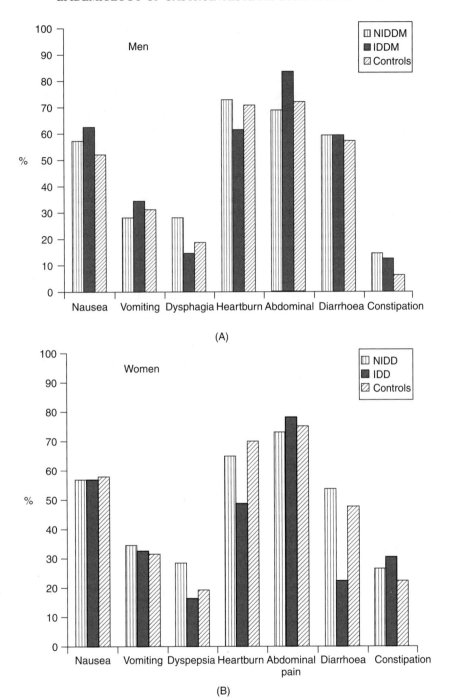

Figure 1.2   Gastrointestinal symptoms in a population of 624 subjects with *insulin-dependent diabetes* mellitus (IDDM), *non-insulin-dependent* diabetes mellitus (NIDDM), and community controls. (a) Data in men. (b) Data in women. From Janatuinen *et al.* [26], with permission

frequent in diabetics than in controls, and the symptoms nausea, diarrhoea or constipation and faecal incontinence were independently associated with diabetes (Figure 1.2).

In conclusion, there is evidence that gastrointestinal symptoms are linked with diabetes mellitus, but the prevalence over and above the general population is at most only modestly increased. Some studies have failed to detect an association between diabetes and gastrointestinal symptoms, but several confounders may have obscured the findings. For example, it is well documented that chronic gastrointestinal symptoms are common in non-diabetics in the community, presumably due to functional gastrointestinal disorders such as the irritable bowel syndrome [33,34]. Moreover, the presence of diabetic complications and possibly long-term glycaemic control appear to be important factors in symptom onset [31,32]. This may explain the difficulty in establishing a firm link between diabetes and chronic gastrointestinal complaints in population-based studies.

Natural history of gastrointestinal symptoms in diabetes mellitus

Community studies suggest that in the general population there is a considerable turnover of individuals reporting gastrointestinal symptoms [35,36]. Moreover, longitudinal studies in the USA [35] and Sweden [36], applying a postal questionnaire on two separate occasions, have demonstrated that the number of subjects who developed gastrointestinal symptoms in a given period of time paralleled the number of subjects who lost them [32, 35–38]. Unfortunately, almost no data exist on the natural history of gastrointestinal symptoms in diabetes, and whether factors such as glycaemic control or the development of autonomic neuropathy influence development and regression of motor dysfunction or disturbed sensation and symptoms is unknown. Indeed, it has been uncertain how many diabetic patients have gastrointestinal symptoms transiently and how many experience them for prolonged periods.

Talley et al. evaluated the natural history of lower gastrointestinal tract symptoms in diabetes, and assessed potential predictors of symptom change in 540 subjects with predominantly type 2 diabetes [39]. The prevalence of abdominal pain, constipation, diarrhoea and faecal incontinence was stable over a three year period, but 4–27% in these symptom groups experienced symptom turnover. Change in symptom status was not associated with change in self-rated glycaemic control or the type or duration of diabetes. Baseline complications of diabetes and psychological factors were variably associated with turnover of symptom groupings, but a consistent pattern did not emerge. Studies of the natural history of upper gastrointestinal symptoms and their relationship to glycaemic control are not available but, based on cross-sectional studies, glycaemic control may be more important in this subset [31,32].

Potential confounders of gastrointestinal symptoms in diabetes mellitus

Here only a brief overview of factors that may alter or bias any association between gastrointestinal symptoms and diabetes will be discussed.

Disordered motor function

In patients with long-standing type 1 and type 2 diabetes, the prevalence of delayed gastric emptying of a nutrient meal is reported to range from 27% to 40% [40–42] and the prevalence is similar in insulin-dependent and non-insulin-dependent diabetes mellitus (see Chapter 4) [43,44]. In a minority of patients (less than 10%) with long-standing diabetes, gastric emptying is accelerated [42–44]. In newly diagnosed patients with type 2 diabetes, gastric emptying of carbohydrates has been reported to be accelerated [45,46], although others have not confirmed these findings [47]. On the other hand, no data exist on the prevalence of deranged gastric emptying in patients with newly diagnosed type 1 diabetes. Manometric abnormalities were found in 81 of 84 patients with either type 1 or type 2 diabetes who completed a 3 hour fast and 2 hour postprandial motility evaluation [48]. Although some have suggested a link between gastric motor disorder and symptoms [41], most have not found a strong correlation between symptoms and either delayed [42] or accelerated gastric emptying [45]. Hence, this is a weak predictor of symptom status overall.

Delayed small bowel and colonic transit have also been reported in 20–70% of patients with long-standing diabetes mellitus (see Chapter 5) [41,49]. However, while no gastrointestinal symptoms correlated with delayed small intestinal transit, constipation (defined as less than three bowel movements/week) was significantly associated with delayed colonic transit [49].

Autonomic neuropathy and visceral sensory dysfunction

Traditionally, gastrointestinal symptoms have been attributed to disordered motor function resulting from autonomic (vagal) neuropathy [50,51]. More recently, impaired sensory function has been implicated as a trigger for gastrointestinal symptoms in dyspeptic patients [52,53]. However, the predictive value of these abnormalities for the induction of chronic gastrointestinal symptoms is unknown.

Glycaemic control

A number of studies have shown that acute changes in blood glucose concentrations can have a profound effect on motor function throughout the gastrointestinal tract in both normal subjects and patients with diabetes mellitus [54]. Recent studies have demonstrated that the blood glucose concentration may also modulate the perception of sensations arising from the gastrointestinal tract [56–58]. However, there is relatively little information about the mechanisms mediating the effects of the blood glucose concentration on gastrointestinal motility. While some studies have implicated impaired glycaemic control in the genesis of chronic gastrointestinal symptoms [24,31], this remains controversial.

Psychological factors

Psychological factors may play a role in the generation and maintenance of gastrointestinal symptoms in the general population [59]. Psychological factors are associated with both the symptoms of irritable bowel syndrome (IBS) and health care seeking by IBS sufferers [59,60]. For example, patients with IBS have higher frequencies of psychiatric diagnoses and personality disturbances, such as neuroticism, than healthy volunteers [60–62]. Further, those who see doctors for their IBS symptoms (consulters) appear to be psychologically more disturbed than those who did not seek medical attention (nonconsulters) [62,63].

Psychological disorders are common in diabetics [64–70] and psychological distress and poor glycaemic control are closely associated [65,70–72]. It has thus been suggested that depression and hyperglycaemia may exacerbate one another [68]. In patients with type 1 diabetes, abnormal anxiety ratings could be identified in up to 13% and psychological abnormalities were related to age and social class, but not to duration of diabetes or glycaemic control [73]. Moreover, in elderly patients with type 2 diabetes (mean age 70 years), mental distress (defined as an elevated score in a 12-item version of the General Health Questionnaire) and depression were associated with peripheral neuropathy [74], which may reflect worse metabolic control in the group who had depression. The presence of affective and anxiety disorders has also been associated with gastrointestinal motility abnormalities in diabetic [75] and non-diabetic [76] subjects. Thus, out of 15 patients with diabetes mellitus who were found to have contraction abnormalities in the oesophageal body, such as an increased amplitude or abnormal motor response to swallowing, 13 (87%) had a psychiatric diagnosis [75].

It remains uncertain whether and to what extent psychological factors account for gastrointestinal symptoms in type 1 or type 2 diabetes mellitus, as this has not been systematically studied. Psychological distress could be the result of having a chronic illness and hence any association with symptoms could be spurious. However, Clouse and Lustman [17] found that psychiatric disturbances were more strongly related to gastrointestinal symptoms than autonomic neuropathy.

Helicobacter pylori infection

Helicobacter pylori causes chronic histological gastritis which can progress to gastric atrophy. *H. pylori* is now established to be a cause of chronic peptic ulcer and is classified as a class 1 carcinogen by the World Health Organisation [77]. An impaired immune response in diabetes that alters both humoral [78] and cellular [79–82] immunity, and the high prevalence of upper gastrointestinal symptoms described in some studies, have led to speculation that *H. pylori* may be linked to diabetes [83]. In a recent Italian study, patients with diabetes with dyspepsia had a higher prevalence of *H. pylori* infection compared to dyspeptic controls [84]. In another study, De Luis *et al.* reported that the seroprevalence of *H. pylori* increased with increasing duration of diabetes in patients with type 1 diabetes [85]. However, others have failed to demonstrate any association between *H. pylori* and gastrointestinal symptoms in diabetes [86–88]. Moreover, no studies have adequately assessed whether cure of *H. pylori* reverses upper gastrointestinal symptoms in diabetes.

Quality of life

Health-related quality of life (HRQL)

HRQL refers to patients' subjective accounts of functioning and/or overall well-being in relation to health status, and encompasses emotional and physical functioning. While clinical medicine usually gauges the severity of illness and success/failure of treatment via strictly objective criteria, HRQL measures are assessed directly from patient reports. Increasingly, the concept that patient perceptions of illness and/or wellness do not necessarily correlate with objective measures of morbidity is becoming accepted [89]. Also, HRQL has critical implications, both for the individual and, when the person is unable to perform his/her daily functions, for society. Measures of function and well-being have been shown to predict both health-care expenditures and mortality [90]. Lastly, HRQL data can provide physicians with vital information on the efficacy of any given treatment regimen.

Measurement of HRQL

Work exploring HRQL has exploded in scope and interest over the past decade (Table 1.2). Two approaches to assessing HRQL in medical illness have emerged: global and disease-specific [91]. Global HRQL measures assess daily functioning and emotional well-being without reference to specific disease symptoms (e.g. impact of illness upon communication skills). Disease-specific HRQL measures assess the impact of very specific symptoms or problems upon functioning or

Table 1.2   HRQL studies assessing gastrointestinal symptoms

Reference	Gastrointestinal disorder	Subjects (n)	HRQL instrument(s)	Gastric emptying assessed
Cutts et al., 1996 [98]	Severe dyspepsia	27	SIP, MMPI, MBHI	Yes, but not reported
Enck et al., 1999 [96]	Upper GI symptoms	5581	PGWB, IDLI	No
Farup et al., 1998 [129]	Diabetic gastroparesis	269	SF-36	Yes
Glia and Lindberg, 1997, [107]	Functional constipation	102	PBWB, GSRS	Yes (Transit Time)
Havelund et al., 1999 [109]	Heartburn without esophagitus	245	PGWB, GSRS	No
Heymann-Monnikes, 2000 [132]	Irritable bowel syndrome	24	GQLI, Beck Depression Inventory, State–Trait Anxiety Inventory, Health and Illness-related Locus of Control Quest., Irrational Beliefs Quest. 'List of Complaints'	No
Drossman et al., 2000 [102]	Functional bowel disorders	156	SIP, IBS–QOL	No
Drossman et al., 2000 [134]	Functional bowel disorders	211	SIP, IBS–QOL, SCL-90 Beck Depression Inventory, five others	No
Koloski et al., 2000 [95]	Functional bowel disorders	2910	SF-12, Eysenck Personality Quest Sphere, Delusions–Symptoms–States Inventory (DSSI)	No
Mathias et al., 1998 [115]	Functional bowel disease	100	SF-36, Visual Analogue Scale	No
O'Keefe et al., 1995 [117]	Functional bowel disorders	533	SF-36	No
Revicki et al., 1998 [108]	gastrooesophageal reflux disease	533	SF-36	No
Revicki et al., 1999 [110]	gastrooesophageal reflux disease	1351	SF-36, PGWB	No
Rockwood et al., 2000 [105]	Faecal incontinence	190	Faecal Incontinence QOL Scale SF-36	No
Sailer et al., 1998 [118]	Faecal incontinence	209	GQLI	No
Sailer et al., 1998 [119]	Benign anorectal disorders	325	GQLI	No
Silvers et al., 1998 [112]	Diabetic gastroparesis	269	SF-36	Yes
Soykan et al., 1997 [113]	Gastroparesis	17	SF-36	Yes
Soykan et al., 1998 [111]	Gastroparesis	146	MBHI, SCL-90, CES-D Depression Scale, Visual Analogue Scale	Yes
Snijders et al., 1998 [116]	AIDS	62	Diary Cards, Interview	No

Table 1.2 (*continued*)

Reference	Gastrointestinal disorder	Subjects (*n*)	HRQL instrument(s)	Gastric emptying assessed
Talley *et al.*, 1999 [106]	Functional dyspepsia	101	Nepean Dyspepsia Index, SF-36, Beck Depression Inventory, State–Trait Inventory, Bowel Symptom Questionnaire Global Assessment	No
Wiklund *et al.*, 1998 [103]	gastrooesophageal reflux disease, dyspepsia		Quality of Life in Reflux and Dyspepsia, GSRS, SF-36	No
Wong *et al.*, 1998 [101]	Irritable bowel syndrome	12	IBS Questionnaire	No
Sailer *et al.*, 1998 [119]	Benign anorectal disorders	325	GQLI	No

GQLI, Gastrointestinal Quality of Life Index; GSRS, Gastrointestinal Symptom Rating Scale; IBS–QOL, Irritable Bowel Syndrome Quality of Life assessment; IDLI, Interference with Daily Life Index; MBHI, Millon Behavioral Health Inventory; MMPI, Minnesota Multiphasic Personality Inventory; PGWB, Psychological General Well-being Index; SF, short form; SIP, Sickness Impact Profile; QOL, quality of life; Quest., questionnaire; GI, gastrointestinal.

well-being, e.g. level of social embarrassment due to having a colostomy. No gold standard exists in terms of assessing HRQL in gastrointestinal disease and researchers disagree on the best approach [92].

In terms of type of HRQL instruments and diabetes, Jacobson and colleagues compared global vs. disease-specific measures in patients with type 2 diabetes [93]. These researchers concluded that, when examining the impact of acute complications and/or regimens on HRQL, a disease-specific measure was most appropriate. A global measure (Medical Outcomes Study Short Form or MOS SF-36) was deemed most useful for examining relationships between patients' experience of living with diabetes and other chronic diseases. Likewise, Anderson *et al.* [94] found that, in a sample of 255 type 2 diabetic patients, exploring 'within-disease' parameters was best assessed via a disease-specific instrument, while relationships 'between' patient experiences of living with diabetes and HRQL and other diseases were best captured via global measures. Several studies examining the impact of HRQL upon patients with upper gastrointestinal distress (typically dyspepsia) have utilised global measures, usually the SF-36 or some variant of that scale [89,95]. Similarly, a larger-scale study [96] investigated HRQL in patients with upper gastrointestinal symptoms from seven European countries, USA, Canada and Japan. This work concluded that, of the 5581 respondents (27% of whom also were diagnosed with diabetes, hypertension or asthma), the presence of gastrointestinal symptoms was associated with impaired well-being and daily life, as measured via the Psychological General Well-being Index (PGWB) and Interference with Daily Life Index (IDLI). Subjects with upper gastrointestinal symptoms (particularly ulcer-like symptoms) manifested poorer scores on these HRQL measures.

Others have opted to use batteries of assessment, encompassing both global and disease-specific measures [97,98]. For example, Talley *et al.* [97] applied a battery of validated measures, which included a short form of the Medical Outcomes Survey (SF-12), a Brief Symptom Inventory and gastrointestinal symptoms. The authors found that patients with functional dyspepsia had poorer mental health, social functioning and health perception, compared with patients with other conditions who presented for upper endoscopy.

Disease-specific measures in gastrointestinal diseases have been developed for several disease entities, including inflammatory bowel disease [99], IBS [100–102], gastro-oesophageal reflux disease (GORD) [103,104], faecal incontinence [105] and functional dyspepsia [106], with varying degrees of psychometric validation. However, no disease-specific quality of life measure exists for gastrointestinal dysfunction in diabetes.

Specific gastrointestinal symptoms and HRQL

Several gastrointestinal symptoms have been specifically related to a deranged HRQL (Table 1.2). Patients with constipation have lower general HRQL scores than healthy controls [107], as have patients with heartburn [108–110]. Appropriate treatment of gastro-oesophageal reflux disease decreased heartburn and in turn increased HRQL scores [108–110]. Nausea and vomiting in patients with severe dyspepsia or gastroparesis was also associated with a decrease in HRQL [98,111]. Patients who were successfully treated for their symptoms showed a significant enhancement of HRQL [98,111–113]. The severity of abdominal pain in patients with functional bowel disease correlates with impaired HRQL and increased levels of psychological distress [114]. When abdominal pain scores improved after treatment, so also did HRQL, as evaluated by the use of the SF-36 [115]. There was also a significant correlation between the change in scores on the IBS–QOL, a disease-specific quality of life scale for patients with IBS, and average daily pain level over two 14 day periods [101]. The IBS–QOL scores discriminated responders to treatment from non-responders for the pain level parameter. Finally, even mild diarrhoea (assessed via diary cards and interview) was perceived as having a debilitating effect on HRQL (assessed via interview) in patients infected with HIV [116]. In a random sample of elderly patients, role functioning scale scores discriminated patients with diarrhoea from asymptomatic controls [117].

The impact of faecal incontinence, an important complication of diabetes (see Chapter 6), on HRQL was investigated by Sailor *et al.* [118,119], using the Gastrointestinal Quality of Life Index [GIQLI]. They evaluated HRQL in patients with faecal incontinence, compared with those with haemorrhoids or fissure in ano, and healthy controls. Patients with faecal incontinence manifested the lowest HRQL scores, compared to both medical and healthy control groups [117]. Subgroups of patients with faecal incontinence and severe constipation had the poorest HRQL scores [119].

Diabetes and HRQL

As part of the Medical Outcomes Study, that determined the impact of nine different chronic illnesses upon HRQL, Stewart *et al.* [90] used the Short Form (SF-20) of the General Health Survey to evaluate HRQL ratings in 9385 patients, 844 of whom had diabetes (92% were type 2 diabetics and 44% had one or more physician-reported complications). Diabetic patients in this study reported lower HRQL scores than control patients with other chronic conditions. Also, after controlling for sex, age, income and education, subjects with diabetes reported significantly lower scores on all summary scales (physical, role, social func-tioning, health perceptions) except for mental health. Moreover, gastrointestinal disorders had a more negative impact on HRQL than all other conditions with the exception of heart disease [90]. Others have reported similar findings [120,121].

Jacobson *et al.* [93] assessed HRQL in 240 diabetic patients (54% were type 2 diabetics) and controlled for age, marital status, education, illness duration and severity of complications. Compared with patients with type 1 diabetes, patients with type 2 diabetes reported less of an impact of diabetes and fewer worries about their illness on the diabetes-specific quality-of-life scale, the DQOL, used in the Diabetes Control and Complications Trial (DCCT), as well as better social functioning on the SF-36.

Gastrointestinal complications of diabetes and HRQL

A study of diabetic patients undergoing transplantation [122] indicated that, of all the factors likely to compromise HRQL, the single most important one was gastrointestinal dysfunction. Drenth and Engel suggested that symptoms of nausea, vomiting, bloating/distension, early satiety and abdominal pain likely all play a role in this perception [123]. Talley *et al.* evaluated quality of life using the SF-36 and gastrointestinal symptoms in 209 outpatients and 892 community subjects with diabetes; quality of life scores were decreased in dia-betics with gastrointestinal symptoms, and decreased markedly with increased numbers of gastrointestinal symptoms [124] (Figure 1.4). Moreover, gastroin-testinal symptoms were significantly associated with poorer quality of life after adjusting for age, gender, smoking, alcohol use and type of diabetes [124]. Siddique *et al.* evaluated upper gastrointestinal symptoms and quality of life using the SF-12 in 483 community subjects with self-reported diabetes and 422 age- and gender-matched controls in the USA [125]. They observed that upper gastrointestinal symptoms were associated with more impaired physi-cal and mental health summary scores; on the other hand, individuals with diabetes and no gastrointestinal symptoms had quality of life scores similar to healthy subjects. Early satiety and nausea were the strongest predictors of physical and mental health score differences, respectively, in those with and without diabetes.

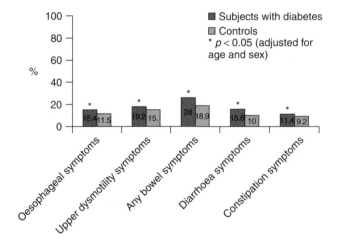

Figure 1.3 Prevalence of gastrointestinal symptom complexes in a population-based study: predominantly type 2 diabetes ($n = 423$) and controls ($n = 8185$). From Bytzer *et al.* [31], with permission

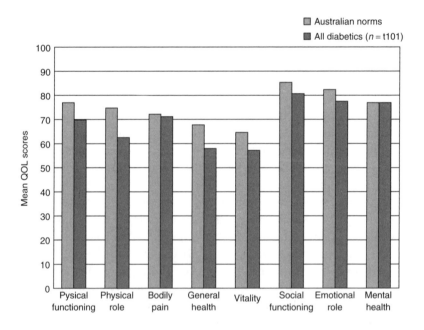

Figure 1.4 A comparison of quality of life scores across SF-36 subscales in subjects with diabetes and normal Australian population data. From Talley *et al.* [124], with permission

Glycaemic control and changes in HRQL

Testa and Simonson [126], attempting to overcome the uncontrolled nature of earlier studies, conducted a randomised, controlled, double-blind study of the short-term impact of glycaemic control upon HRQL in patients with type 2 diabetes. They concluded that treatment, and subsequent good glycaemic controls was associated with improved HRQL (measured using a visual analogue scale) and a number of health economic indices related to work (e.g. less absenteeism, greater work productivity, fewer bed days and fewer restricted activity days). Additionally, these researchers concluded that the rate of HRQL deterioration due to increasing symptoms was progressive with worsening glycaemic control, suggesting, on the other hand, that improvement of glycaemic control also might facilitate the improvement of the HRQL.

Prokinetic therapy in diabetes and quality of life

Studies assessing prokinetic therapy for gastrointestinal symptoms and HRQL in both diabetic patients and those with alternative aetiologies have proliferated over the last decade [97,110,111,127]. A number of these studies have assessed HRQL in addition to traditional symptom improvement indices. Cutts *et al.* [98] found that one year of treatment with prokinetic therapy (cisapride or domperidone) resulted in improved HRQL as measured by the Sickness Impact Profile (SIP), as well as symptom improvement in a group of patients with severe dyspeptic symptoms of both diabetic and idiopathic aetiologies. Soykan *et al.* [111] followed 146 patients with 'gastroparesis' symptoms and delayed gastric emptying, treated with prokinetic therapy and other treatment modalities for six years after initial diagnosis. They assessed psychological and HRQL (by visual analogue scale) parameters, as well as gastric emptying and gastrointestinal symptoms, and found that 74% responded favourably to prokinetic therapy. Also, those patients with a presumed viral aetiology had greater symptom resolution and improved HRQL, as compared to their idiopathic counterparts. The same group of researchers investigated the use of oral domperidone in the treatment of 17 patients with a documented delay in gastric emptying [113]. They found that domperidone therapy (average 23.3 months) significantly reduced nausea, vomiting, abdominal pain and bloating and resulted in enhanced HRQL (measured via select questions from the SF-36) in 88% of the patients treated, with minimal side effects (three patients developed gynaecomastia). Of the 15 patients re-evaluated at follow-up, gastric emptying of a solid meal was significantly accelerated to a normal rate. However, none of the studies cited above compared their samples to matched controls, and Cutts *et al.* did not document delayed gastric emptying (Table 1.2).

Rashed *et al.* [128] examined autonomic functioning as a determinant of quality of life improvement in a group of seven patients with diabetic gastroparesis, in an uncontrolled study. These investigators compared patients in an open label trial of domperidone for 12 months, assessing gastrointestinal symptoms via the Total Symptom Score (TSS), a summed index gathered from patient reports, HRQL via the SIP and autonomic functioning, reported as the total autonomic score (TAS), previously described [129]. Patients showed a significant improvement of 56% in the total symptom score at baseline vs. 12 months. SIP scores improved in six of seven patients, with a median improvement level of 22%, from baseline to one year. Autonomic functioning status at baseline correlated significantly with the SIP Psychosocial Dimension scale (measuring emotional behaviour, communication, social interaction, and alertness behaviour). Hence, in the small sample of diabetic gastroparesis patients, domperidone use was associated with improvement in both gastrointestinal symptoms and HRQL. However, in patients with impaired autonomic functioning, the level of HRQL manifested less improvement. These findings may have implications for selection of diabetic patient subgroups that may benefit from prokinetic therapy.

These data were substantiated in the recent multi-centre examination of the effect of treatment with domperidone on HRQOL in diabetic gastropathy [112,130]. Silvers et al. [112] and Farup et al. [130] reported on use of domperidone therapy in a sample of patients with insulin-treated diabetes and symptoms of gastroparesis. These researchers conducted a four-week, double-blind, placebo-controlled study and found that patients who responded favourably to domperidone experienced significantly improved gastrointestinal symptom relief and HRQL (measured via the SF-36) compared to placebo. In a long-term follow-up of idiopathic gastroparesis, 12 patients (all of whom had taken prokinetic drugs at some point) of presumed viral aetiology reported improved HRQL (measured via the SF-20), compared to the remainder with gastroparesis [127]. These results suggest that prokinetic therapy is useful in the treatment of gastrointestinal symptoms in both diabetic and idiopathic subgroups of patients. Domperidone therapy may potentially be most efficacious in those diabetic patients with delayed gastric emptying who have preserved autonomic function [131].

In addition to prokinetic therapies and HRQL, gastric electrical stimulation is currently being investigated in multi-centre trials across the USA and internationally [132,133]. Preliminary results indicate that, over a 24 month treatment of 28 patients with severe dyspepsia (primary symptoms of intractable nausea and vomiting), gastric pacing was associated with significant changes in sympathetic cholinergic function, decreased gastrointestinal symptoms and HRQL [134]. Recent approval of this treatment modality of gastric pacing as a Humanitarian Use Device by the US Food and Drug Administration will allow further exploration of this treatment for patients who do not respond to, or cannot tolerate, available drug therapies.

In conclusion, measurement of health-related quality of life provides the physician with another tool with which to monitor a patient's progress during long-term treatment for chronic disease, such as diabetes mellitus. This type of assessment also provides a vehicle for communication between physician and patient—a means for the physician to understand the phenomenological 'experience' of the disease and promote treatment. In diabetic patients with gastrointestinal symptoms, which can further complicate self-management and so easily lead to discouragement and frustration, this may prove to be one of the most valuable applications of HRQL information.

References

1. Katz LA, Spiro HM. Gastrointestinal manifestations of diabetes. *N Engl J Med* 1966; **275**: 1350–61.
2. Goyal RK, Spiro HM. Gastrointestinal manifestations of diabetes mellitus. *Med Clin N Am* 1971; **55**: 1031–44.
3. Taub S, Mariani A, Barkin JS. Gastrointestinal manifestations of diabetes mellitus. *Diabetes Care* 1979; **2**: 437–47.
4. Feldman M, Schiller LR. Disorders of gastrointestinal motility associated with diabetes mellitus. *Ann Intern Med* 1983; **98**: 378–84.
5. Atkinson M, Hosking DJ. Gastrointestinal complications of diabetes mellitus. *Clin Gastroenterol* 1983; **2**: 633–50.
6. Yang R, Arem R, Chan L. Gastrointestinal tract complications of diabetes mellitus. *Arch Intern Med* 1984; **144**: 1251–6.
7. Niakan E, Harati Y, Comstock JP. Diabetic autonomic neuropathy. *Metabolism* 1986; **35**: 224–34.
8. Nompleggi D, Bell SJ, Blackburn GL, Bistrian BR. Overview of gastrointestinal disorders due to diabetes mellitus: emphasis on nutritional support. *J Parent Ent Nutr* 1989; **13**: 84–91.
9. Rothstein RD. Gastrointestinal motility disorders in diabetes mellitus. *Am J Gastroenterol* 1990; **85**: 782–5.
10. Locke GR III. Epidemiology of gastrointestinal complications of diabetes mellitus. *Eur J Gastroenterol Hepatol* 1995; **7**: 711–16.
11. Talley NJ, Hammer J, Giles N, Jones MP, Horowitz M. Measuring gastrointestinal symptoms in diabetes: development and validation of the Diabetes Bowel Symptom Questionnaire. *Gastroenterology* (abstr) 2001 (in press).
12. Horowitz M, Fraser R. Disordered gastric motor function in diabetes mellitus. *Diabetologia* 1994; **37**: 543–51.
13. Horowitz M, Wishart JM, Jones KL, Hebbard GS. Gastric emptying in diabetes: an overview. *Diabet Med* 1996; **13**: S16–22.
14. Rothman KJ. A proposal to calculate publication equivalents. *Epidemiology* 1999; **10**: 664–5.
15. Rundles RW. Diabetic neuropathy: general review with report of 125 cases. *Medicine* 1945; **24**: 111–60.
16. Hodges FJ, Rundles RW, Hanelin J. Roentgenologic study of the small intestine II. Dysfunction associated with neurologic disease. *Radiology* 1947; **49**: 659–73.
17. Clouse RE, Lustman PJ. Gastrointestinal symptoms in diabetic patients: lack of association with neuropathy. *Am J Gastroenterol* 1989; **84**: 868–72.
18. Ko GT, Chan WB, Chan JC, Tsang LW, Cockram CS. Gastrointestinal symptoms in Chinese patients with type 2 diabetes mellitus. *Diabet Med* 1999; **16**: 670–74.
19. Maxton DG, Whorwell PJ. Functional bowel symptoms in diabetes—the role of autonomic neuropathy. *Postgrad Med J* 1991; **67**: 991–3.
20. Dandona P, Fonseca V, Mier A, Beckett AG. Diarrhea and metformin in a diabetic clinic. *Diabetes Care* 1983; **6**: 472–4.

21. Keshavarzian A, Iber FL. Gastrointestinal involvement in insulin-requiring diabetes mellitus. *J Clin Gastroenterol* 1987; **9**: 685–92.

22. Maser RE, Pfeifer MA, Dorman JS, Kuller LH *et al.* Diabetic autonomic neuropathy and cardiovascular risk. Pittsburgh epidemiology of diabetes complications study III. *Arch Intern Med* 1990; **150**: 1218–22.

23. Enck P, Rathmann W, Spiekermann M, Czerner D *et al.* Prevalence of gastrointestinal symptoms in diabetic patients and non-diabetic subjects. *Z Gastroenterol* 1994; **32**: 637–41.

24. Dyck PJ, Kratz KM, Karnes JL, Litchy WJ *et al.* The prevalence by staged severity of various types of diabetic neuropathy, retinopathy and nephropathy in a population-based cohort: the Rochester Diabetic Neuropathy Study. *Neurology* 1993; **43**: 817–24.

25. Schvarcz E, Palmér M, Ingberg CM, Åman J, Berne C. Increased prevalence of upper gastrointestinal symptoms in long-term type 1 diabetes mellitus. *Diabet Med* 1996; **13**: 478–81.

26. Janatuinen E, Pikkarainen P, Laakso M, Pyorala K. Gastrointestinal symptoms in middle-aged diabetic patients. *Scand J Gastroenterol* 1993; **28**: 427–32.

27. Spångéus A, El-Salhy M, Suhr O, Eriksson J, Lithner F. Prevalence of gastrointestinal symptoms in young and middle-aged diabetic patients. *Scand J Gastroenterol* 1999; **34**: 1196–202.

28. Ricci JA, Siddique R, Stewart WF, Sandler RS *et al.* Upper gastrointestinal symptoms in a U.S. national sample of adults with diabetes. *Scand J Gastroenterol* 2000; **35**: 152–9.

29. Maleki D, Locke GR III, Camilleri M, Zinsmeister AR *et al.* Gastrointestinal tract symptoms among persons with diabetes mellitus in the community. *Arch Intern Med* 2000; **160**: 2808–16.

30. Hammer J, Willson T, Horowitz M, Talley NJ. Prevalence and determinants of chronic gastrointestinal symptoms in diabetes mellitus. *Gastroenterology* 1999; **116**: A63.

31. Bytzer PM, Talley NJ, Hammer J, Young LJ *et al.* Gastrointestinal symptoms in diabetes mellitus are associated with both poor glycaemic control and diabetic complications. *Am J Gastroenterol* 2002; **97**: 604–11.

32. Bytzer PM, Talley NJ, Leemon M, Young LJ *et al.* Prevalence of gastrointestinal symptoms associated with diabetes mellitus: a population-based survey of 15 000 adults. *Arch Intern Med* 2001; **161**: 1989–96.

33. Thompson WG, Heaton KW. Functional bowel disorders in apparently healthy people. *Gastroenterology* 1980; **79**: 283–88.

34. Talley NJ, Zinsmeister AR, Van Dyke C, Melton LJ III. Epidemiology of colonic symptoms and the irritable bowel syndrome. *Gastroenterology* 1991; **101**: 927–34.

35. Talley NJ, Weaver AL, Zinsmeister AR Melton LJ III. Onset and disappearance of gastrointestinal symptoms and functional gastrointestinal disorders. *Am J Epidemiol* 1992; **136**: 1–13.

36. Agréus L, Svärdsudd K, Nyrén O, Tibblin G. Irritable bowel syndrome and dyspepsia in the general population: overlap and lack of stability over time. *Gastroenterology* 1995; **109**: 671–80.

37. Weir RD, Backett EM. Studies of the epidemiology of peptic ulcer in a rural community: prevalence and natural history of dyspepsia and peptic ulcer. *Gut* 1968; **9**: 75–83.

38. Talley NJ. Why do functional gastrointestinal disorders come and go? *Dig Dis Sci* 1994; **39**: 673–77.

39. Talley NJ, Howell S, Jones MP, Horowitz M. Predictors of turnover of lower gastrointestinal symptoms in diabetes mellitus. *Am J Gastroenterol* 2002; **97**: 3087–94.

40. Horowitz M, Maddox AF, Wishart JM, Harding PE *et al*. Relationships between oesophageal transit and solid and liquid gastric emptying in diabetes mellitus. *Eur J Nucl Med* 1991; **18**: 229–34.

41. Wegener M, Börsch G, Schaffstein J, Luerweg C, Leverkus F. Gastrointestinal transit disorders in patients with insulin-treated diabetes mellitus. *Dig Dis* 1990; **8**: 23–6.

42. Keshavarzian A, Iber FL, Vaeth J. Gastric emptying in patients with insulin-requiring diabetes mellitus. *Am J Gastroenterol* 1987; **82**: 29–35.

43. Horowitz M, Harding PE, Maddox AF, Wishart JM *et al*. Gastric and oesophageal emptying in patients with type 2 (non-insulin-dependent) diabetes mellitus. *Diabetologia* 1989; **32**: 151–9.

44. Nowak TV, Johnson CP, Kalbfleisch JH, Roza AM *et al*. Highly variable gastric emptying in patients with insulin-dependent diabetes mellitus. *Gut* 1995; **37**: 23–9.

45. Phillips WT, Schwartz JG, McMahan CA. Rapid gastric emptying of an oral glucose solution in type 2 diabetic patients. *J Nucl Med* 1992; **33**: 1496–500.

46. Schwartz JG, Green GM, Guan D, McMahan CA, Phillips WT. Rapid gastric emptying of a solid pancake meal in type 2 diabetic patients. *Diabetes Care* 1996; **19**: 468–71.

47. Jones KL, Horowitz M, Carney BI, Wishart JM *et al*. Gastric emptying in 'early' non-insulin-dependent diabetes mellitus. *J Nucl Med* 1996; **37**: 1643–8.

48. Kim CH, Kennedy FP, Camilleri M, Zinsmeister AR, Ballard DJ. The relationship between clinical factors and gastrointestinal dysmotility in diabetes mellitus. *J Gastrointest Motil* 1991; **3**: 268–72.

49. Iber FL, Parveen S, Vandrunen M, Sood KB *et al*. Relation of symptoms to impaired stomach, small bowel, and colon motility in long-standing diabetes. *Dig Dis Sci* 1993; **38**: 45–50.

50. Mearin F, Malagelada J-R. Gastroparesis and dyspepsia in patients with diabetes mellitus. *Eur J Gastroenterol Hepatol* 1995; **7**: 717–23.

51. Horowitz M, Edelbroek M, Fraser R, Maddox A, Wishart J. Disordered gastric motor function in diabetes mellitus. Recent insights into prevalence, pathophysiology, clinical relevance, and treatment. *Scand J Gastroenterol* 1991; **26**: 673–84.

52. Holtmann G, Goebell H, Talley NJ. Gastrointestinal sensory function in functional dyspepsia. *Gastroenterology* 1995; **109**: 331–2.

53. Samsom M, Salet GAM, Roelofs JMM, Akkermans LMA *et al*. Compliance of the proximal stomach and dyspeptic symptoms in patients with type 1 diabetes mellitus. *Dig Dis Sci* 1995; **40**: 2037–42.

54. Hebbard GS, Sun WM, Dent J, Horowitz M. Acute hyperglycaemia increases proximal gastric compliance. *Gastroenterology* 1994; **106**: A509.

55. Schvarcz E, Palmér M, Åman J, Lindkvist B, Beckman K-W. Hypoglycaemia increases the gastric emptying rate in patients with type 1 diabetes mellitus. *Diabet Med* 1993; **10**: 660–63.

56. Hebbard GS, Sun WM, Dent J, Horowitz M. Hyperglycaemia affects gastric motor and sensory function in normal subjects. *Eur J Gastroenterol Hepatol* 1996; **8**: 211–17.

57. Hebbard GS, Samsom M, Sun WM, Dent J, Horowitz M. Hyperglycaemia affects proximal gastric motor and sensory function during small intestinal nutrient infusion. *Am J Physiol* 1996; **271**: G814–19.

58. Chey WD, Kim M, Hasler W, Owyang C. Hyperglycaemia alters perception of rectal distension and blunts the recto-anal inhibitory reflex in healthy volunteers. *Gastroenterology* 1995; **108**: 1700–708.

59. Drossman DA, McKee DC, Sandler RS, Mitchell CM *et al*. Psychosocial factors in the irritable bowel syndrome: a multivariate study of patients and non-patients with irritable bowel syndrome. *Gastroenterology* 1988; **95**: 701–8.

60. Whitehead WE, Bosmajian L, Zonderman AB, Costa PT Jr, Schuster MM. Symptoms of psychological distress associated with irritable bowel syndrome. Comparison of community and medical clinic samples. *Gastroenterology* 1988; **95**: 709–14.

61. Talley NJ, Phillips SF, Bruce B, Twomey CK *et al*. Relation among personality and symptoms in non-ulcer dyspepsia and the irritable bowel syndrome. *Gastroenterology* 1990; **99**: 327–33.

62. Zighelboim J, Talley NJ. What are functional bowel disorders? *Gastroenterology* 1993; **104**: 1196–201.

63. Drossman DA, Richter JE, Talley NJ, Thompson WG *et al*. (eds). *The Functional Gastrointestinal Disorders: Diagnosis, Pathophysiology and Treatment—A Multinational Consensus*. Little, Brown: Boston, 1994

64. Skenzay JA, Bigler ED. Psychological adjustment and neuropsychological performance in diabetic patients. *J Clin Psychol* 1985; **41**: 391–6.

65. Lustman PJ, Grifith LS, Clouse RE *et al.*. Psychiatric illness in diabetes mellitus: relationship to symptoms and glucose control. *J Nerv Ment Dis* 1986; **174**: 736–42.

66. Popkin MK, Callies AL, Lentz RD *et al.*. Prevalence of major depression, simple phobia, and other psychiatric disorders in patients with long-standing type 1 diabetes mellitus. *Arch Gen Psychiat* 1988; **45**: 64–70.

67. Wilkinson G, Borsey DQ, Leslie P, Newton RW *et al*. Psychiatric morbidity and social problems in patients with insulin-dependent diabetes mellitus. *Br J Psychiat* 1988; **153**: 38–43.

68. Rubin RR, Peyrot M. Psychological problems and interventions in diabetes. A review of the literature. *Diabetes Care* 1992; **15**: 1640–57.

69. Lustman PJ, Griffith LS, Gavard JA, Clouse RE. Depression in adults with diabetes. *Diabetes Care* 1992; **15**: 1631–9.

70. Gavard JA, Lustman PJ, Clouse RE. Prevalence of depression in adults with diabetes. An epidemiological evaluation. *Diabetes Care* 1993; **16**: 1167–78.

71. Mazze RS, Lucido D, Shamoon H. Psychological and social correlates of glycaemic control. *Diabetes Care* 1984; **7**: 360–66.

72. Lustman PJ, Frank BL, McGill JB. Relationship of personality characteristics to glucose regulation in adults with diabetes. *Psychosom Med* 1991; **53**: 305–12.

73. Winocour PH, Main CJ, Medlicott G, Anderson DC. A psychometric evaluation of adult patients with type 1 (insulin-dependent) diabetes mellitus: prevalence of psychological dysfunction and relationship to demographic variables, metabolic control and complications. *Diabetes Res* 1990; **14**: 171–6.

74. Viinamäki H, Niskanen L, Uusitupa M. Mental well-being in people with non-insulin-dependent diabetes. *Acta Psychiatr Scand* 1995; **92**: 392–7.

75. Clouse RE, Lustman PJ, Reidel WL. Correlation of oesophageal motility abnormalities with neuropsychiatric status in diabetics. *Gastroenterology* 1986; **90**: 1146–54.

76. Clouse RE, Lustman PJ. Psychiatric illness and contraction abnormalities of the oesophagus. *N Engl J Med* 1983; **309**: 1337–42.

77. Talley NJ, Zinsmeister AR, Weaver A, DiMagno EP *et al*. Gastric adenocarcinoma and *Helicobacter pylori* infection. *J Natl Cancer Inst* 1991; **83**: 1734–9.

78. Diepersloot RJA, Bouter KP, Beyer WEP, Hoekstra JBL, Masurel N. Humoral immune response and delayed type hypersensitivity to influenza vaccine in patients with diabetes mellitus. *Diabetologia* 1987; **30**: 397–401.

79. Nolan CM, Beaty HN, Bagdale JD. Further characterisation of the impaired bactericidal function of granulocytes in patients with poorly controlled diabetes. *Diabetes* 1978; **27**: 889–94.

80. Glass EJ, Stewart J, Matthews DM, Collier A *et al*. Impairment of monocyte 'lectin-like' receptor activity in type 1 (insulin-dependent) diabetic patients. *Diabetologia* 1987; **30**: 228–31.

81. Hussein MJ, Alviggi L, Millwand BA, Leslie RDG *et al*. Evidence that the reduced number of natural killer cells in type 1 (insulin-dependent) diabetes mellitus may be genetically determinated. *Diabetologia* 1987; **30**: 907–11.

82. Ohno Y, Aoki N, Nishimura A. *In vitro* production of interleukin-1, interleukin-6, and tumor necrosis factor-α in insulin-dependent diabetes mellitus. *J Clin Endocrinol Metab* 1993; **77**: 1072–7.

83. Oldenburg B, Diepersloot RJA, Hoekstra JBL. High seroprevalence of *Helicobacter pylori* in diabetes mellitus patients. *Dig Dis Sci* 1996; **41**: 458–61.

84. Marrollo M, Latella G, Melideo D, Iannarelli R *et al*. *Helicobacter pylori* and peptic lesions prevalence is increased in diabetes mellitus patients. *Gastroenterology* 1997; **112**: A212.

85. De Luis DA, de la Calle H, Roy G, de Argila CM *et al*. *Helicobacter pylori* infection and insulin-dependent diabetes mellitus. *Diabetes Res Clin Pract* 1998; **39**: 143–6.

86. Gasbarrini A, Ojetti V, Pitocco D, De Luca A *et al*. *Helicobacter pylori* infection in patients affected by insulin-dependent diabetes mellitus. *Eur J Gastroenterol Hepatol* 1998; **10**: 469–72.

87. Dore MP, Bilotta M, Malaty HM, Pacifico A *et al*. Diabetes mellitus and *Helicobacter pylori* infection. *Nutrition* 2000; **16**: 407–10.

88. Xia HH, Talley NJ, Kam EP, Young LJ *et al*. *Helicobacter pylori* infection is not increased or linked to upper gastrointestinal symptoms in diabetes mellitus. *Am J Gastroenterol* 2001; **96**:1039–46.

89. Dimenas E, Glise H, Hallerback B, Hernqvist H *et al*. Quality of life in patients with upper gastrointestinal symptoms: an improved evaluation of treatment regimens? *Scand J Gastroenterol* 1993; **28**: 681–7.

90. Stewart AL, Greenfield S, Hays RD. Functional status and well-being of patients with chronic conditions. *J Am Med Assoc* 1989; **262**: 907–13.

91. Gill TM, Feinstein AR. A critical reappraisal of the quality of quality-of-life measurements. *J Am Med Assoc* 1994; **272**: 619–26.

92. Moyer CA, Fendrick AM. Measuring HRQL in patients with upper gastrointestinal disease. *Dig Dis Sci* 1998; **16**: 315–24.

93. Jacobson Am, Groot M, Samson JA. The evaluation of two measures of quality of life in patients with type 1 and type 2 diabetes. *Diabetes Care* 1994; **17**: 269–272.

94. Anderson RM, Fitzgerald JT, Wisdom K, Davis WK, Hiss RG. A comparison of global vs. disease-specific quality-of-life measures in patients with NIDDM. *Diabetes Care* 1997; **20**: 299–305.

95. Koloski NA, Talley NJ, Boyce PM. The impact of functional gastrointestinal disorders on quality of life. *Am J Gastroenterol* 2000; **95**: 67–71.

96. Enck P, Dubois D, Marquis P. Quality of life in patients with upper gastrointestinal symptoms: results from the Domestic/International Gastroenterology Surveillance Study (DIGEST). *Scand J Gastroenterol* 1999; **231**(suppl): 48–54.

97. Talley NJ, Weaver AL, Zinsmeister AR. Impact of functional dyspepsia on quality of life. *Dig Dis Sci* 1995; **40**: 584–9.

98. Cutts TF, Abell TL, Karas JG, Kuns J. Symptom improvement from prokinetic therapy corresponds to improved quality of life in patients with severe dyspepsia. *Dig Dis Sci* 1996; **41**: 1369–78.

99. Guyatt G, Mitchell A, Irvine EJ, Singer J *et al*. A new measure of health status for clinical trials in inflammatory bowel disease. *Gastroenterology* 1989; **96**: 804–10.

100. Patrick DL, Drossman DA, Frederick IO, Discesare J, Puder KL. Quality of life in persons with irritable bowel syndrome: development of a new measure. *Dig Dis Sci* 1998; **43**: 400–411.

101. Wong E, Guyatt GH, Cook DJ, Griffith LE, Irvine EJ. Development of a questionnaire to measure quality of life in patients with irritable bowel syndrome. *Eur J Surg* 1998; **583**(suppl): 50–56.

102. Drossman DA, Patrick DL, Whitehead WE, Toner BB *et al.* Further validation of the IBS–QOL: a disease-specific quality-of-life questionnaire. *Am J Gastroenterol* 2000; **95**: 999–1007.

103. Wiklund IK, Junghard O, Grace E, Talley NJ *et al.* Quality of life in reflux and dyspepsia patients. Psychometric documentation of a new disease-specific questionnaire (QOLRAD). *Eur J Surg* 1998; **583** (Suppl): 41–9.

104. Dimenas E, Glise H, Hallerback B, Hernqvist H *et al.* Well-being and gastrointestinal symptoms among patients referred to endoscopy owing to suspected duodenal ulcer. *Scand J Gastroenterol* 1995; **30**: 1046–52.

105. Rockwood TH, Church JM, Fleshman JW, Kane RL *et al.* Fecal incontinence quality of life scale. *Dis Colon Rectum* 2000; **43**: 9–17.

106. Talley NJ, Verlinden M, Jones M. Validity of a new quality of life scale for functional dyspepsia: a United States multicenter trial of the Nepean Dyspepsia Index. *Am J Gastroenterol* 1999; **94**: 2390–7.

107. Glia A, Lindberg G. Quality of life in patients with different types of functional constipation. *Scand J Gastroenterol* 1997; **32**: 1083–9.

108. Revicki DA, Wood M, Maton PN, Sorensen S. The impact of gastroesophageal reflux disease on health-related quality of life. *Am J Med* 1998; **104**: 252–8.

109. Havelund T, Lind T, Wiklund I, Glise H *et al.* Quality of life in patients with heartburn but without esophagitis: effects of treatment with omeprazole. *Am J Gastroenterol* 1999; **94**: 1782–9.

110. Revicki DA, Crawley JA, Zodet MW, Levine DS, Joelsson BO. Complete resolution of heartburn symptoms and health-related quality of life in patients with gastro-oesophageal reflux disease. *Aliment Pharmacol Ther* 1999; **13**: 1621–30.

111. Soykan I, Sivri B, Sarosiek I, Kiernan B, McCallum RW. Demography, clinical characteristics, psychological and abuse profiles, treatment and long-term follow-up of patients with gastroparesis. *Dig Dis Sci* 1998; **43**: 2398–404.

112. Silvers D, Kipnes M, Broadstone V, Patterson D *et al.* Domperidone in the management of symptoms of diabetic gastroparesis: efficacy, tolerability, and quality-of-life outcomes in a multicenter controlled trial. DOM-USA Study Group. *Clin Ther* 1998; **20**: 438–53.

113. Soykan I, Sarosiek I, McCallum RW. The effect of chronic oral domperidone therapy on gastrointestinal symptoms, gastric emptying, and quality of life in patients with gastroparesis. *Am J Gastroenterol* 1997; **92**: 976–80.

114. Drossman DA. Do psychosocial factors define symptom severity and patient status in irritable bowel syndrome? *Am J Med* 1999; **107**(5A): 41–50S.

115. Mathias JR, Clench MH, Abell TL, Koch KL *et al.* Effect of leuprolide acetate in treatment of abdominal pain and nausea in premenopausal women with functional bowel disease: a double-blind, placebo-controlled, randomized study. *Dig Dis Sci* 1998; **43**: 1347–55.

116. Snijders F, de Boer JB, Steenbergen B, Schouten M *et al.* Impact of diarrhoea and faecal incontinence on the daily life of HIV-infected patients. *AIDS Care* 1998; **10**: 620–37.

117. O'Keefe EA, Talley NJ, Zinsmeister AR, Jacobsen SJ. Bowel disorders impair functional status and quality of life in the elderly: a population-based study. *J Gerontol Med Sci* 1995; **50**: M184–9.

118. Sailer M, Bussen D, Fuchs KH, Thiede A. Quality of life in patients with fecal incontinence. *Langenbecks Arch Chir Suppl Kongressbd* 1998; **115**: 973–5.

119. Sailer M, Bussen D, Debus ES, Fuchs KH, Thiede A. Quality of life in patients with benign anorectal disorders. *Br J Surg* 1998; **85**: 1716–9.

120. Glasgow RE, Ruggiero L, Eakin EG, Dryfoos J, Chobanian L. Quality of life and associated characteristics in a large national sample of adults with diabetes. *Diabetes Care* 1997; **20**: 562–7.

121. Mazze RS, Lucido D, Shamoon H. Psychological and social correlates of glycemic control. *Diabetes Care* 1984; **7**: 360–66.

122. Hathaway DK, Abell TL, Cardoso S, Hartwig MS *et al.* Improvement in autonomic and gastric function following pancreas–kidney vs. kidney-alone transplantation and the correlation with quality of life. *Transplantation* 1994; **57**: 816–22.

123. Denth JPH, Engel LGJB. Diabetic gastroparesis: a critical reappraisal of new treatment strategies. *Drugs* 1992; **44**: 537–53.

124. Talley NJ, Young L, Hammer J, Leemon M *et al.* Impact of chronic gastrointestinal symptoms in diabetes mellitus on health-related quality of life. *Am J Gastroenterol* 2001; **96**: 71–6.

125. Siddique R, Ricci JA, Stewart WF, Sloan S, Farup CE. Quality of life in a US national sample of adults with diabetes and motility-related upper gastrointestinal symptoms. *Dig Dis Sci* 2002; **47**: 683–9.

126. Testa MA, Simonson DC. Health economic benefits and quality of life during improved glycemic control in patients with type 2 diabetes mellitus. *J Am Med Assoc* 1998; **280**: 1490–96.

127. Bityutskiy LP, Soykan I, McCallum RW. Viral gastroparesis: a subgroup of idiopathic gastroparesis—clinical characteristics and long-term outcomes. *Am J Gastroenterol* 1997; **92**: 1501–4.

128. Rashed H, Abell TL, Cardoso S, Cutts T *et al.* Autonomic function testing correlates with response to domperidone therapy in patients with diabetes mellitus and the symptoms of gastroparesis. *Diabetes* 1997; **381** A.

129. Aggarwal A, Cutts T, Abell TL, Cardoso S *et al.* Predominant symptoms in the irritable bowel syndrome may correlate with specific abnormalities of the autonomic nervous system. *Gastroenterology* 1994; **106**: 945–50.

130. Farup CE, Leidy NK, Murray M, Williams GR *et al.* Effect of domperidone on the health-related quality of life of patients with symptoms of diabetic gastroparesis. *Diabetes Care* 1998; **21**: 1699–706.

131. Prakash A, Wagstaff AJ. Domperidone: a review of its use in diabetic gastropathy. *Drugs* 1998; **56**: 429–45.

132. Familoni BO, Abell TL, Voeller G, Salem A, Gaber O. Electrical stimulation at a higher frequency than basal rate in human stomach. *Dig Dis Sci* 1997; **42**: 885–91.

133. Rashed H, Luo J, Cutts T, Abell TL. Practitioner-rated score (ADAPS) correlates with symptom severity in patients with severe dyspepsia treated with long-term device, prokinetics and behavioural treatment. *Neurogastroenterol Motil* 2000; **12**: 492.

2

Effects of Diabetes Mellitus on Gastrointestinal Function in Animal Models

Andrew A. Young and **Gaylen L. Edwards**

Introduction

This chapter describes the use of, and features of, animal models that are most commonly used in studies of gastrointestinal function relating to diabetes mellitus. In animal studies of gastrointestinal function in diabetes mellitus, most information has been generated using insulinopenic rats with severe hyperglycaemia; around one-third of the literature has been generated using BB rats (autoimmune spontaneous diabetic) and two-thirds using streptozotocin (STZ; chemically-induced) diabetic models. In the choice of these animal models, an assumption appears to have been often made that hyperglycaemia *per se*, or at least some aspect of the metabolic disturbance secondary to insulin lack, is the aetiopathologic insult. A common hypothesis is that neurotoxicity of the

Gastrointestinal Function in Diabetes Mellitus. Edited by Michael Horowitz and Melvin Samsom
© 2004 John Wiley & Sons, Ltd ISBN: 0-471-89916-X

autonomic nervous system, secondary to this metabolic insult, is responsible for the gastrointestinal effects of diabetes. This hypothesis is described here as the 'autonomic neuropathic' hypothesis. Evidence of autonomic neuropathy and the potential role of such neuropathy is discussed in conjunction with a synopsis of normal autonomic control of the gut.

Central nervous structures, especially those in the brain stem, that are implicated in the normal autonomic control of gastrointestinal function, and the impact on those structures of agents commonly used to induce diabetes, are also discussed. The importance of this information relates primarily to the fact that over two-thirds of the literature regarding gastrointestinal dysfunction in diabetes is derived from chemically-induced models in which, alarmingly, much of the reported gut dysfunction could be an artifact of selective damage to central structures. It is now recognised that there are major differences in gastrointestinal function between animals in which β-cell damage was caused by chemical means and those in which damage was a result of an autoimmune process. These differences prompt an examination of the extent to which gastrointestinal dysfunction in some models is a consequence of diabetes *per se*, perhaps applicable to human disease, as opposed to being a consequence of damage to specific central structures. The latter part of this chapter addresses the endocrine derangements in rodent diabetes, specifically discussing what is primary, what is secondary to gut dysfunction and what may be artifactual. A 'neurocrine' alternative to the neuropathic hypothesis of diabetes-associated gut dysfunction is proposed, that focuses on the possibility that absolute or relative deficiency of the pancreatic β-cell hormone, amylin, may be of importance in the aetiology of disordered gastrointestinal function in diabetes.

Purposes and choices of diabetic animal models

It is the purpose of many animal models to inform us of pathogenic and pathophysiological aspects of human disease. To accomplish this, it is not necessary for the animal model to exhibit the full panoply of signs present in the human condition. Indeed, in some cases a close concordance in animals of a constellation of clinical signs may reflect aetiologies that are not relevant to, and do not fully inform us of, human diseases. Furthermore, the predominance of one or other model in the literature is not necessarily indicative of its fidelity to human disease. For example, the approximately four-fold higher use of STZ compared to BB rats almost certainly reflects the facility with which these different models are produced and maintained, and not their similitude to human type 1 diabetes. Most models have attributes which favour their use in different circumstances.

Table 2.1 lists several commonly used animal models of diabetes mellitus, and includes the metabolic attributes associated with each. The majority of the literature relating to gastrointestinal dysfunction in these models is based on studies in insulinopenic rodents, mainly rats, characterised by severe hyperglycaemia.

Table 2.1 Commonly used animal models of diabetes mellitus

Animal Model	Total insulinopenia (insulin lack)	Subtotal insulinopenia (insulin deficiency), hyposecretion	Hyperphagia, insulin excess, peripheral insulin resistance	Dyslipidaemia, vascular disease	Severe hyperglycaemia	Moderate hyperglycaemia	Ketosis, hyperglucagonaemia	Easy to obtain or induce	Easy to maintain or manage	Aetiology	Papers
Pancreatectomy[1]	•				•					Surgical	•••
BB rat[1]	•				•		•			Autoimmune	•••
NOD mouse[1]	•				•		•			Autoimmune	•••
STZ rat[1]		•			•		•	•	•	Cytotoxicity via GLUT2	•••
Alloxan rat/mouse/etc[1]	•				•		•	•	•	Cytotoxicity via GLUT2	•••
Gold thioglucose[2]			•			•			•	Neurotoxic to glucosensors	•••
Monosodium glutamate[2]			•			•			•	Neurotoxic to glucosensors	•••
VMH lesioning[2]			•			•			•	Surgical	•••
ob/ob mouse[2]			•			•		•	•	Leptin deficiency	•••
db/db mouse[2]			•			•		•	•	Leptin receptor deficiency	•••
Zucker rat[2]			•	•		•		•	•	Leptin receptor deficiency	•••
ZDF rat[2]		•	•	•	•				•	Leptin receptor, secretory	•••
OLET F rat[2]			•			•			•	CCK receptor deficiency	•••
LAN corpulent rat[2]			•	•		•			•	Unknown	•••

[1] Models of type 1 (insulinopenic) diabetes.
[2] Models of type 2 diabetes mellitus.

Insulinopenic diabetic animals used as models of human type 1 diabetes mellitus have either spontaneous (genetically predisposed autoimmune) disease, such as in the Bio-Breeding (BB) rat or non-obese diabetic (NOD) mouse, or have been exposed to β-cell toxins such as streptozotocin (STZ) or alloxan, to induce insulitis chemically.

Rodent models of obesity, insulin resistance and type 2 diabetes, all of which exhibit spontaneous hyperphagia, include genetic models such as the *ob/ob* mouse, *db/db* mouse, Fatty Zucker rat (defective leptin signalling due to absent ligand or impaired receptor function) and OLETF rat (defective receptor for the satiogenic hormone CCK) or have been exposed to agents such as monosodium glutamate (MSG) and gold thioglucose (GTG) that are toxic to central glucosensitive neurones. Destruction of these neurones, important in appetite regulation, results in hyperphagia, obesity and animals showing many features of human type 2 diabetes. The utility of these models in understanding the pathogenesis and pathophysiology of human diabetes has been considerable.

Bio-Breeding (BB) rat

The genetic basis of the islet-specific autoimmune disease in the BB rat, and how that process relates to the aetiology in human disease, is poorly understood.

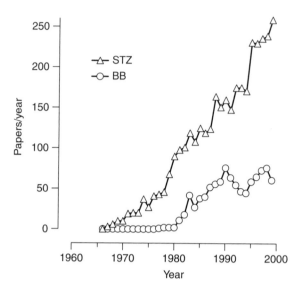

Figure 2.1 Comparison of annual publications using streptozotocin and BB rat models of insulinopenic diabetes mellitus since first use

Nevertheless, a highly desired attribute of the BB rat is the degree to which it mimics the natural history of human type 1 diabetes, including the development of diabetic complications [1,2]. The BB rat has been used to study many sequelae of the human disease [3], including retinopathy [4,5] and neuropathy [6–8], which develop more rapidly than in the STZ rat. However, the BB rat appears comparatively resistant to diabetic nephropathy [9] and angiopathy [3] and accordingly has not been widely used in studies of these pathologies (Figure 2.1). The BB rat has been widely used to test emergent therapies, such as islet transplants [10–12] and drugs for diabetic complications. The insulin-deficiency in the BB rat appears to be more profound, and metabolic control more disturbed, than in the STZ rat. It might therefore be concluded that the BB rat is a preferred model of human disease. However, a limitation in the use of the BB rat is that it is difficult to produce and resource-intensive to maintain after the onset of diabetes. Moreover, the onset of diabetes is not certain or predictable in individual animals.

The Spontaneous Diabetic Wistar BB (BBDP/*Wor*) rat was developed in 1974 following the observation of spontaneous diabetes of unknown aetiology in an outbred colony of Wistar rats at Bio-Breeding Laboratories, Ontario, Canada. In 1977, these animals were brought to Worcester, where Butler *et al.* [13] began inbreeding BB rats at the University of Massachusetts Medical Centre (laboratory code *Wor*) [14]. The aim was to develop an inbred model with good fecundity and a high incidence of diabetes. Selection for breeding did not occur until after the onset of hyperglycaemia [14]. Genetic studies [13] showed that diabetic × diabetic mating resulted in the fixing of recessive diabetogenic genes and enabled mating prior to the onset of hyperglycaemia [14]. A predictable and large fraction (up to 91%) of the ensuing litter could be expected to spontaneously develop diabetes [15], and in some circumstances the autoimmune process can be initiated with a dose of STZ that is ordinarily sub-diabetogenic in other rats. If the insulinopenia and autoimmune processes of human type 1 diabetes are to be closely mimicked, then the BB rat or NOD mouse may be preferred over other models.

The non-obese diabetic (NOD) mouse merits mention at this stage [16], since in the spontaneity of its autoimmune insulitis, it is similar in many respects to the BB rat. This animal model is widely used in studies of autoimmune processes, and as a model for the pathogenesis of human type 1 diabetes. However, it is not featured in studies of gastrointestinal dysfunction, and will, therefore, receive scant coverage here.

Streptozotocin-treated (STZ) rat

Type 1 (insulin-dependent) diabetes may be pharmacologically induced via a number of agents that selectively destroy pancreatic β-cells. Streptozotocin (STZ) and alloxan are the most commonly used drugs and have been used in many species, including non-human primates, dogs, cats, rabbits, rodents and pigs. More than 50 STZ analogues have been produced. Less selective β-cell toxins include organic metal-binding compounds and derivatives of ascorbic acid and uric acid [17], and the rodenticide pyriminil (Vacor) [18,19].

Streptozotocin, or streptozocin (US adopted name), commonly abbreviated as STZ, is an antibiotic produced by *Streptomyces achromogenes* (variety 128) isolated from a soil sample taken at Blue Rapids, Kansas, by an Upjohn salesman in 1959. In highly purified form, STZ has been shown to exert antitumoral activity in leukaemia, carcinosarcoma and other neoplastic models. In 1963, Rakeiten *et al.* [20] reported that intravenous streptozotocin was diabetogenic in dogs and rats. STZ is also diabetogenic in the hamster, monkey, mouse and guinea pig [17], but causes no more than mild glucose intolerance in humans [21]. Susceptibility to the diabetogenic and toxic effects of STZ, therefore, varies widely between species. In some species, the lethal and diabetogenic doses are very similar.

In contrast to the BB rat, the streptozotocin-induced diabetic rat is easily produced upon demand. However, the β-cell destruction invoked with STZ is cytotoxic and not autoimmune, and is less complete. Moreover, STZ can affect tissues other than β-cells, as discussed below. The STZ-diabetic rat is easier to treat and can be maintained in better metabolic control than the BB rat. This may relate to a subtotal β-cell toxicity of the drug. Reports of reversion of STZ-induced diabetes in rats [22,23], and our own observations that insulin requirement is higher following multiple (vs. a single) treatment with STZ are indicative of the survival of some β-cells. Furthermore, STZ-treated rats (in contrast to BB rats) can survive for days to months after the onset of diabetes without insulin injections.

As a model of pathological and metabolic processes associated with human hyperglycaemia, the STZ-treated rat is very convenient. Rats can be purchased and STZ-treated as required, and the difficulties associated with breeding from diabetes-prone females, detecting diabetes in offspring, and unpredictable conversion to diabetes (as occurs with the BB rat) can be largely avoided; diabetes can be invoked easily and on a desired date. Histologically, the insulitis induced by STZ is indistinguishable from that produced by alloxan [24], and similar in some respects to that observed in autoimmune insulitis. The use of STZ allows the investigator to study a reproducible type of diabetes in a variety of species and to use smaller animal models for economy of care. The STZ rat has been used to develop antidiabetic drugs and therapies, such as islet transplants [25,26]. Models using STZ-induced type 1 diabetes have been used to study the aetiopathogenesis of retinopathy [4,5], angiopathy [27] and neuropathy [28–30]. The STZ diabetic rat has also been used to study nephropathy [31–33], but it should be recognised in this context that STZ can be nephrotoxic in rats. A major issue that will be discussed in some detail is the neurotoxic effect of STZ and other agents used to induce diabetes chemically, focusing on effects on central GLUT2-containing neurones that are involved in gastrointestinal function.

Gastrointestinal function and the autonomic nervous system

Neural interactions with the gastrointestinal system and pancreas occur via the autonomic nervous system. This control of gastrointestinal functions (motility and secretion) is shared by all three divisions of the autonomic nervous system, the parasympathetic nervous system via vagal and pelvic nerves, the sympathetic system via the mesenteric nerves, and the enteric nervous system intrinsic to the walls of the intestine.

Parasympathetic innervation

The parasympathetic system innervates the proximal gastrointestinal tract via the Xth cranial (vagus) nerve and the anad gastrointestinal tract via pelvic nerves. Preganglionic motor fibres of the efferent vagus arise primarily in the dorsal motor nucleus of the vagus (DMV), the nucleus ambiguus (NA), the retrofacial nucleus, and the nucleus retroambiguus (NRA), all situated in the medulla oblongata. Preganglionic motor neurons of the pelvic nerve arise in the central grey matter of the sacral spinal cord in a region analogous to the intermediolateral cell column in the thoracolumbar cord [34]. The best-characterised neurotransmitter in these preganglionic fibres is acetylcholine, but other neurotransmitters are also present, including enkephalin, substance P, somatostatin and gastrin, which are also found in the preganglionic parasympathetic neurons. Acetylcholine, released from preganglionic motor neurons, acts primarily upon postganglionic nicotinic receptors (some muscarinic receptors) in ganglia that are closely associated with the end organ, and are often difficult to differenti-ate from those of the enteric nervous system. Postganglionic fibres project onto effector organs (glands or smooth muscle) in the gastrointestinal tract. Most postganglionic fibres also contain acetylcholine, which usually acts on atropine-blockable muscarinic receptors to produce an effect. Postganglionic fibres, which are often difficult to distinguish from enteric nervous system fibres, also contain neuropeptides, including somatostatin and vasoactive intestinal peptide.

Sympathetic innervation

Sympathetic innervation of the gastrointestinal tract via the coeliac and mesen-teric nervosa arises in cholinergic preganglionic fibres in the intermediolateral cell column of the thoracolumbar spinal cord from approximately T10 to L2 [34]. As in the parasympathetic system, acetylcholine released from these fibres typically activates nicotinic receptors on postganglionic neurons in paraverte-bral ganglia. Most postganglionic sympathetic fibres use norepinephrine as their major transmitter. However, some fibres to sweat glands and skeletal muscle contain acetylcholine. Most postganglionic sympathetic fibres cosecrete addi-tional neurotransmitters/neuromodulators, such as neuropeptide Y, somatostatin and ATP. The sympathetic nervous system has a lesser influence over gastroin-testinal function than the vagus (parasympathetic). Sympathetic effects typically include inhibition of gastrointestinal activity, such as relaxation of intestinal smooth muscle and inhibition of secretion.

The enteric nervous system

The enteric nervous system consists of an extensive network of nerves lining the gut that are as numerous as the nerves in the spinal cord. Enteric neu-rons consist of those in the myenteric plexus (more involved in motility) lying between the longitudinal and circular muscle layers of the gut, and the sub-mucosal plexus (more involved in secretion and absorption), found beneath the mucosal layer. Neurotransmitters in the enteric nervous system include acetylcholine, but also biogenic amines (serotonin, dopamine and histamine), amino acids (γ-aminobutyric acid), neuropeptides such as dynorphin, vasoac-tive intestinal peptide (VIP), substance P and motilin, and nitric oxide (NO). Dynorphin and VIP are reported to inhibit gastrointestinal motility [35] while substance P and motilin increase it [35]. Neuropeptides and neurotransmitters are almost always co-localised within the same neurone. It has been suggested that in general neuropeptides modulate activity over a longer time domain, while neurotransmitters tend to operate over shorter time domains, with some excep-tions (acetylcholine evokes fast excitatory postsynaptic potentials, but serotonin and substance P evoke slow excitatory postsynaptic potentials in the myenteric plexus [35]. A combination of excitatory and inhibitory influences, acting over different time domains, contributes to an aggregate postsynaptic effect within the enteric nervous system.

Some recent work suggests that disturbances in nitric oxide signalling may be implicated in gastric dysfunction. The presence of glucose (0%, 10%, 20%) in the gavage dose-dependently slowed the rate of gastric emptying in wild-type mice, and showed that the glucose content of the gavage needed to be controlled (20%) in subsequent experiments. In mice with a gene deletion of neural nitric oxide synthase (nNOS$^-$), there was a marked prolongation of emptying. The delay in gastric emptying observed in nNOS$^-$ mice, NOD diabetic mice and STZ mice was similar. Insulin treatment reversed the delayed emptying observed in the NOD and STZ mice. In the nNOS$^-$ mice, the effect of non-adrenergic non-cholinergic stimulation to relax excised pylorus was absent, suggesting a local tissue cause of delayed emptying. Phosphodiesterase 5 (PDE5) is found in high abundance in the pylorus, and hydrolyses the effector molecule of NO, cyclic GMP. A drug that inhibits PDE5, sildenafil (Viagra), and enhances the effector molecule, reversed the slowed gastric emptying observed in nNOS$^-$ mice [36]. These experiments raised the possibility that some aspect of the diabetic state is associated with disturbances in the NO signalling system, and that the latter could underlie slowed gastric emptying.

In addition to its acknowledged motor function, the enteric nervous system may also serve a sensory function. Neurones that are potentially glucose-responsive, in that they possess many of the markers of pancreatic β-cells, have been identified in the ileum [37]. By immunolocalisation they were shown to express $K_{ir6.2}$, the inwardly-rectifying potassium channel, and SUR1, the sulpho-nylurea receptor, characteristic of pancreatic β-cells. Similarly, these cells were depolarised with tolbutamide and hyperpolarised with diazoxide. How activation of these cells relates to localised or general gut function is currently unknown.

Gastrointestinal functions disturbed in animal diabetes

Gastric emptying

Disturbances of gastric emptying are reported to be a common feature of human diabetes. However, the literature in this area is acknowledged to be confusing [38] and is reviewed more thoroughly in Chapter 4. General issues in assessing gastric emptying include:

1. The absence of population-based studies to define 'normal' emptying, i.e. most studies are done in patients.

2. Failure to characterise metabolic status. Many reports do not distinguish between type 1 and type 2 diabetes. Further, very few assessments of gastric emptying are reported in association with controlled plasma glucose concentrations, which is important since hyperglycaemia itself can slow the rate of emptying [39].

3. Failure to assess autonomic function. Many do not assess the presence of autonomic neuropathy, reportedly associated with gastroparesis and delayed gastric emptying [40].

Thus, while many reports cite that type 1 diabetic patients show delayed ($\sim 40\%$) or normal emptying, some authors report that patients with type 1 diabetes may show accelerated gastric emptying [41–43]. Other studies in type 1 diabetic humans report instances of both accelerated and delayed emptying [44].

The clinical picture in 'early' type 2 diabetes mellitus and insulin resistance appears less confused. Studies more consistently report an acceleration of gastric emptying [45–49]. This may partly be technically related, given that most of these data come from one group which monitored principally liquid emptying. Others who measured solid emptying [50] did not see acceleration.

There is less disagreement regarding diabetes-associated changes in gastric emptying in animal models of diabetes mellitus. The BB rat model of autoimmune type 1 diabetes [51–53] exhibits accelerated gastric emptying (Figure 2.2). Most studies using STZ rats also report accelerated gastric emptying [52,54–57], although two studies report a slowing [58,59]. In one of these, slowing was present only during the first week after induction of diabetes [58]. There is a single study of gastric emptying rates in insulinopenic mice that uses both NOD and STZ models [36]. In that study, in which a fixed glucose load was gavaged, both models exhibited slowed gastric emptying.

Most studies performed in animal models of insulin resistance and type 2 diabetes report an acceleration of gastric emptying. The diabetic Fatty Zucker model

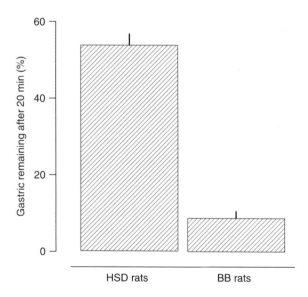

Figure 2.2 Fraction of phenol red tracer recoverable from the stomach of BB (autoimmune type 1 diabetic) rats compared to Harlan Sprague–Dawley (non-diabetic) rats 20 min after gavage with an acaloric gel

of type 2 diabetes [60], the LA/N corpulent rat [61] and a hyperphagic model [62] exhibited accelerated emptying. Thus, gastric emptying appears accelerated in hyperphagic, insulin-resistant rats and in most insulinopenic rodent models.

Gastric acid secretion

STZ diabetic rats most often show increased gastric acid secretion [63,64] and increased rates of ulceration [65–71]. This effect is exacerbated by fasting [67] and is reversed by hyperglycaemia [72] but not by insulin replacement [73]. It thus appears that insulin lack is not the ulcerogenic stimulus, and raises the possibility that absence of gastric-inhibitory factors (e.g. amylin, PYY, GLP-1), which may be absent or reduced in diabetes, could be implicated. In contrast to the majority finding of acid hypersecretion, one study noted no difference between diabetic and non-diabetic animals in pentagastrin-stimulated acid secretion [74], and one study described a reduction in acid secretion in alloxan-treated rats [75]. A direct, toxic effect of STZ on gastric mucosa has been proposed as a mechanism of increased ulceration in STZ diabetes. However, this does not explain why autoimmune type 1 diabetic BB rats [76] and autoimmune non-obese diabetic (NOD) mice [77] in which the gastric mucosa is not an immune target, also show a marked increase in gastric erosions. The constancy of findings of acid hypersecretion and ulceration in insulinopenic diabetes invoked by diverse insults (chemical and autoimmune) indicates that this gastrointestinal disturbance is a direct consequence of the diabetes, and perhaps of β-cell deficiency.

Central control of gastric acid secretion is mediated via a cholinergic pathway that includes the nucleus tractus solitarius (NTS), area postrema (AP), dorsal motor nucleus of the vagus [78,79] and capsaicin-sensitive vagal afferents [80]. Insulin stimulation of gastric acid secretion [81] appears to depend upon its hypoglycaemic effect. Increasing plasma glucose concentration inhibits gastric acid secretion [82,83], including that stimulated by insulin [84] and amino acids [85]. In contrast, glucagon-induced inhibition of gastric acid secretion appears to be independent of its effect on plasma glucose [86]. Amylin, which has a high density of receptors in the area postrema/nucleus tractus solitarius [87], is a potent inhibitor of gastric acid secretion [88], independent of changes in plasma glucose [89] and prevents gastric erosion in response to a number of irritants [90–92]. These effects appear to be specific to amylin, since they can be prevented by prior administration of the amylin receptor antagonist AC187 (unpublished). Studies using microinjection of D-glucose into different brain regions indicate that the effects of glucose to inhibit gastric acid secretion appear to be localised to structures around the nucleus tractus solitarius [80]. It is possible that amylin deficiency could be implicated in a propensity to ulceration in some forms of diabetes. It is unclear whether such a propensity exists in type 1 diabetic adults. However, type 1 diabetic children are reported to have a three- to four-fold elevation in rate of peptic disease [93].

Pancreatic exocrine secretion

Defective pancreatic exocrine function coexists with diabetes in some genetic models. One example is the Otsuka Long-Evans Tokushima fatty (OLETF) rat [94,95], in which the major deficiency is a defective CCK-A receptor [96]. Another example is the BETA2/neuroD-deficient mouse, in which there is a reduction in number of β-cells (leading to diabetes) and a failure to secrete zymogen granules from acinar cells [97]. There is scant evidence, however, of exocrine pancreatic dysfunction in humans [98] or animals. One paper reported that the composition of CCK-stimulated exocrine secretion is altered in STZ rats, while secretin-stimulated secretion was normal [99]. Another paper described a reduced secretin effect in perfused pancreas from STZ and alloxan rats [100], and another described a reduced secretin effect that is restored by intrahepatic islet transplantation [101]. In rats in which differing severities of diabetes were induced by graded injections of STZ, basal and caerulein-stimulated flow rates of pancreatic juice and protein output were similar in the control and in all three groups of diabetic rats [102]. Thus far, it appears that there is no consistently recognised defect in exocrine pancreatic function in animal models of diabetes.

Hyperglycaemia (but not hyperinsulinaemia) suppresses CCK-stimulated exocrine secretion from the pancreas in humans [103,104]. The concordance of inhibition of exocrine secretion and circulating pancreatic polypeptide (a marker of vagal activation) suggests that inhibition of pancreatico-biliary secretion during hyperglycaemia is vagal-cholinergic [105,106]. The β-cell hormone, amylin, potently inhibits CCK-stimulated pancreatic enzyme secretion [107] and has been shown to exert gastrointestinal effects via the vagus [108]. It is possible that the effects of hyperglycaemia on pancreatic exocrine secretion are mediated partly via glucose-stimulated amylin secretion (not via glucose-stimulated insulin secretion, since insulin does not have a direct effect on exocrine function [103]).

Intestinal mucosal function

Changes in intestinal mucosal function are observed in diabetic rodents, but it is unclear whether these are intrinsic and contributory to the disease process, or are secondary to the disease. For example, the BB rat exhibits enzymatic (i.e. apparently purposeful) glycosylation of the intestinal brush border enzyme amino-oligopeptidase soon after the onset of diabetes, with reversal of this pattern with vigorous insulin treatment. In contrast, this is not evident in the STZ rat [109], which typically has less severe diabetes, as previously discussed. A similar change and reversal in the BB rat has also been observed with intestinal sucrase-α-dextrinase [110]. Large increases in intestinal acyl-CoA:cholesterol acyltransferase (ACAT) and cholesterol esterase, implicated in cholesterol absorption from the gut, were also observed in the STZ diabetic rat, and these elevations were reversed with insulin-mediated improvement of glycaemic control [111]. It thus appears likely, from these studies, that diabetes-associated changes in gut enzyme expression represent a response to some aspect of the diabetic state, since they occur in both chemically-induced and genetic models, and are reversible with vigorous treatment of the diabetes.

Diet, as well as susceptibility to diabetes, increases expression of gut transporters (sodium–glucose co-transporter and GLUT5) and proglucagon mRNA in the BB rat [112], indicating that expression of these genes could be a response to an altered nutritive state, rather than being genetically determined. STZ treatment also increased gut glucose transporter and co-transporter expression [113] and increased expression of the Na^+-K^+-ATPase engine that drives sodium–glucose co-transport [114]. Proglucagon expression was also increased in the STZ diabetic rat [115]. The presence of parallel changes in both BB and STZ rat models again suggests that these changes represent a reaction to the diabetic state. Increased proglucagon expression and subsequent oversecretion of glucagon-like peptide-2 (GLP-2; a gut growth stimulant [116]) in STZ diabetic rats accounts for intestinal overgrowth observed in this model [117–119] and could account for some of the increased intestinal brush border enzyme expression observed in diabetic animals. Possible mechanisms accounting for hyperexpression of proglucagon and hypersecretion of GLP-2 from intestinal L-cells are discussed under 'glucagon-like peptide-2'. Diabetic animals exhibit increased capacity for glucose uptake from the gut [120,121], consistent with the observed changes in brush border enzyme expression. The observation that similar changes can be invoked by glucose administration for 4 h or more [122] suggests that this is glucose-driven.

Diabetes-associated changes in intestinal mucosal neurotransmitters are also observed in a number of animal models. In the submucosal plexus of hyperglycaemic (but not normoglycaemic) BB rats, somatostatin-containing neurons were reduced, and in the myenteric plexus galanin-containing nerve fibres were increased [123]. In the STZ rat, responsiveness of intestinal smooth muscle to acetylcholine and substance P was reduced [124].

Autonomic neuropathy in diabetic gastrointestinal dysfunction

As discussed elsewhere in this book, disordered gastrointestinal motility has long been recognised as a frequent feature in diabetic patients who also exhibit neuropathy [125]. Disturbances in gastrointestinal function have been estimated by some to have a prevalence of $\sim 30\%$ (range 5–60% [126–128]). Both peripheral and autonomic [126–128] neuropathy are frequent complications of diabetes mellitus. Since the autonomic nervous system (ANS) plays a prominent role in the regulation of gut motility, a prevailing hypothesis has been that autonomic neuropathic dysfunction could account for much of this disturbance.

Involvement of different autonomic branches

Although the sympathetic, parasympathetic and enteric divisions of the autonomic nervous system are each reported to show microscopic, neurochemical and functional changes during diabetes [129–132], there is debate as to how they might be implicated in diabetes-associated dysfunction. Motor disturbances associated with autonomic neuropathy include dilation of the oesophagus, gastrointestinal stasis, accumulation of digesta and constipation, mainly signs associated with vagal (parasympathetic) dysfunction. There are also reports of faecal incontinence, related to decreased sphincter pressure, and diarrhoea. These latter signs may be more related to loss of sympathetic tone, or possibly a relative increase in a neuropeptide, such as motilin. The enteric division appears to be most important to intrinsic (local) gastrointestinal control, providing more specific commands to the musculature to effect altered motility, while the parasympathetic and sympathetic divisions transmit general commands to the enteric nervous system.

Mechanisms of autonomic neuropathy

The best-characterised signs of damage to the autonomic nervous system during diabetes are morphological [129, 131, 133–135]. For example, the number of myelinated axons in the vagosympathetic trunk is decreased in diabetic rats [131], as is the number of neurones in dorsal root ganglia and peripheral postganglionic sympathetic nerves. There are also signs characteristic of neuroaxonal dystrophy [136], indicative of degeneration–regeneration cycles. In addition to alterations in numbers and morphology of axons, the tissue around the axons is also often disturbed. For example, there is a thickening of the endoneurium [128], which may sensitise axons to damage from increased pressure or decreased oxygen and glucose availability. Endoneural thickening may be further exacerbated by perineural vascular changes that have been noted in diabetic animals. It is thus possible that axonal damage may be secondary to disorders in tissue surrounding the neurons. It is of interest that autonomic neuropathy can be prevented or partially reversed by rigorous glycaemic control [137], suggesting that hyperglycaemia *per se* is of major aetiological importance in autonomic neuropathy.

Sorbitol accumulation

One hypothesis regarding the pathogenesis of autonomic neuropathy is that hyperglycaemia, by promoting increased intraneuronal glucose, results in an increase in production of sorbitol from glucose by aldose reductase. The sorbitol accumulation leads to decreased myo-inositol, reduced Na^+/K^+-ATPase, impaired nerve conduction [138] and, ultimately, a structural change in neurons. Aldose reductase inhibitors are effective at preventing structural neuronal damage in animal models of diabetes [139–141]. However, in patients with autonomic neuropathy, sorbitol accumulation and reduced myoinositol are not as evident as in animal models, and aldose reductase inhibitors and replacement of myoinositol appear to be of doubtful clinical benefit.

Impaired peptide secretion or synthesis

The secretion of a number of neuroendocrine substances may be decreased in diabetes. Glucagon, pancreatic polypeptide, gastrin, somatostatin and gastric inhibitory peptide levels are reportedly reduced in the gastrointestinal tract of diabetic patients [129, 133–135]. Since in animal studies there appears to be discordance between tissue levels and circulating concentrations [142], the significance of decreased levels of these peptides remains unclear; it is possible that a loss of these neuroendocrine substances contributes to the pathologies observed in autonomic neuropathy. Disturbances in systemic secretion of GLP-1, amylin and peptide YY in diabetes are covered under 'Neuroendocrine explanations for diabetic gastrointestinal dysfunction (p. 47)'.

Disturbances of axonal transport

Deficiencies in amino acid transport, subsequent protein synthesis and intra-axonal transport, noted in animal models of diabetes, could result in a failure to deliver macromolecules, such as neurofilament, to the distal ends of axons and dendrites [129–132, 138]. Retrograde axonal transport is also affected and thus important signals from the periphery, such as growth factors, would not reach the cell body. It appears that neuropathy is initiated distally and progresses toward the cell body.

Inflammatory processes

Inflammatory responses may account for some damage to autonomic neurons; inflammatory infiltrates have been observed in the autonomic ganglia of diabetic patients. This immune response, the genesis of which is unknown, could ultimately result in neuronal damage and death.

Microangiopathy

A feature of neuropathy in many experimental models of diabetic neuropathy is resistance to ischaemic conduction block, i.e. nerves from diabetic animals conduct traffic for a longer time after total ischaemia, consistent with the idea that nerves have adapted to chronic hypoxia. Such changes can be induced by chronic hypoxia *per se* [143]. Endoneural hypoxia induced by angiopathy has been recognised as a feature of STZ rats [144]; neurovascular disturbances are reported in diabetic rats [145] and humans [146].

Neuropathy in the STZ diabetic rat

Most of the literature regarding autonomic and gastrointestinal dysfunction has been generated using the STZ rat, which is now discussed. Many studies have reported morphological, neurochemical and functional disturbances in nerves following streptozotocin administration to rodents.

Morphological changes, consisting chiefly of dystrophic axonopathy, are mainly restricted to the alimentary tract [137], particularly the ileal mesenteric nerves and sympathetic ganglia [28,147,148]. These changes can be reversed with intensive insulin treatment [148] or islet transplantation [137]. Degeneration of mesenteric nerves and ganglia is seen in the ileum, and is not evident in the colon [149]. There are some changes, however, in the colon of the STZ rat, such as an increase in adrenergic and serotonergic neurone number [150].

Neurochemical changes in STZ rats, as with morphological changes, are most pronounced in the ileum, particularly the myenteric plexus. There is an increase in VIP mRNA [151], increased VIP content [152,153] and an increase in VIP containing nerves [154]. The increase in VIP, which paradoxically is associated with reduced neuronal VIP release [155], may reflect selective damage to VIP-containing fibres [156] and can be prevented with insulin treatment. Another neurotransmitter that is elevated in the myenteric plexus of the ileum is neuropeptide Y [152,154], while substance P is unchanged [134,152,153]. Adrenergic fibres [150] are reduced, as is CGRP content [134,152], possibly associated with selective loss of CGRPergic neurones [157]. The pyloric sphincter, in contrast to the ileum, shows a loss of most neuropeptides, including CGRP, met-enkephalin, neuropeptide Y, substance P and VIP [158].

Functional neurologic changes in the STZ rat are less evident than morphologic and neurochemical changes. Decreases in cardiovascular vagal and sympathetic tone have been reported [159,160], as has decreased sympathetic and parasympathetic action at salivary glands [161]. Although adrenergic and cholinergic responses of gastric smooth muscle were not altered in fundus strips [162], large changes in ATP release from strips of stomach from STZ rats suggested that purinergic autonomic innervation may have been altered.

General applicability of neuropathic changes

The question arises as to whether neuropathic changes in STZ rats are secondary to the diabetic process or are attributable to a direct neurotoxic effect of STZ.

Observations of similar perturbations in animal models of diverse aetiology would argue that at least some of these phenomena are generally diabetes-associated, and are less likely to be an STZ artifact. For example, alterations in the rate of axonal transport are seen in both STZ and BB rats [163], and reductions in pain threshold are seen in models where diabetes was induced by STZ, genetics (as in the sand rat, *Psammomys obesus*) or by galactose feeding [164]. Reversal of neuropathic changes following intensive glycaemic control also argues that at least some aspects of neuropathy are related to the metabolic state and are not entirely due to the initial cytotoxic insult. There are no descriptions of potential neurotoxic effects of subdiabetic doses of STZ; paradoxically, low-dose STZ appears to protect against kainic acid-induced neurotoxicity [165], and diabetogenic doses, while they do not induce acute peripheral nerve defects, paradoxically protect against defects induced by acrylamide [166]. However, in view of the potential for direct effects of STZ on nerve tissue, it may be that more secure conclusions can be drawn with models, such as the BB rat.

Neuropathy in the diabetic BB rat

Autoimmune diabetic BB rats have been used extensively as a model of autonomic neuropathy. Functional nerve impairment has been characterised by reduced conduction velocity [8,167,168], also manifest in the optic nerve as slowing of visual evoked potentials [169] and some components of retrograde axonal transport [132]. Brismar proposed that reduced sodium permeability and axoplasmic sodium concentrations may principally account for slowed conduction velocity [170]. Morphological evidence of neuropathy in BB rats includes axonal degeneration, irregularity of myelin sheaths and Mullerian degeneration [139,171,172]. It has been proposed that periodic hypoglycaemia in BB rats may induce Wallerian degeneration and reduced conduction velocity, primarily in motor pathways, including anterior horn cells, while abnormalities associated with chronic hyperglycaemia include sensory (afferent) axonopathy [172]. Abnormalities in urinary bladder contraction in chronically hyperglycaemic BB rats, for example, appear to be attributable to afferent axonopathy in pelvic and hypogastric autonomic nerves [173]. Other evidence of autonomic involvement in the neuropathy observed in BB rats includes morphological descriptions of reduced sympathetic fibre numbers in atrial myocardium [174], dystrophic changes in mesenteric nerves [175], the sympathetic chain (paravertebral thoracic ganglion cells, preganglionic myelinated fibres of the white ramus, and postganglionic unmyelinated fibres of the grey ramus communicans) [131,176], and reduced R–R variability [6].

Central vs. peripheral neuropathy

In addition to peripheral autonomic neuropathy, neurons within the central nervous system are also reported to be damaged in animal models of diabetes, including areas such as the paraventricular nucleus of the hypothalamus and the dorsal motor nucleus of the vagus, both of which are important in controlling those parts of the autonomic nervous system that innervate the gut. Because preganglionic fibres of the autonomic nervous system originate in the dorsal motor nucleus of the vagus nerve (DMV) and the nucleus ambiguus (NA), neuropathic lesions at these sites can be expected to affect gastrointestinal function. This also applies to defects in pathways that project onto these areas, such as the paraventricular nucleus of the hypothalamus, the amygdala and the nucleus of the tractus solitarius, which project onto neurons in the DMV [177]. Examples of brain regions associated with specific gut functions include the DMV, activation of which increases antral and pyloric contractions [178]. The lateral reticular formation, the pons (implicated in defecation [177]), the infralimbic and prelimbic cortex (an area that decreases gastric tone [177,179]) mediate emotive influences on gut function. Emotive effects on gut function were recognised by Cannon [180] and other early physiologists [181].

The brain stem and gastrointestinal function

A pathway that includes the nucleus tractus solitarius (NTS), the area postrema (AP) and the dorsal motor nucleus of the vagus nerve (DMV) [182], appears to be particularly important in controlling several gut functions. As with the innervation of other viscera, such as heart and lungs, gastrointestinal connections into the brain stem appear to be comparatively simple. There is a vague viscerotopic organisation of the NTS, in that distension of different viscera evoke activity in different parts of the nucleus [183,184]. Vagal afferents appear to terminate in the NTS [185,186], which projects to the DMV [187]. The DMV projects vagal efferents back to the stomach [186]. The area postrema is also driven by gastrointestinal and vagal stimuli [185,188], perhaps via reciprocal connections with the NTS [189].

The significance of the area postrema in this neuronal loop is its sensitivity to circulating stimuli. The area postrema is situated at the posterior margin of the fourth cerebral ventricle in the hindbrain, and is one of a family of circumventricular organs where fenestrated capillaries permit direct communication of circulating peptides with receptors on nerve cells, i.e. it functions as a sensory organ of the brain. The numerous receptors for peptide hormones described at the area postrema include those for IGF-2 [190], insulin [191,192], glutamate [193], serotonin [194], substance P (NK1) [195], arginine-vasopressin [196–198], imidazoline [199,200], angiotensin [201,202], glucagon-like peptide-1 [203–205], neuropeptide Y4 [206], pancreatic polypeptide [207,208], cholecystokinin [209,210], pituitary adenylate cyclase activating peptide [211], atrial natriuretic peptide [212], dopamine 3 [213], melatonin [214], PTH/PTHrP [215], hCG/LH [216], oxytocin [217], VIP/secretin [218–220], nicotine [221], somatostatin [222], histamine 2 [223], gastrin-releasing peptide [224], calcitonin [225] and amylin [87,226].

It has recently been discovered, using slice preparations of the area postrema, that the same neurones that respond to the insulin-modulating hormones, amylin and GLP-1, are also responsive to glucose [227]. The identification of glucose-sensitive neurones in the area postrema [228,229] supports the concept that this organ has a fuel-sensing function that will ultimately contribute to hormonal responses important in fuel homeostasis, especially those gastrointestinal functions important for defence against hypoglycaemia [229]. Interestingly, while the area postrema is implicated in the behavioural (feeding) response to 2 deoxyglucose-induced glucoprivation, it does not appear to be necessary for adrenomedullary responses [230].

Effect of diabetogenic chemicals on brain stem structures

The central role of the above-mentioned hindbrain structures in the regulation of gastrointestinal function demands that they be examined when considering possible aetiologies of disturbed gastrointestinal function in diabetes. Alarmingly, it appears that most, if not all, chemical agents used to produce diabetes in animal models selectively destroy or damage those hindbrain structures that control enteric function, and these are discussed further below. Major differences in gastrointestinal function in animals in which β-cell destruction was invoked by chemical means, use those in which it resulted from autoimmune destruction, raises substantial concerns about the extent to which gastrointestinal dysfunction in some models is an artifactual consequence of damage to specific central structures, rather than a general consequence of diabetes, perhaps applicable to human disease. As summarised below, steptozotocin (STZ), gold-thioglucose (GTG), monosodium glutamate (MSG) and alloxan all affect the function of neurones in the area postrema.

Streptozotocin (STZ) consists of 1-methyl-nitrosourea linked to C_2 of D-glucose [231], and is usually a mixture of α- and β-isomers. The observation that some non-metabolised glucose analogues, including 3-O-methyl-D-glucose and 2-deoxy-D-glucose, dose-dependently protect against STZ-induced β-cell toxicity [24], suggests a glucose-specific recognition site. The observation that STZ is selectively toxic in gluconeogenic tissues (β-cells, liver and kidney) is consistent with it being carried preferentially by the GLUT-2 glucose transporter found in those tissues [232–234]. It is believed that the glucose moiety of the α-anomer acts as a carrier for the toxic N-nitroso-N-methylurea moiety [235]. Interestingly, GLUT2 immunoreactivity has been identified in the region of the nucleus tractus solitarius/area postrema/dorsal motor nucleus of the vagus [236], leading to the concept that STZ may be selectively neurotoxic in those brain regions. Consistent with that idea, STZ reduces responses (angiotensin II-mediated pressor responses) that reside in the area postrema [237]. These data suggest that STZ may target the nucleus tractus solitarius/area postrema/DMV, wherein reside glucose- and hormone-sensitive cells that participate in glucoregulatory gut functions.

Gold thioglucose (GTG), which targets central glucose-responsive neurones to invoke hyperphagia and models of obesity and type 2 diabetes, also produces specific lesions in the area postrema [238–240]. Gold thioglucose changes feeding behaviour in sham-operated but not in area postrema-lesioned rats [241], indicating that the feeding-associated neurones upon which GTG acts, reside in, or are dependent upon, the area postrema.

Monosodium glutamate (MSG), which targets central glucose-sensitive neurones to invoke hyperphagia, also induces lesions in circumventricular organs, including the area postrema [242–244]. Changes in ingestive behaviour with monosodium glutamate are prevented by prior ablation of the area postrema [245], similar to the situation with gold thioglucose. Further evidence that MSG affects function at the area postrema comes from studies with GLP-1 which binds to [204] and activates [205,246] that structure *in vivo*. The inhibitory effect of GLP-1 on food intake is negated by treatment with monosodium glutamate [247], consistent with MSG having disabled GLP-1 action at the area postrema.

Alloxan treatment causes destruction in the area postrema [248] and, when administered centrally, reduces the hyperphagic response to glucoprivation [249] in the same way that total lesions of the area postrema block the hyperphagic response to glucoprivation [230].

Conclusions: neuropathic hypothesis

Despite ample evidence of morphologic and functional changes in nerves of rodent models of type 1 diabetes mellitus, it is not clear to what extent these changes underly the gastrointestinal dysfunction evident in these animals. Coincidence of neuropathic and gastrointestinal changes does not necessarily prove a causal association between autonomic neuropathy and gastrointestinal dysfunction in diabetes. Alternatively, recently recognised neuroendocrine disturbances in diabetes, especially of the β-cell hormone amylin, provide an alternative to the neuropathic hypothesis, and this will be discussed in the next section. Finally, it appears that diabetogenic agents used to invoke diabetes in many animal models also damage central brain regions involved in normal gastrointestinal control. The utility of these animal models of diabetes in understanding diabetes-associated changes in gut function in humans warrants further examination.

Neuroendocrine explanations for diabetic gastrointestinal dysfunction

The pancreatic β-cell defect is most profound in models of type 1 diabetes, and most work done on the gastrointestinal sequelae of diabetes, as cited in this chapter, has been done using type 1 models of diabetes. However, type 2 diabetes mellitus, with a prevalence of 7.7% in the NHANES II study, is ~10 times more prevalent, compared with the 0.74% cumulative incidence (~ prevalence) of type 1 diabetes mellitus [250]. From that viewpoint, type 2 diabetes mellitus has a greater impact in terms of human disease. An attempt will be made to include what data exists for gastrointestinal dysfunction in animal models of type 2 diabetes.

In considering primary endocrine changes associated with type 1 diabetes mellitus, it should be recognised that the central pathogenic event is a selective and near-absolute autoimmune destruction of pancreatic β-cells. Other cell types in the islets, and other tissues, are preserved. The only confirmed hormones currently known to be specific to pancreatic β-cells are insulin and amylin [251]. Recent evidence also suggests that C-peptide, cleaved from proinsulin during intracellular processing and co-secreted with insulin, may also be biologically active [252], so this molecule is briefly discussed. Other proteins secreted from the β-cell, such as pancreastatin (derived from chromogranin-A [253]) are also secreted from many other tissues [254] and are not absolutely deficient in insulinopenic diabetes.

It is therefore only insulin, C-peptide and amylin that disappear following the selective destruction of β-cells. The implications of this statement are profound; all diabetes-associated sequelae are somehow related to the absence of these (and/or other possibly undiscovered) hormones, whether directly or indirectly (such as via hyperglycaemia or advanced glycosylation end-products). Since insulin has minimal direct effect on gut function, until recently the most plausible explanation linking β-cell destruction to changes in gastrointestinal functions was a neuropathic effect secondary to hyperglycaemia. With the recent discovery of multiple physiological gastrointestinal effects of the second β-cell hormone, amylin [255], a plausible alternate explanation of gut dysfunction following β-cell loss has emerged. That is, instead of being due to insulin lack, some gut dysfunction in insulinopenic diabetes may instead be due to the loss of its co-secreted partner, amylin. For this reason, special emphasis is given in the following section to amylin's gastrointestinal actions. This does not discount the possibility that other β-cell-specific secreted proteins of gastrointestinal significance (and a clear role for C-peptide deficiency) could emerge in the future.

While insulin and amylin are essentially absent in type 1 diabetes, in states of impaired glucose tolerance and early type 2 diabetes, each of these hormones may in fact be hypersecreted [256,257]. The states of impaired glucose tolerance and early type 2 diabetes mellitus are further characterised by resistance to the effects of insulin, or 'insulin-resistance'. The ZDF rat is a model of insulin resistance, with some strains developing type 2 diabetes. These animals, which hypersecrete from pancreatic β-cells, exhibit both hyperinsulinaemia and hyperamylinaemia. In addition to their insulin resistance, they also show a resistance to the effect of amylin to slow gastric emptying [258].

With worsening of glucose tolerance, the clinical course progresses to a state of reduced (but non-zero) secretion for each, insulin and amylin, that is no longer modulated by nutrient stimuli [259,260]. In some aspects, the resultant effect in type 2 diabetes may be similar to that in type 1 diabetes in that through loss of sensitivity, loss of secretion or both, insulin and amylin action is lost. In this way, insulin-dependent and amylin-dependent sequelae may be shared in type 1 and type 2 diabetes.

In other respects, the pathophysiology is different and may prove to result in different gastrointestinal sequelae. In those species that develop type 2 diabetes, amylin oversecretion may paradoxically participate in end-stage secretory failure; insoluble hypersecreted amylin may form toxic islet amyloid [261,262], leading to disruption of islet architecture and a secretory defect [263].

Insulin and glucose

Many gastrointestinal reflexes are glucose-sensitive, reflecting their often unrecognised glucoregulatory (restricting elevations of glucose during hyperglycaemia) and counter-regulatory functions (promoting elevation of glucose during hypoglycaemia). Glucose-sensitive effects include inhibition of food intake, control of gastric emptying rate, and regulation of gastric acid secretion and pancreatic enzyme secretion (collectively control of digestive rate). Some gastrointestinal manifestations of diabetes may therefore be secondary, and compensatory, to markedly disturbed plasma glucose concentrations.

Via its powerful hypoglycaemic actions, insulin may indirectly evoke gastrointestinal actions if plasma glucose is permitted to fall.

Since insulin is lacking, it may be initially tempting to attribute gastrointestinal sequelae of insulinopenic diabetes directly to such deficiency. However, the evidence that insulin directly affects gastrointestinal function in animals is sparse. While insulin can affect some brain structures implicated in gastrointestinal function, such as the area postrema [191,192] and dorsal motor nucleus of the vagus [264], insulin does not affect gastric emptying if blood glucose is kept constant [265,266] Similarly, the effect of insulin to stimulate gastric acid secretion [81] appears to be only a consequence of its glucose-lowering effect, since increasing and decreasing plasma glucose concentration appears to result in obligatory inhibition and stimulation of gastric acid secretion [82–85]. The effect of glucose on acid secretion appears to be mediated via vagal afferents [267] and the nucleus tractus solitarius [80]. In contrast, the effect of glucagon to counteract the gastric secretory effect of insulin appears to be independent of plasma glucose [86].

Insulin has been reported to stimulate sodium–glucose co-transport in the rat jejunum [268]. But there is no evidence that this function is impaired in insulinopenic animal models; indeed, in BB [112] and STZ rats [113], mRNA for gut-specific GLUT5 and co-transporters is increased.

Amylin

Considerable comment is devoted to amylin in this chapter, since its absence, like that of insulin, is a primary event in insulinopenic diabetes, and because it has multiple physiological effects on the gastrointestinal tract. By these arguments, its absence is likely to be involved in at least some of the gastrointestinal dysfunction that accompanies diabetes.

Amylin [255] is a 37-amino acid peptide that is localised with insulin in secretory granules, and secreted with it from the pancreatic β-cell in response to nutrient stimuli [269]. In humans, amylin circulates at basal plasma levels of 4–8 pM, rising to levels of 20–25 pM post-prandially [260,270]. Amylin-like immunoreactivity is also present in the amygdala and other brain regions [271] and in the spinal cord. Amylin shows some structural similarity to CGRP [255], the calcitonins (especially teleost calcitonins [272]) and adrenomedullin [273].

The role of amylin as a neuroendocrine hormone participating in fuel homeostasis has been elusive, the subject of much debate, and is still often misunderstood. Earlier hypotheses on the possible physiological and pathophysiological roles of amylin were guided by the historical order in which biological actions were discovered. A potent effect to inhibit insulin-stimulated glycogen formation in isolated skeletal muscle in rats [274,275] but not impair insulin action in fat [276], as well as effects to increase lactate turnover [277], blunt first-phase insulin secretion [278], and stimulate the renin–angiotensin system [279], mirrored many of the features of insulin-resistance and contributed to the hypotheses that amylin may be involved in the pathogenesis of insulin resistance [280] and syndrome X [281]. Amylin antagonists were considered as a potential treatment in insulin-resistant patients. It now appears that these actions occur at either supraphysiological concentrations, or represent a feature of the animal, but not human, response to amylin agonists.

In the rat, the first physiological effect of amylin identified using selective antagonists was the inhibition of insulin secretion [282–284], i.e. administration of amylin antagonists augmented insulin secretion, consistent with the idea that a tonic (physiological) inhibition of insulin secretion had been removed. A similar effect of an amylin antagonist to disinhibit insulin secretion was observed in humans [285]. The inhibition by amylin of β-cell secretion thus appears similar to the situation in other neuroendocrine tissues where secreted products feed back to limit secretion at the cell of origin.

It has emerged in recent years that several of the most potent of nearly 60 reported biological actions of amylin [286] are gastrointestinal effects that appear to collectively restrict nutrient influx and promote glucose tolerance. These include inhibition of gastric emptying, inhibition of food intake, inhibition of digestive functions (pancreatic enzyme secretion, gastric acid secretion and bile ejection), and inhibition of nutrient-stimulated glucagon secretion. The manner in which these actions are now believed to collectively regulate the rate of nutrient appearance (R_a) is shown in Figure 2.3, juxtaposed with one of the multiple peripheral insulin effects, which collectively promote fuel storage and rate of nutrient disappearance (R_d). It can thus be seen how the pancreatic β-cell evokes complimentary effects on both R_a and R_d in fuel homeostasis.

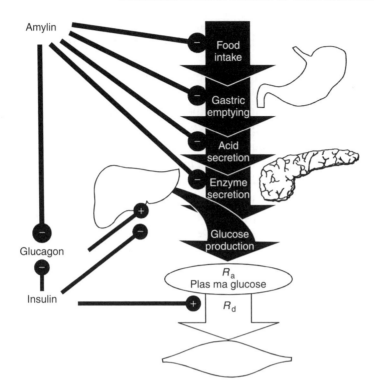

Figure 2.3 Diagram of fuel fluxes through amylin-regulated processes, illustrating the proposed physiologic role of the β-cell hormone amylin, and how its function in regulating R_a (nutrient appearance) compliments that of insulin, which regulates R_d (nutrient disappearance/storage)

Amylin and gastric emptying

In rats, amylin is the most potent of any known mammalian peptide in slowing gastric emptying [287,288]. A similar potency in slowing gastric emptying has been observed in man with the human amylin analogue pramlintide [289]. The observation that amylin inhibits gastric emptying in rats at concentrations that normally circulate suggests that this action is physiological. Plasma concentrations of pramlintide that exert gastric effects in diabetic humans are similar to amylin concentrations in non-diabetic humans, further supporting the idea that inhibition of gastric emptying is a physiological effect of this hormone.

Evidence of an effect of (and physiological significance of) endogenous hormones can also often be inferred from observations made after the administration of selective antagonists. For example, prior administration of the selective amylin antagoinst, AC187, to non-fasted or hyperamylinaemic rats [61] accelerated gastric emptying. This result is consistent with the removal of a tonic amylinergic constraint on gastric emptying, also supporting a physiological effect. Accelerated gastric emptying is also observed in the absence of any administered agents in β-cell-deficient (amylin-deficient) BB rats [52,287], further supporting the idea that endogenous amylin tonically restrains the rate of stomach emptying.

One interpretation of disturbed gastric function observed in STZ rats is that it could reflect the absence of β-cell signals, such as amylin, that have gastrointestinal activity. However, in view of the possible toxicity of STZ to area postrema neurones and other GLUT2-containing brain structures that influence gastric function, we should be cautious about this interpretation in these and other chemically-induced diabetic models. This caveat is unlikely to apply, however, when the β-cell insult is immunological, for example, and not accompanied by brain stem lesions.

Paradoxically, gastric emptying is also reported to be accelerated in the ZDF rat model of type 2 diabetes [60] [Gedulin; unpublished], shown elsewhere to be hyperamylinaemic. A mechanism that might explain accelerated gastric emptying in such hyperamylinaemic models, including LA/N corpulent rats [61] and Fatty Zucker rats [60], is a recently-described phenomenon of amylin resistance. In hyperamylinaemic Fatty Zucker rats, there was an 8.3-fold reduction in amylin sensitivity compared to lean controls for gastric emptying [258]. Why amylin resistance occurs, or whether other amylinergic responses become insensitive to amylin, is presently unknown. It appears, however, that rats that have become resistant to amylin retain sensitivity to exendin-4, indicating preservation of effector mechanisms [Gedulin et al., unpublished].

The significance of gastric emptying rate on constancy of plasma nutrient levels, briefly discussed here, is covered more fully in Chapter 8. The concept that release of carbohydrate and other nutrients from the stomach into the intestine is a regulated process is supported by observations in normal subjects of a comparatively constant efflux of calories from the stomach; between 1.6 [290] and 2.1 [291] kcal/min (~ 400–530 mg of glucose/min), maintained over a range of ingested glucose concentrations and glucose loads [291]. This constancy of efflux in the face of large variations in magnitude of delivered nutrient load is indicative of feedback control of nutrient release. The above rates of carbohydrate release are approximately equal to the rate of peripheral glucose disposal attainable with physiological insulin concentrations [292], fitting with the idea that nutrient supply and nutrient disposal are co-regulated. The intermediaries responsible for such co-regulation have been unclear; gastric inhibitory polypeptide (GIP), proposed as a candidate [293], has only a weak action to inhibit gastric emptying [294]. Instead, it appears that amylin and GLP-1, secreted in response to carbohydrate-containing meals, and potently inhibiting gastric emptying [294], may mediate glucoregulatory control of gastric emptying [287].

Amylin inhibition of gastric emptying (Figure 2.4) depends upon an intact vagus nerve [108], is annulled by lesions of the area postrema [295] and is reversed by hypoglycaemia [265]. The area postrema has a high density of

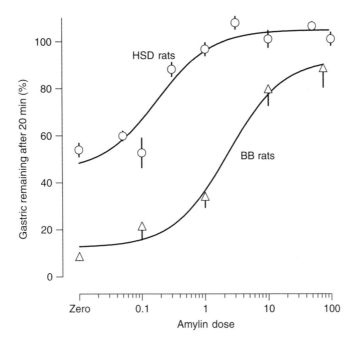

Figure 2.4 Inhibition of gastric emptying in non-diabetic Sprague–Dawley (HSD) and diabetic BB rats, in which accelerated gastric emptying is manifested as a low fraction of gavaged load being present 20 min after gavage ($p < 0.001$ at zero dose) [287] with permission from Young *et al.*; $n = 5$–8/dose for HSD rats and 3–10/dose for BB rats

amylin receptors [296]. In brain-slice preparations, most neurones in the area postrema are amylin-sensitive [227]. Almost all amylin-sensitive neurones in the area postrema are also glucose-sensitive (and amylin-insensitive neurones were also glucose-insensitive) [227]. GLP-1-sensitivity also correlated with glucose-sensitivity in area postrema brain slices.

An amylin agonist (pramlintide), several GLP-1 agonists and exendin-4 are being explored as potential therapies for the treatment of diabetes, with inhibition of gastric emptying being recognised as a mode of therapeutic action. However, diabetic subjects are frequently treated with insulin, and are at risk for insulin-induced hypoglycaemia. Oral supplementation with carbohydrates is the main mode of rescue from insulin-induced hypoglycaemia. Therapies that inhibited emptying of the stomach could thus potentially impede such rescue attempts. However, in distinction to this potential hazard, a recently-discovered feature of the agents is that their inhibition of gastric emptying is overridden during hypoglycaemia [265,297,298]. The implication from this override, hitherto demonstrated in animal stimuli, is that the gastric inhibitory effect will carry no or little additional risk of insulin-induced hypoglycaemia.

The findings that gastric inhibitory effects can be localised to the area postrema/nucleus tractus solitarius region, together with the findings of dual peptide- and glucose-sensitivity in the same neurones, leads to the proposition that hypoglycaemic override resides in the inherent response properties of those neurones. Other glucoregulatory gastrointestinal reflexes, such as inhibition of acid and pancreatic enzyme secretion, may also be driven by cells in this area and be similarly disabled as part of a generalised gut counter-regulatory response to hypoglycaemia [299]. The concept of the gut as an organ of metabolic control is yet to be widely accepted, and antidiabetic drugs that moderate nutrient uptake as a mode of therapy have only begun to emerge. A potential advantage such therapies hold over those that enhance insulin action, is their general glucose dependence and low propensity to (*per se*) induce hypoglycaemia.

Other gastrointestinal actions of amylin

Digestive secretions, alterations in which could affect absorptive function, include exocrine pancreatic secretion (Figure 2.5), gastric acid secretion and

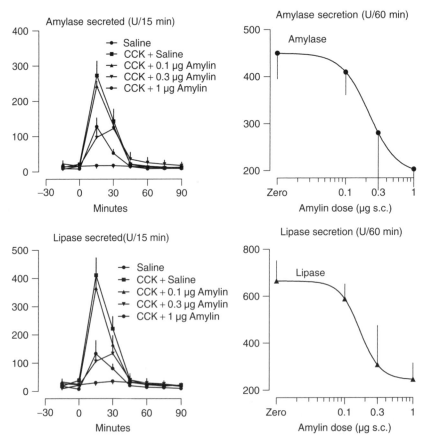

Figure 2.5   Effect of amylin to inhibit exocrine pancreatic secretion in Sprague–Dawley rats cannulated via the pancreatic duc. From Gedulin *et al.* [107] with permission

biliary function, and are discussed here. Amylin inhibited cholecystokinin-stimulated secretion of amylase and lipase from the exocrine pancreas in the anesthetised rat by up to 70% [107] with a potency consistent with this being a physiological action. Studies of exocrine pancreatic function in animal diabetes appear to be restricted to STZ rats, where CCK-stimulated enzyme secretion is greater [99] but stimulation due to secretin appears depressed [100,101] or unchanged [99]. The effects of insulin-deficient and amylin-deficient diabetes (e.g. autoimmune diabetes uncomplicated by brain stem toxicity) on exocrine pancreatic function have not been reported.

Gastric acid is important in breaking down dietary macromolecules into absorbable moieties. Modulation of acid secretion may thereby influence postprandial nutrient uptake. While there appear to be no reports that quantify the relationship between acid secretion and rates of nutrient assimilation, there is evidence that type 1 diabetes, in animal models at least, is characterised by disturbed acid regulation. STZ-treated rodents exhibit gastric mucosal lesions [66,68,70,73], a condition that is not reversed by insulin replacement [73]. A direct effect of STZ on the gastric mucosa has been proposed, and as discussed above, STZ damage to brain stem structures could also be involved. This explanation does not, however, accommodate why NOD mice with isolated autoimmune β-cell destruction also exhibit gastric erosions [77]. Gastric erosions in isolated β-cell deficiency instead supports the possibility that the loss of a β-cell product, such as amylin, could result in the loss of a physiological gastroprotective action. The observation that type 1 diabetic (i.e. amylin- as well as insulin-deficient) children have a three- to four-fold elevation in rate of peptic disease [93] also supports this notion.

Amylin given intracerebroventricularly [300] or peripherally [301] inhibited gastric acid secretion (Figure 2.6) by up to 93%. The acid inhibitory effects

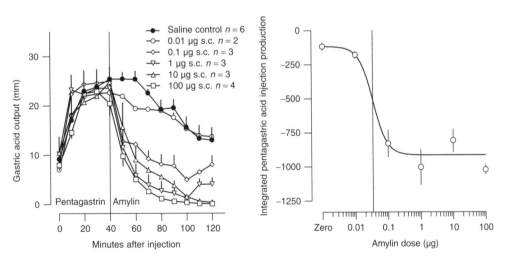

Figure 2.6 Effect of amylin to inhibit pentagastrin-stimulated gastric acid secretion. From Gedulin *et al.* [323] with permission

are also manifest as protection against erosions and mucosal damage in rats administered ethanol [302], indomethacin [303], reserpine or serotonin [304]. The acid inhibitory and gastroprotective effects appear to be equipotent and physiological [301,302] and to be mediated via amylin receptors, since the effects can be blocked with the amylin receptor anatagonist AC187. Other amylin agonists, including CGRP [305–311] and calcitonins [305, 308–310, 312, 313], also inhibit gastric acid secretion and gastric lesions. The mode of action appears predominantly central rather than directed to parietal cells [314,315]. Involvement of central amylinergic neurones in the area postrema/nucleus tractus solitarius [227,296] in this response appears likely. Agents applied locally to the area postrema result in changes in gastric acid secretion [316–319].

Amylin's effect in inhibiting exocrine pancreatic secretion, and its effect in inhibiting gastric acid secretion, are mechanistically aligned with the effect of amylin agonists (salmon calcitonin and CGRP) in inhibiting bile ejection [320–322], in that each of these actions is consistent with a coordinated regulation of digestive function.

Other metabolic actions of amylin

Several studies have documented an effect of amylin in inhibiting food intake in rodents [324,325]. The potency of amylin's inhibition of food intake is comparable to that of its gastric effect and is amplified in the presence of cholecystokinin [326], a situation that normally follows the ingestion of a mixed meal. Amylin's satiety effect appears to reside, at least partly, in the area postrema/nucleus tractus solitarius [327] but does not involve vagal afferents [328]. The proposal that endogenous amylin may contribute to the control of food intake is supported by an increase in food intake [329] and body fat [330] after administration of the selective antagonist AC187 alone. A role of endogenous amylin is further supported by an increase in body weight in amylin gene knockout mice [331,332]. While type 1 and type 2 diabetic patients administered insulin alone typically increase body weight, patients with type 1 and type 2 diabetes co-administered the amylin analogue pramlintide showed decreases in body weight [333].

In addition, amylin has profound effects to inhibit glucagon secretion, which are relevant to the disturbances of glucagon secretion observed in insulinopenic diabetes, and are covered in the following section.

Glucagon

Relative or absolute hyperglucagonaemia, especially in response to arginine [334,335], is an important feature of human diabetes likely to be responsible for the excessive glucose production and fasting hyperglycaemia present during diabetes [336]. Relative glucagon excess appears to be necessary for ketoacidosis during loss of metabolic control [337]. Diabetic BB rats exhibit a dysregulation of glucagon secretion similar to that present in humans, including inappropriately normal immunoreactive glucagon in the presence of hyperglycaemia, absolute hyperglucagonaemia with severe ketosis, and hyper-responsiveness to exogenous arginine *in vivo* [338]. A similar pattern is present in isolated preparations from BB rats [339,340]. STZ-treated models of diabetes also typically show an enhanced glucagon response to arginine. This has been observed in perfused pancreas of STZ-treated [341] and alloxan-treated [342] rats, and in dispersed α-cells of STZ-treated hamsters [343].

In contrast to the hyperglucagonaemia observed in profoundly insulinopenic diabetes, normal or reduced glucagon responses to arginine administration have been reported in chemically induced diabetes in rodents [344], such as in the neonatal STZ model of type 2 diabetes [345]. Comparatively normal glucagon responses were also seen in humans who took a β-cell-toxic rodenticide [346], raising the possibility that the characteristics of glucagon secretion may differ in forms of diabetes according to specificity of the insult.

In animal models of type 1 diabetes, the magnitude of glucagon hypersecretion associates somewhat with the severity of β-cell deficiency [338], promoting the idea that hyperglucagonaemia is attributable to loss of a tonic inhibitory influence on α-cell secretion. Insulin is reported to inhibit pancreatic α-cell secretion of glucagon [347], a so-called 'glucagonostatic' effect. The exaggerated glucagon secretion in type 1 diabetes has been proposed to reflect the loss of such a restraining influence of insulin on pancreatic α-cells [348], and reports of high basal glucagon secretion, hyper-responsiveness to arginine stimulation, and blunted responses to hypoglycaemia in different insulinopenic animal models [341,343,349–351] further support the idea that α-cell secretion is driven inversely to β-cell secretion. Similarly, stimulation of glucagon secretion at low plasma glucose concentrations may also partly reflect the loss of a paracrine inhibitory action from glucose-mediated insulin secretion [352]. This mechanism may be exemplified by observations of a diminished glucagon response to glucopenia in animals in which 'glucose competence' is low (there is little modulation of insulin secretion in response to changes in plasma glucose). Examples are the Otsuka Long Evans Tokushima Fatty rat [353], the Fatty Zucker rat [351] and the neonatal STZ rat [354].

The potential effect of amylin lack as a contributor to disturbances in glucagon secretion has only recently been addressed. In rats, amylin potently inhibits arginine-stimulated secretion of glucagon [355] (Figure 2.7). The dose–response for this effect [356], and observations that administration of neutralizing anti-amylin antibody and AC187 can increase circulating glucagon concentrations [357], support the physiological nature of this effect. Glucagonostatic effects of amylin are only manifest *in vivo*, and do not occur in isolated perfused pancreas or isolated islets [358], pointing to an extrapancreatic central mechanism. As with other amylinergic effects, inhibition of glucagon secretion is glucose-dependent, and does not occur at low glucose concentrations [358].

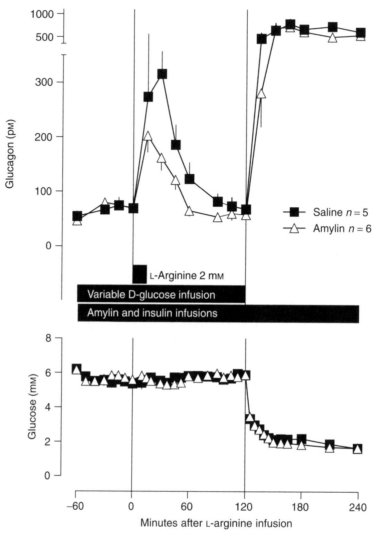

Figure 2.7   Selective glucagonostatic effect of amylin in rats, showing inhibition of arginine-induced glucagon secretion but preservation of hypoglycaemia-induced counter-regulatory secretion. From Silvestre *et al.* [358] with permission

C-Peptide

There is recent evidence that C-peptide, a product cleaved from proinsulin during processing, and co-secreted with insulin, may also be biologically active [252]. C-peptide is absent in insulinopenic diabetes. C-peptide can activate various cellular responses, including the Na^+/K^+-ATPase [359] and nitric oxide synthase [360], and its replacement in diabetic patients has been reported to benefit autonomic neuropathy [361], nephropathy [362] and haemodynamics [363].

Glucagon-like peptide-1

Glucagon-like peptide-1 (GLP-1) is a 30 amino acid peptide derived from the larger precursor, proglucagon. Proglucagon is a 160 amino acid peptide expressed predominantly in α-cells of the pancreatic islets, and in L-cells in terminal ileum and large bowel. Proteolytic cleavage in the pancreatic α-cells yields glucagon [proglucagon (33–61)], while different cleavage in intestinal cells yields predominantly glicentin [proglucagon (1–69)], GLP-1 [proglucagon (78–107)] and GLP-2 [proglucagon (126–158)] [364].

GLP-1 has a number of actions relevant to metabolic control, some of which are mediated via the gastrointestinal tract. From this point of view, alterations in GLP-1 concentrations or in GLP-1 activity in diabetic states are relevant to discussion of gastrointestinal function in diabetes. Additionally, GLP-1 has been of interest in diabetes since it was proposed as an antidiabetic therapy. Interest in developing GLP-1 as an antidiabetic agent followed its identification as an insulinotropic agent [365–367] which, unlike sulphonylurea drugs, stimulated insulin secretion only in the presence of normal or elevated plasma glucose concentrations [368,369]. The glucose dependence of its insulinotropic effect promised to confer some protection from the potential side effects of hypoglycaemia. Unfortunately, GLP-1 exhibits a half-life of ~ 5 min in man [370], principally due to its rapid degradation to GLP-1 [9–36] amide by the hormone dipeptidyl peptidase IV [371,372]. This rapid degradation of GLP-1 has impeded its development as an antidiabetic agent.

Glucagon-like peptide-1 and gastric emptying

GLP-1 has been shown to slow emptying of the stomach in rodents [294] with a potency that approaches that of amylin. It also exhibits gastric slowing in humans [373–377]. The importance of this action in glucose control (vs. its well-known insulinotropic effect, for example), was recognised when Dupre *et al.* described its postprandial benefit in insulin-deficient patients [376]. The significance of regulation of gastric emptying on glycaemic excursions has also been affirmed in insulin-replete subjects [378,379]. Some authors propose that the gastric effect predominates in postprandial glucose control [379]. As with amylin and some other modulators of gastric emptying, the effects of GLP-1 in slowing gastric emptying are glucose-dependent, in that they are overridden during insulin-induced hypoglycaemia [297], at least in animals.

Glucagon-like peptide-1 concentrations in diabetes

In human type 2 diabetes, GLP-1 has been reported to be low and to not increase normally after a meal [380–383]. Comparable animal data in models of type 2 diabetes are lacking. A relative deficiency of GLP-1 (a gastric slowing agent) in type 2 diabetes could theoretically contribute to a propensity to accelerated gastric emptying, discussed above. However, measurements of GLP-1 secretion and gastric emptying in the same individual, which would support this idea, have not been performed.

Expression of the proglucagon gene and prohormone are unchanged by diabetes in NOD mice and ZDF rats [384], except that in ZDF rats, mRNA was somewhat depleted in the small bowel and increased in the large bowel. STZ rats were reported to have elevated GLP-1 content in the colon [385]. In another study, there was a 3.5-fold elevation of GLP-1 content in the ileum of STZ diabetic rats on days 8–22 after the onset of diabetes [115].

There was an elevation of plasma GLP-1 concentration in poorly controlled STZ rats relative to non-diabetic controls [386]. This elevation was not due to differences in intestinal L-cell function, since luminal perfusion of fats in duodenum and ileum resulted in indistinguishable increments in plasma GLP-1 concentration [387]. The implication, therefore, is that differences in plasma concentration were likely to be due to differences in secretagogue stimuli at the L-cells in the gut lumen. However, there appear to be no studies to support this implication in metabolic disease models of changes in gut motility beyond the stomach. It is possible that increased plasma GLP-1 could be a consequence of accelerated gastric emptying into the duodenum; although duodenal content of GLP-1 is 50-fold lower than in the ileum [387], GLP-1 output following perfusion of either of these two segments is similar, implying that a factor from the duodenum could feed forward to stimulate large bowel GLP-1 release. GIP, which is found in the highest concentrations in the proximal bowel, potently stimulates GLP-1 release [388], as does CGRP, and these peptides have been postulated as humoral mediators of GLP-1 secretion following nutrient stimulation at the proximal bowel. The type 1 diabetic human data are contrary to the animal model data in regard to GLP-1 levels. GLP-1 secreted in response to food ingestion was universally decreased in type 1 diabetic patients, even though gastric emptying T50s were similar [389].

In metabolic disease characterised by hormonal excess (e.g. the hyperinsulinaemia and hyperamylinaemia of obesity), there is often resistance to hormonal action. The insulinotropic effects of GLP-1 cannot be determined in STZ rats, where there is no insulin secretion to amplify. Other effects, e.g., on gastric emptying, have not been studied in that model. In models of type 2 diabetes, there appears to be no evidence of resistance to the hormonal effects of GLP-1. The potency of GLP-1 to inhibit gastric emptying in type 2 diabetic ZDF rats was similar to that in non-diabetic controls [Gedulin, unpublished].

Other gastrointestinal actions of GLP-1 include inhibition of gastric acid secretion [373,390–393] and pancreatic [373] and gastric [394] enzyme secretion. These effects appear to be central [395], mediated via the vagus nerve [396–398] and a somatostatin-dependent pathway [399]. However, the inhibitory gastropancreatic effects of GLP-1 are modest in rats and dogs in comparison to the effects of other gut peptides [294,400,401], and in one human study, effects in inhibiting acid secretion were not evident at all [402]. Potential changes in these GLP-1-mediated actions have not been reported in diabetic models.

Other metabolic actions of glucagon-like peptide-1

Centrally delivered GLP-1 acutely decreases food and/or water intake in rats and other species [403–410]. However, the role of GLP-1 as a physiologically relevant peripheral satiety agent has been disputed due to its induction of conditioned taste aversion (i.e. GLP-1 invoked a 'sickness' rather than a 'satiety' response) [411–414]. Further, its acute anorectic effect is reported to fade rapidly [409] and, peripherally administered (as opposed to ICV-injected), GLP-1 failed to inhibit food intake in rats [403–405,415]. The lack of apparent change in body weight or ingestive behaviour in GLP-1 receptor knockout mice [416,417] has cast further doubt on its role as an endogenous satiety agent.

On the other hand, the effect of GLP-1 to induce conditioned taste aversion is dissociable from effects to reduce food and water intake [418–420] and, despite modest effects in rodents, in humans peripherally-infused GLP-1 increased sensations of satiety and fullness and decreased energy intake [421–424]. A physiological role of endogenous GLP-1 was further supported by a report that exendin (9–39), a GLP-1 antagonist, enhanced food intake in non-fasted animals [403]. This result supported the interpretation that the effect of the antagonist was a disinhibition of a tonic GLP-1 signal that was therefore physiologically relevent. The inference of physiological relevance of GLP-1 was further supported by an increase in body weight following semi-chronic administration of exendin (9–39). However, it is worth mentioning that other workers have not been able to replicate an increase in food intake during treatment with exendin (9–39) [425] [Bhavsar *et al.*, unpublished]. A long-lasting GLP-1 analogue, when delivered peripherally, was capable of inhibiting food intake and decreasing body weight in the MSG-lesioned hyperphagic rat model of type 2 diabetes [426]. These results suggest that GLP-1 acts to inhibit food intake via other than the glucoresponsive hypothalamic neurones that are destroyed by MSG. GLP-1 reduced feeding in obese Zucker rats [427], indicating that, as with gastric emptying, responsiveness to this peptide is preserved in this profoundly insulin-resistant animal model.

Glucagon-like peptide-1 insulinotropic and glucagonostatic effects

The first described biological action of GLP-1, and that which prompted its investigation as an antidiabetic therapy [365], was its amplification of nutrient-stimulated insulin secretion. This 'insulinotropic' effect of GLP-1 has been observed in a number of systems, including isolated islets [428–434] the isolated perfused pancreas [366,366,368,435–438] or the whole organism, including rats [431,439–441], dogs [442], minipigs [443] and humans [444–448]. This effect of GLP-1 to amplify insulin secretion is present only during euglycaemia and hyperglycaemia, and generally not during hypoglycaemia, and hence has been described as 'glucose-dependent' [365,368,369,441,449].

Exaggerated secretion of glucagon, especially in response to protein-containing meals [450] has been implicated in the excess gluconeogenesis and propensity to ketoacidosis in insulinopenic diabetes [451]. GLP-1 is reported to suppress glucagon secretion [452,453], its so-called 'glucagonostatic' effect, which may have clinical benefit. In studies of the isolated perfused pancreas of the rat, Rodriguez-Gallardo *et al.* observed that a GLP-1 agonist inhibited arginine-stimulated glucagon secretion from the pancreases of normal rats, but of insulin-deficient (STZ) rats in which an insulinotropic effect was precluded by the absence of β-cells. They proposed that the glucagonostatic effect of GLP-1 is secondary to a paracrine effect of β-cell products to inhibit α-cell secretion [454]. This mechanism is supported by reports of high basal glucagon secretion, hyper-responsiveness to arginine stimulation, and blunted responses to hypoglycaemia in different insulinopenic models [341,343,349–351], which collectively fit with the idea of α-cell secretion being inversely by β-cell secretion. However, contrary to the conclusion that GLP-1 exerts only an indirect glucagonostatic effect is an observation that, in insulin-deficient dogs, infusions resulting in 40 pM GLP-1 suppressed the pre-existing diabetic hyperglucagonaemia and reduced the hyperglycaemia somewhat [455].

Some authors report no abnormalities in glucagon secretion in the neonatal STZ model of type 2 diabetes [345]. Other authors describe a diminished glucagon response to glucopenia in, for example, the Otsuka Long Evans Tokushima Fatty rat [353], the Fatty Zucker rat [351] and the neonatal STZ rat [354]. Insulinotropic and glucagonostatic effects of GLP-1 were similar in non-diabetic and neonatal STZ rats [456]. Indeed, the isolated perfused pancreas of Fatty Zucker rats appears to be more sensitive to GLP-1 than do the pancreases of lean controls [457]. Variability of effects observed in different animal models may reflect the differing extents to which insulin resistance (e.g. induced by hyperphagia) vs. comparative insulinopenia (e.g. induced by β-cell toxins) contribute to the metabolic derangement.

In summary, GLP-1 tissue content and secretion may be altered in some models of type 1 and type 2 diabetes. Several gut functions are either directly or indirectly responsive to GLP-1 in the direction of reduced nutrient uptake. However, it is currently unclear to what extent changes in GLP-1 secretion contribute to changes in gastrointestinal function in diabetic animal models, or to what extent changes in gastrointestinal function may be responsible for altered GLP-1 secretion.

Glucagon-like peptide-2

Glucagon-like peptide-2 (GLP-2), like GLP-1, is a gut-derived cleavage prod-uct of proglucagon [458]. Its secretion thus tends to follow that of GLP-1, and changes in plasma levels, e.g. in animal models of diabetes, may mirror those of GLP-1. After STZ treatment, in addition to GLP-1, other cleavage products of proglucagon, including glucagon-like peptide-2 (GLP-2), glicentin and oxyntomodulin are also increased [459]. Bowel mass is also increased in this animal model [459], probably reflecting the fact that GLP-2, released from terminal ileum and large bowel in response to incompletely absorbed luminal nutrient, promotes small bowel epithelial (crypt cell) proliferation [116]. GLP-2 can be seen as part of a slowly acting feedback control loop, i.e. excess nutrient reaching the distal small bowel triggers a trophic response in proximal gut that results in more absorptive capacity and a reduction in nutrient reaching the distal small bowel. The presence of elevated GLP-2 in STZ rats could account for the bowel overgrowth observed in diabetes [459]. GLP-2 also stimulates the synthesis of dipeptidyl peptidase IV [460], the main enzyme implicated in breakdown of GLP-1 and GLP-2.

GLP-2 is reported to have some effects on electrical activity of the stomach, inhibiting interdigestive gastroduodenal motility in the gastric pouch of vagally denervated (but not intact) dogs [461], and inhibiting antral motility invoked by insulin-induced hypoglycaemia [462]. While synergy with GLP-1 was reported, GLP-2 alone had little effect on fasting small bowel motility [463]. GLP-2 inhibits food intake when injected centrally [464], but not peripherally, and does not inhibit gastric emptying at doses up to 300 μg/kg in rats [Gedulin, unpublished]. GLP-2 binds to specific receptors and not to GLP-1 receptors, and does not exhibit a GLP-1-like spectrum of actions. It has no haemodynamic effects [465], no pulmonary surfactant effects [466], no effect on intestinal somatostatin release [467], no effect on insulin-stimulated glucose uptake in adipocytes [468], no effect on basal H^+ and cAMP production in parietal cells (where, incidentally, another proglucagon product, oxyntomodulin acted) [469] and no insulinotropic activity [470].

In summary, the gastrointestinal effects of GLP-2 appear to be mainly trophic, and may secondarily contribute to changes in bowel mass and morphology in animal models of diabetes.

Gastric inhibitory peptide

Gastric inhibitory peptide (GIP) is a 42 amino acid peptide found predominantly in the K-cells of duodenum and jejunum, from where it is released in response to intraluminal carbohydrates, fats and amino acids [364]. Originally named gastric inhibitory peptide (GIP), the discovery of a more interesting action, amplification of insulin secretion, resulted in a name change to glucose-dependent insulinotropic peptide (also GIP). Expression of GIP gene and hormone in the bowel of NOD mice and ZDF rats is indistinguishable in diabetic and non-diabetic controls [384]. In ob/ob and db/db mice, plasma concentrations are elevated 15- and six-fold [471] and small bowel weight is increased. In steroid-induced and alloxan-induced diabetic rats, plasma GIP is elevated, but not duodenal GIP content [472], indicating changes in release rather than in synthesis. Plasma GIP is elevated in STZ mice [473]. Increases in secretion of GIP in diabetic models are consistent with accelerated nutrient flux into the duodenum. There is no evidence of reduced GIP effect (GIP resistance) in these models; insulinotropic and glucagonotropic effects of GIP are similar in non-diabetic and diabetic (neonatal STZ) rats [456]. Given that GIP is believed to be a minor incretin in comparison to GLP-1, there appears to be no reason to implicate GIP in diabetes-related changes in gastrointestinal function.

Cholecystokinin

Cholecystokinin (CCK), so named for its first-described action of stimulating gallbladder contraction, exists in forms that are 83, 58, 39, 33 and eight amino acids long. CCK was subsequently found to stimulate pancreatic enzyme secretion, inhibit gastric emptying, inhibit gastric acid production, stimulate insulin secretion (in some species, e.g. rats) and initiate satiety [364]. CCK is found in neurones, especially in the cerebral cortex, and in intestinal I-cells, from which it is released principally in response to fatty acids and some amino acids. In addition, its release is stimulated by a peptide secreted into the gut lumen, luminal CCK-releasing factor (LCRF) whose active 41 amino acid fragment is digested by trypsin following CCK-stimulated pancreatic secretion [474]. The absence or presence of undigested LCRF thereby exerts feedback control of proteolytic activity in the gut lumen. Central alloxan administration diminishes the hypophagic effect of CCK in food-deprived rats [249]. In the STZ rat, the pancreatic acinar cell response to CCK [475], CCK-stimulated amylase secretion [99] and CCK-stimulation of insulin secretion [228] are impaired. The satiety, insulinotropic and exocrine trophic and zymogen roles of CCK are exemplified in Otsuka Long-Evans Tokushima Fatty (OLETF) rats, which express little or no CCK-A receptor [96,476]. These animals become, respectively, hyperphagic and unresponsive to central CCK [477,478], hyperglycaemic [478], have impaired insulin secretion [94,479], and develop acinar atrophy [480] and loss of zymogen response to CCK [94,95]. The glucoregulatory effects of CCK are further exemplified by the observation that CCK antagonists worsen the diabetogenic effect of alloxan in mice [481].

Secretin

Secretin, the first peptide hormone discovered, has 27 amino acids and is secreted from the proximal small intestine in response to intraluminal acid. Its principal actions, inhibiting gastric acid secretion and gastric emptying and stimulating pancreatic bicarbonate secretion, point to a role in controlling the acidity of the gut lumen [364]. There is little evidence that secretin-mediated functions are disturbed in animal models of diabetes. While in NOD mice, duodenal secretin cells are more numerous [482], secretin-induced secretion of protein from exocrine pancreas is normal in the STZ rat [99] and secretin-mediated inhibition of gastric emptying is not impaired in hyperglycaemic Zucker rats who otherwise exhibit accelerated gastric emptying [60].

Gastrin-releasing peptide

Gastrin-releasing peptide (GRP), the analogue of an endocrine hormone in birds, and bombesin from the skin of frogs, only exists in the mammalian gut as a neurotransmitter in the myenteric plexus. It has potent effects to stimulate gastrin release and acid production, and to inhibit gastric emptying, and is probably a key component of local peptone-stimulated acid secretion [364]. GRP content of the duodenum in NOD mice [483] and the stomach in STZ rats [484] is normal. Plasma concentrations are not generally changed in humans with diabetes [485] but do increase during hypoglycaemia [486].

Somatostatin

Somatostatin, so-named because of its first described action to inhibit growth hormone secretion, circulates in 14 amino acid and 28 amino acid forms in D-cells of the gastric antral mucosa, small intestinal mucosa, pancreatic islets, and extensively as a neurotransmitter throughout the central and peripheral nervous systems. Most circulating somatostatin is the 28 amino acid form released from small intestinal D-cells, mainly in response to fat and protein [364]. Acidification of the gastric lumen also stimulates somatostatin release. The most pronounced effects of somatostatin are inhibition of neurotransmitter and hormonal (acetyl-choline, CCK, enteroglucagon/GLP-1, GIP, gastrin, glucagon, insulin, amylin, pancreatic polypeptide, peptide YY, secretin, VIP and growth hormone) as well as exocrine (gastric acid, pepsin and histamine, pancreatic enzymes and bicar-bonate, hepatic bicarbonate, and intestinal water and electrolyte) secretion. Other effects include inhibition of growth in a range of tissues.

Most studies addressing somatostatin biology during experimental diabetes have been conducted in STZ rats. Somatostatin is increased in the circulation [487–491], gastric mucosa [484,492–494], salivary gland [495] and pancreas [494,496–499] (with exaggerated arginine-stimulated release [500–502]) following STZ-induction of diabetes.

Some authors have observed normalisation of STZ-induced hypersomato-statinaemia following treatment with insulin [488,495,503,504], that gastric somatostatin excess is reversed by islet transplant [505], and that insulin lack and somatostatin excess are proportional [496]. One interpretation is that insulin directly inhibits somatostatin secretion, and that insulin lack accounts for hypersomatostatinaemia in STZ-diabetc animals. Other explanations for STZ-induced hypersomatostatinaemia include slower hepatic clearance [506].

While insulinopenia in BB rats is similar to, or more severe than, that in STZ rats, somatostatin profiles are profoundly different (see 'Intestinal mucosal function', p. 39). There is an increase in number of D-cells in STZ-treated animals, but in the BB rat, D-cells decrease in number [507–509], and islet somatostatin is lower [504,509,510] or normal [511]. In the BB rat, the somatostatin content of a stomach/pancreas/duodenum/spleen preparation was not different from normal [512], and brain and gut somatostatin are normal [509].

There is some indication that neural control of somatostatin secretion may be altered in STZ-treated animals; splanchnic nerve stimulation does not appear to suppress somatostatin secretion as much in STZ rats as in normal rats [513]. So it is possible that hindbrain toxicity of STZ, more than insulin lack, accounts for hypersomatostatinaemia in STZ-treated rats, and for the differences between this and autoimmune (BB) models of insulinopenia. In contrast to descriptions of altered plasma levels, evidence for a disturbed response to somatostatin in animal models of diabetes is sparse. There are fewer somatostatin receptors on pancreatic acinar cells in the STZ rat [514], but this could be a downregulatory consequence of hypersomatostatinaemia in this model. Islets from diabetic BB rats, which are hyperresponsive to arginine, respond to somatostatin with a normal suppression of endocrine secretion [515].

Peptide YY

Peptide YY is co-localised with GLP-1 in intestinal L-cells. As with GLP-1, PYY tends to be hyposecreted in animal models of type 2 diabetes. In the *ob/ob* mouse, the numbers of PYY- and enteroglucagon-immunoreactive cells in the colon are decreased relative to controls [516]. In the colon of obese diabetic mice (*Umea/Bom-ob*), the levels of PYY were significantly lower than in lean controls [517]. In the colon of NOD mice, a model of type 1 diabetes, the concentrations of PYY were also lower in prediabetic and diabetic NOD mice than in controls [518]. The reasons for reduced expression and secretion are not known.

PYY slows gastric emptying in humans [519,520], dogs [521] and rats [522,523]; this effect appears to be mediated via a vagally dependent central mechanism. PYY inhibits other gastric functions besides gastric emptying, including gastric acid secretion [524–532] and pancreatic exocrine secretion [533]. PYY exhibits a similar spectrum of gastrointestinal actions to amylin but, unlike amylin, has no significant insulinostatic or glucagonostatic effect [534,535]. PYY may contribute to metabolic control, as does amylin, via limiting nutrient uptake from the gut. As with amylin, some of the disturbances in gut function in diabetes may be attributable to lack of PYY action.

Conclusions: neuroendocrine disturbance

As in our consideration of neuropathy in diabetic animals, we are faced with differences between chemically-induced and autoimmune models in the spectrum of endocrine change. Most remarkable in this regard is the hypersomatostatinaemia present in STZ rats that appears not to be a feature in autoimmune BB rats. On the other hand, there are also changes that are common in both chemically-induced and autoimmune classes of diabetic model. In both these models of type 1 diabetes, and in models of insulinopenic type 2 diabetes, a primary defect is relative or absolute deficiency in both insulin and amylin. While insulin itself appears somewhat inert in the gastrointestinal system, this is not the case with its partner hormone amylin, which has potent effects on several gut functions. In this chapter, an emphasis is, therefore, placed upon the proposal that some of the alterations in gut function in animal models of diabetes may be attributable to changes in amylin effect.

Summary

The most plausable and most accepted hypothesis in the past to explain gastrointestinal dysfunction in diabetes has been the proposal that autonomic neuropathy has disturbed the normal regulation of gut function. But there are recently identified disturbances in several of the neurohormones found in gut in different diabetic states. Several of these, including amylin, GLP-1 and PYY have effects on gut function, and should now be considered in explanations of diabetes-associated changes in gut function. Some changes in gut function may prove to be an artifact of neurotoxicity of STZ at specific locations in the brain that are important in the regulation of gut function, emphasising the point that the choice of animal model is critical if artifacts are to be avoided and relevance to human disease is to be maintained.

References

1. Nordin BE, Need AG, Morris HA, Horowitz M, Robertson WG. Evidence for a renal calcium leak in postmenopausal women. *J Clin Endocrinol Metab* 1991; **72**: 401–7.
2. Sima AA, Chakrabarti S, Garcia-Salinas R, Basu PK. The BB-rat—an authentic model of human diabetic retinopathy. *Curr Eye Res* 1985; **4**: 1087–92.
3. Wright JR Jr, Yates AJ, Sharma HM, Thibert P. Pathological lesions in the spontaneously diabetic BB Wistar rat: a comprehensive autopsy study. *Metabolism* 1983; **32**: 101–5.
4. Armstrong D, al-Awadi F. Lipid peroxidation and retinopathy in streptozotocin-induced diabetes. *Free Radic Biol Med* 1991; **11**: 433–6.
5. Papachristodoulou D, Heath H. Ultrastructural alterations during the development of retinopathy in sucrose-fed and streptozotocin-diabetic rats. *Exp Eye Res* 1977; **25**: 371–84.
6. McEwen TA, Sima AA. Autonomic neuropathy in BB rat. Assessment by improved method for measuring heart-rate variability. *Diabetes* 1987; **36**: 251–5.
7. Sima AA. Can the BB-rat help to unravel diabetic neuropathy? *Neuropathol Appl Neurobiol* 1985; **11**: 253–64.
8. Sima AA, Hay K. Functional aspects and pathogenetic considerations of the neuropathy in the spontaneously diabetic BB-Wistar rat. *Neuropathol Appl Neurobiol* 1981; **7**: 341–50.

9. Brown DM, Steffes MW, Thibert P, Azar S, Mauer SM. Glomerular manifestations of diabetes in the BB rat. *Metabolism* 1983; **32**: 131–135.

10. Lanza RP, Borland KM, Staruk JE, Appel MC, Solomon BA, Chick WL. Transplantation of encapsulated canine islets into spontaneously diabetic BB/Wor rats without immunosuppression. *Endocrinology* 1992; **131**: 637–42.

11. Woehrle M, Pullmann J, Bretzel RG, Federlin K. Prevention of recurrent autoimmune diabetes in the BB rat by islet transplantation under the renal capsule. *Transplantation* 1992; **53**: 1099–102.

12. Pipeleers D, Pipeleers-Marichal M, Markholst H, Hoorens A, Kloppel G. Transplantation of purified islet cells in diabetic BB rats. *Diabetologia* 1991; **34**: 390–96.

13. Butler L, Guberski DL, Like AA. Genetic analysis of the BB/W diabetic rat. *Can J Genet Cytol* 1983; **25**: 7–15.

14. Guberski D. Diabetes-prone and diabetes-resistant BB rats: animal models of spontaneous and virally induced diabetes mellitus, lymphocytic thyroiditis, and collagen-induced arthritis. *ILAR News* 1994; **35**: 29–37.

15. Butler L, Guberski DL, Like AA. Changes in penetrance and onset of spontaneous diabetes in the BB/Wor rat. In Shafrir E (ed.), *Frontiers in Diabetes Research: Lessons from Animal Diabetes III*, 3rd edn. Smith-Gordon; London, 1991: 50–53.

16. Shafrir E. Diabetic animals with autoimmune etiology: NOD mice. In Shafrir E (ed.), *Lessons from Animal Diabetes III*. Smith-Gordon; London, 1991; 54–98.

17. Rerup CC. Drugs producing diabetes through damage of the insulin secreting cells. *Pharmacol Rev* 1970; **22**: 485–518.

18. Karam JH, Lewitt PA, Young CW *et al*. Insulinopenic diabetes after rodenticide (Vacor) ingestion: a unique model of acquired diabetes in man. *Diabetes* 1980; **29**: 971–8.

19. Lee TH, Doi K, Yoshida M, Baba S. Morphological study of nervous system in Vacor-induced diabetic rats. *Diabetes Res Clin Pract* 1988; **4**: 275–9.

20. Rakieten N, Rakieten ML, Nadkarni MV. Studies on the diabetogenic actions of streptozotocin (NSC37919). *Cancer Chemother Rep* 1963; **29**: 91.

21. Stolinsky DC, Bull FE, Pajak TF, Bateman JR. Trial of 1-(2-chloroethyl)-3-cyclohexyl-1-nitrosourea (CCNU; NSC-79037) in advanced bronchogenic carcinoma 1,2,3. *Oncology* 1975; **31**: 288–92.

22. Arison RN, Ciaccio EI, Glitzer MS, Cassaro JA, Pruss MP. Light and electron microscopy of lesions in rats rendered diabetic with streptozotocin. *Diabetes* 1967; **16**: 51–6.

23. Junod A, Lambert AE, Orci L, Pictet R *et al*. Studies of the diabetogenic action of streptozotocin. *Proc Soc Exp Biol Med* 1967; **126**: 201–5.

24. Ganda OP, Rossini AA, Like AA. Studies on streptozotocin diabetes. *Diabetes* 1976; **25**: 595–603.

25. Cole DR, Waterfall M, Ashworth L, Bone AJ, Baird JD. Metabolic control in streptozotocin diabetic rats following transplantation of microencapsulated pancreatic islets. *Horm Metab Res* 1993; **25**: 553–6.

26. Finegood DT, Tobin BW, Lewis JT. Dynamics of glycemic normalization following transplantation of incremental islet masses in streptozotocin-diabetic rats. *Transplantation* 1992; **53**: 1033–7.

27. Waber S, Meister V, Rossi GL, Mordasini RC, Riesen WF. Studies on retinal microangiopathy and coronary macroangiopathy in rats with streptozotocin-induced diabetes. *Virchows Arch B Cell Pathol* 1981; **37**: 1–10.

28. Schmidt RE, Plurad SB, Modert CW. Experimental diabetic autonomic neuropathy characterization in streptozotocin-diabetic Sprague–Dawley rats. *Lab Invest* 1983; **49**: 538–52.

29. Mattingly GE, Fischer VW. Peripheral neuropathy following prolonged exposure to streptozotocin-induced diabetes in rats: a teased nerve fiber study. *Acta Neuropathol (Berl)* 1983; **59**: 133–8.

30. Monckton G, Pehowich E. Autonomic neuropathy in the streptozotocin diabetic rat. *Can J Neurol Sci* 1980; **7**: 135–42.

31. Niwa T, Miyazaki T, Katsuzaki T, Tatemichi N, Takei Y. Serum levels of 3-deoxyglucosone and tissue contents of advanced glycation end products are increased in streptozotocin-induced diabetic rats with nephropathy. *Nephron* 1996; **74**: 580–85.

32. Cooper ME, Allen TJ, Macmillan P, Bach L *et al.* Genetic hypertension accelerates nephropathy in the streptozotocin diabetic rat. *Am J Hypertens* 1988; **1**: 5–10.

33. Cohen MP, Klein CV. Glomerulopathy in rats with streptozotocin diabetes. Accumulation of glomerular basement membrane analogous to human diabetic nephropathy. *J Exp Med* 1979; **149**: 623–31.

34. Loewy AD. Anatomy of the autonomic nervous system: an overview. In Loewy AD, Spyer KM (eds.), *Central Regulation of Autonomic Functions*. Oxford University Press: New York, 1990.

35. Furness JB, Costa M. Identification of transmitters of functionally defined enteric neurones. In Wood JD (ed.), *The Gastrointestinal System, vol 1, Motility and Circulation, Section 6*. Bethesda, MD American Physiological Society: 1989; 387.

36. Watkins CC, Sawa A, Jaffrey S *et al.* Insulin restores neuronal nitric oxide synthase expression and function that is lost in diabetic gastropathy. *J Clin Invest* 2000; **106**: 373–84.

37. Liu M, Seino S, Kirchgessner AL. Identification and characterization of glucoresponsive neurons in the enteric nervous system. *J Neurosci* 1999; **19**: 10305–17.

38. Horowitz M, Fraser R. Disordered gastric motor function in diabetes mellitus. *Diabetologia* 1994; **37**: 543–51.

39. Fraser RJ, Horowitz M, Maddox AF, Harding PE *et al.* Hyperglycaemia slows gastric emptying in type 1 (insulin-dependent) diabetes mellitus. *Diabetologia* 1990; **33**: 675–80.

40. Cavallo-Perin P, Aimo G, Mazzillo A, Riccardini F, Pagano G. Gastric emptying of liquids and solids evaluated by acetaminophen test in diabetic patients with and without autonomic neuropathy. *Riv Eur Sci Med Farmacol* 1991; **13**: 205–9.

41. Nakanome C, Akai H, Hongo M *et al.* Disturbances of the alimentary tract motility and hypermotilinemia in the patients with diabetes mellitus. *Tohoku J Exp Med* 1983; **139**: 205–15.

42. Nowak TV, Johnson CP, Wood CM *et al.* Evidence for accelerated gastric emptying in asymptomatic patients with insulin-dependent diabetes mellitus. *Gastroenterology* 1990; **98**: A378.

43. Fürnsinn C, Leuvenink H, Roden M *et al.* Islet amyloid polypeptide inhibits insulin secretion in conscious rats. *Am J Physiol* 1994; **267**: E300–305.

44. Lipp RW, Schnedl WJ, Hammer HF, Kotanko P *et al.* Evidence of accelerated gastric emptying in longstanding diabetic patients after ingestion of a semisolid meal. *J Nucl Med* 1997; **38**: 814–18.

45. Phillips WT, Schwartz JG, McMahan CA. Rapid gastric emptying of an oral glucose solution in type 2 diabetic patients. *J Nucl Med* 1992; **33**: 1496–500.

46. Phillips WT, Schwartz JG, McMahan CA. Rapid gastric emptying in patients with early non-insulin-dependent diabetes mellitus [letter]. *N Engl J Med* 1991; **324**: 130–31.

47. Mulder H, Ahren B, Sundler F. Islet amyloid polypeptide and insulin gene expression are regulated in parallel by glucose *in vivo* in rats. *Am J Physiol* 1996; **271**: E1008–14.

48. Frank JW, Saslow SB, Camilleri M, Thomforde GM *et al.* Mechanism of accelerated gastric emptying of liquids and hyperglycaemia in patients with type II diabetes mellitus. *Gastroenterology* 1995; **109**: 755–65.

49. Phillips WT, Salman UA, McMahan CA, Schwartz JG. Accelerated gastric emptying in hypertensive subjects. *J Nucl Med* 1997; **38**: 207–11.

50. Jones KL, Horowitz M, Carney BI, Wishart JM *et al.* Gastric emptying in early non-insulin-dependent diabetes mellitus. *J Nucl Med* 1996; **37**: 1643–8.

51. Thompson RG, Gottlieb AB, Organ K, Kolterman OG. The human amylin analogue (AC137) reduces glucose following Sustacal in patients with type II diabetes. *Diabetes* 1995; **44**: 127A.

52. Nowak TV, Roza AM, Weisbruch JP, Brosnan MR. Accelerated gastric emptying in diabetic rodents: effect of insulin treatment and pancreas transplantation. *J Lab Clin Med* 1994; **123**: 110–16.

53. Flint A, Raben A, Astrup A, Holst JJ. Glucagon-like peptide 1 promotes satiety and suppresses energy intake in humans. *J Clin Invest* 1998; **101**: 515–20.

54. Stricker EM, McCann MJ. Visceral factors in the control of food intake. *Brain Res Bull* 1985; **14**: 687–92.

55. Edens NK, Friedman MI. Satiating effect of fat in diabetic rats: gastrointestinal and postabsorptive factors. *Am J Physiol* 1988; **255**: R123–7.

56. Granneman JG, Stricker EM. Food intake and gastric emptying in rats with streptozotocin-induced diabetes. *Am J Physiol* 1984; **247**: R1054–61.

57. Ogata M, Iizuka Y, Murata R, Hikichi N. Effect of streptozotocin-induced diabetes on cyclosporin A disposition in rats. *Biol Pharm Bull* 1996; **19**: 1586–90.

58. Yamano M, Kamato T, Nagakura Y, Miyata K. Effects of gastroprokinetic agents on gastroparesis in streptozotocin-induced diabetic rats. *Naunyn Schmiedebergs Arch Pharmacol* 1997; **356**: 145–50.

59. Chang FY, Doong ML, Chen TS, Lee SD, Wang PS. Altered intestinal transit is independent of gastroparesis in the early diabetic rats. *Chin J Physiol* 1997; **40**: 31–5.

60. Green GM, Guan D, Schwartz JG, Phillips WT. Accelerated gastric emptying of glucose in Zucker type 2 diabetic rats: role in postprandial hyperglycaemia. *Diabetologia* 1997; **40**: 136–142.

61. Gedulin B, Jodka C, Green D, Young A. Effect of amylin receptor antagonist, AC187, on labelled glucose absorption and oral glucose tolerance in corpulent LA/N rats. *Program and Abstracts, American Diabetes Association 29th Research Symposium and the International Congress on Obesity Satellite Conference, August 25–27, Boston, MA,* 1994; p. 40 (abstr 45).

62. Black RM, Conover KL, Weingarten HP. Accelerated gastric emptying in VMH-lesioned rats is secondary to excess weight gain. *Am J Physiol* 1990; **259**: R658–61.

63. Lin CY, Yeh GH, Hsu FC *et al.* Gastric acid secretion in streptozotocin-diabetic female rats. *Chin J Physiol* 1991; **34**: 179–86.

64. Piyachaturawat P, Poprasit J, Glinsukon T, Wanichanon C. Gastric mucosal lesions in streptozotocin-diabetic rats. *Cell Biol Int Rep* 1988; **12**: 53–63.

65. Rosenfeld RG, Attie KM, Frane J *et al.* Growth hormone therapy of Turner's syndrome: beneficial effect on adult height. *J Pediat* 1998; **132**: 319–24.

66. Goldin E, Ardite E, Elizalde JI *et al.* Gastric mucosal damage in experimental diabetes in rats: role of endogenous glutathione. *Gastroenterology* 1997; **112**: 855–863.

67. Takeuchi K, Ueshima K, Ohuchi T, Okabe S. Induction of gastric lesions and hypoglycaemic response by food deprivation in streptozotocin-diabetic rats. *Dig Dis Sci* 1994; **39**: 626–34.

68. Horowitz M, Wishart JM, Need AG, Morris HA, Nordin BE. Biochemical effects of a calcium supplement in postmenopausal women with primary hyperparathyroidism. *Horm Metab Res* 1994; **26**: 39–42.

69. Chabre O, Liakos P, Vivier J *et al*. Gastric inhibitory polypeptide (Gip) stimulates cortisol secretion, cAMP production and DNA synthesis in an adrenal adenoma responsible for food dependent Cushing's syndrome. *Endocr Res* 1998; **24**: 851–6.

70. Hung CR, Huang EY. Role of acid back-diffusion in the formation of mucosal ulceration and its treatment with drugs in diabetic rats. *J Pharm Pharmacol* 1995; **47**: 493–8.

71. Sahajwalla CG, Ayres JW. Multiple-dose acetaminophen pharmacokinetics. *J Pharm Sci* 1991; **80**: 855–60.

72. Arai I, Hirose-Kijima H, Usuki-Ito C, Muramatsu M, Otomo S. Putative role of endogenous insulin in cystamine-induced hypersecretion of gastric acid in rats. *Eur J Pharmacol* 1991; **202**: 213–19.

73. Piyachaturawat P, Poprasit J, Glinsukon T. Gastric mucosal secretions and lesions by different doses of streptozotocin in rats. *Toxicol Lett* 1991; **55**: 21–9.

74. Baydoun R, Dunbar JC. Impaired insulin but normal pentagastrin effect on gastric acid secretion in diabetic rats: a role for nitric oxide. *Diabetes Res Clin Pract* 1997; **38**: 1–8.

75. Ozcelikay AT, Altan VM, Yildizoglu-Ari N, Altinkurt O *et al*. Basal and histamine-induced gastric acid secretion in alloxan diabetic rats. *Gen Pharmacol* 1993; **24**: 121–6.

76. Wright JR Jr, Yates AJ, Sharma HM, Thibert P. Spontaneous gastric erosions and ulcerations in BB Wistar rats. *Lab Anim Sci* 1981; **31**: 63–6.

77. Nishimura M, Yokoyama M, Taguchi T, Kitamura Y. Spontaneous gastric erosions in NOD and KK-A gamma. *Lab Anim Sci* 1983; **33**: 577–9.

78. Gedulin B, Jodka C, Hoyt J, Young A. Evidence for amylin resistance for inhibition of gastric emptying in hyperamylinemic Fatty Zucker rats. *Endocrine Society 81st Annual Meeting Program and Abstracts*, 1999; **217**.

79. Silvestre RA, Rodriguez-Gallardo J, Gutiérrez E, García P *et al*. Failure of amylin to directly affect glucagon release. Study in the perfused rat pancreas. *Diabetologia* 1999; **42**: A146.

80. Sakaguchi T, Sato Y. D-Glucose anomers in the nucleus of the tractus solitarius can reduce gastric acid secretion of rats. *Exp Neurol* 1987; **95**: 525–9.

81. Isenberg JI, Stening GF, Ward S, Grossman MI. Relation of gastric secretory response in man to dose of insulin. *Gastroenterology* 1969; **57**: 395–8.

82. Moore JG. The relationship of gastric acid secretion to plasma glucose in five men. *Scand J Gastroenterol* 1980; **15**: 625–32.

83. Lam WF, Masclee AA, de Boer SY, Lamers CB. Hyperglycemia reduces gastric secretory and plasma pancreatic polypeptide responses to modified sham feeding in humans. *Digestion* 1993; **54**: 48–53.

84. Stacher G, Bauer P, Starker H, Schulze D. Inhibitory effect of an intravenous glucose load on basal and insulin-stimulated gastric acid secretion in man. *Int J Clin Pharmacol Biopharm* 1976; **13**: 107–12.

85. Lam WF, Masclee AA, Muller ES, Lamers CB. Effect of hyperglycemia on gastric acid secretion and gastrin release induced by intravenous amino acids. *Am J Clin Nutr* 1995; **61**: 1268–72.

86. Loud FB, Holst JJ, Rehfeld JF, Christiansen J. Inhibition of gastric acid secretion in humans by glucagon during euglycemia, hyperglycemia, and hypoglycemia. *Dig Dis Sci* 1988; **33**: 530–34.

87. Zaidi M, Pazianas M, Shankar VS *et al*. Osteoclast function and its control. *Exp Physiol* 1993; **78**: 721–39.

88. Hirsch IB. Type 1 diabetes mellitus and the use of flexible insulin regimens. *Am Fam Physician* 1999; **60**: 2343–52, 2355–6.
89. Gedulin BR, Lawler RL, Jodka CM, Young AA. Comparison of effects of amylin, glucagon-like peptide-1 and exendin-4 to inhibit pentagastrin-stimulated gastric acid secretion. *Diabetologia* 1997; **40**(suppl 1): A300.
90. Limb C, Tamborlane WV, Sherwin RS, Pederson R, Caprio S. Acute incretin response to oral glucose is associated with stimulation of gastric inhibitory polypeptide, not glucagon-like peptide in young subjects. *Pediatr Res* 1997; **41**: 364–7.
91. Guidobono F, Pagani F, Ticozzi C, Sibilia V, Netti C. Investigation on the mechanisms involved in the central protective effect of amylin on gastric ulcers in rats. *Br J Pharmacol* 1998; **125**: 23–8.
92. Thompson R, Pearson L, Schoenfeld S, Kolterman O. Pramlintide improves glycemic control in patients with type II diabetes requiring insulin. *Diabetologia* 1997; **40**: A355.
93. Kaufman FR. Role of the continuous glucose monitoring system in pediatric patients. *Diabetes Technol Ther* 2000; **2**(suppl 1): S49–52.
94. Tachibana I, Akiyama T, Kanagawa K *et al*. Defect in pancreatic exocrine and endocrine response to CCK in genetically diabetic OLETF rats. *Am J Physiol* 1996; **270**: G730–37.
95. Otsuki M, Akiyama T, Shirohara H, Nakano S *et al*. Loss of sensitivity to cholecystokinin stimulation of isolated pancreatic acini from genetically diabetic rats. *Am J Physiol* 1995; **268**: E531–6.
96. Funakoshi A, Miyasaka K, Jimi A, Kawanai T *et al*. Little or no expression of the cholecystokinin-A receptor gene in the pancreas of diabetic rats (Otsuka Long-Evans Tokushima Fatty = OLETF rats). *Biochem Biophys Res Commun* 1994; **199**: 482–8.
97. Naya FJ, Huang HP, Qiu Y *et al*. Diabetes, defective pancreatic morphogenesis, and abnormal enteroendocrine differentiation in BETA2/neuroD-deficient mice. *Genes Dev* 1997; **11**: 2323–34.
98. Domschke W, Tympner F, Domschke S, Demling L. Exocrine pancreatic function in juvenile diabetics. *Am J Dig Dis* 1975; **20**: 309–12.
99. Sofrankova A, Dockray GJ. Cholecystokinin- and secretin-induced pancreatic secretion in normal and diabetic rats. *Am J Physiol* 1983; **244**: G370–74.
100. Okabayashi Y, Otsuki M, Ohki A, Nakamura T *et al*. Secretin-induced exocrine secretion in perfused pancreas isolated from diabetic rats. *Diabetes* 1988; **37**: 1173–80.
101. Dodi G, Militello C, Pedrazzoli S, Zannini G, Lise M. Exocrine pancreatic function in diabetic rats treated with intraportal islet transplantation. *Eur Surg Res* 1984; **16**: 9–14.
102. Okabayashi Y, Ohki A, Sakamoto C, Otsuki M. Relationship between the severity of diabetes mellitus and pancreatic exocrine dysfunction in rats. *Diabetes Res Clin Pract* 1985; **1**: 21–30.
103. Lam WF, Gielkens HA, Coenraad M, Souverijn JH *et al*. Effect of insulin and glucose on basal and cholecystokinin-stimulated exocrine pancreatic secretion in humans. *Pancreas* 1999; **18**: 252–8.
104. Lam WF, Masclee AA, Souverijn JH, Lamers CB. Effect of acute hyperglycemia on basal, secretin and secretin + cholecystokinin stimulated exocrine pancreatic secretion in humans. *Life Sci* 1999; **64**: 617–26.
105. Lam WF, Muller ES, Souverijn JH, Lamers CB, Masclee AA. Effect of acute hyperglycaemia on basal and fat-induced exocrine pancreatic secretion in humans. *Clin Sci (Colch)* 1997; **93**: 573–80.
106. Lam WF, Masclee AA, de Boer SY, Souverijn JH, Lamers CB. Effect of acute hyperglycemia on basal and cholecystokinin-stimulated exocrine pancreatic secretion in humans. *Life Sci* 1997; **60**: 2183–90.
107. Gedulin BR, Jodka C, Lawler R, Hoyt JA, Young AA. Amylin inhibits lipase and amylase secretion from the exocrine pancreas in rats. *Diabetes* 1998; **47**: A280.

108. Jodka C, Green D, Young A, Gedulin B. Amylin modulation of gastric emptying in rats depends upon an intact vagus nerve. *Diabetes* 1996; **45**: 235A.

109. Najjar SM, Hampp LT, Rabkin R, Gray GM. Altered intestinal and renal brush border amino-oligopeptidase structure in diabetes and metabolic acidosis: normal and biobreed (BB) rats. *Metabolism* 1992; **41**: 76–84.

110. Najjar SM, Hampp LT, Rabkin R, Gray GM. Sucrase-α-dextrinase in diabetic BioBreed rats: reversible alteration of subunit structure. *Am J Physiol* 1991; **260**: G275–83.

111. Jiao S, Matsuzawa Y, Matsubara K *et al.* Increased activity of intestinal acyl-CoA: cholesterol acyltransferase in rats with streptozocin-induced diabetes and restoration by insulin supplementation. *Diabetes* 1988; **37**: 342–6.

112. Reimer RA, Glen S, Field CJ, McBurney MI. Proglucagon and glucose transporter mRNA is altered by diet and disease susceptibility in 30 day-old biobreeding (BB) diabetes-prone and normal rats. *Pediat Res* 1998; **44**: 68–73.

113. Miyamoto K, Hase K, Taketani Y *et al.* Diabetes and glucose transporter gene expression in rat small intestine. *Biochem Biophys Res Commun* 1991; **181**: 1110–17.

114. Wild GE, Thompson JA, Searles L, Turner R *et al.* Small intestinal Na$^+$, K$^+$-adenosine triphosphatase activity and gene expression in experimental diabetes mellitus. *Dig Dis Sci* 1999; **44**: 407–14.

115. Brubaker PL, So DC, Drucker DJ. Tissue-specific differences in the levels of proglucagon-derived peptides in streptozotocin-induced diabetes. *Endocrinology* 1989; **124**: 3003–9.

116. Tsai CH, Hill M, Asa SL, Brubaker PL, Drucker DJ. Intestinal growth-promoting properties of glucagon-like peptide-2 in mice. *Am J Physiol* 1997; **36**: E77–84.

117. Nordin BE, Wishart JM, Horowitz M, Need AG *et al.* The relation between forearm and vertebral mineral density and fractures in postmenopausal women. *Bone Mine.* 1988; **5**: 21–33.

118. Mayne RG, Armstrong WE, Crowley WR, Bealer SL. Cytoarchitectonic analysis of Fos-immunoreactivity in brainstem neurones following visceral stimuli in conscious rats. *J Neuroendocrinol* 1998; **10**: 839–47.

119. Pillion DJ, Jenkins RL, Atchison JA, Stockard CR *et al.* Paradoxical organ-specific adaptations to streptozotocin diabetes mellitus in adult rats. *Am J Physiol* 1988; **254**: E749–55.

120. Fedorak RN, Gershon MD, Field M. Induction of intestinal glucose carriers in streptozocin-treated chronically diabetic rats. *Gastroenterology* 1989; **96**: 37–44.

121. Fedorak RN, Chang EB, Madara JL, Field M. Intestinal adaptation to diabetes. Altered Na-dependent nutrient absorption in streptozocin-treated chronically diabetic rats. *J Clin Invest* 1987; **79**: 1571–8.

122. Csaky TZ, Fischer E. Intestinal sugar transport in experimental diabetes. *Diabetes* 1981; **30**: 568–74.

123. Buchan AM. Effect of diabetes in the BB Wistar rat on the peptidergic component of the enteric innervation. *Digestion* 1990; **46**(suppl 2): 142–7.

124. Liu HS, Karakida T, Homma S. Acetylcholine and substance P responsiveness of intestinal smooth muscles in streptozotocin diabetic rats. *Jpn J Physiol* 1988; **38**: 787–97.

125. Buzzard F. Illustrations of some less known forms of peripheral neuritis, especially alcoholic monplegia and diabetic neuritis. *Br Med J* 1890; **1**: 1419.

126. Rothstein RD. Gastrointestinal motility disorders in diabetes mellitus. *Am J Gastroenterol* 1990; **85**: 782–5.

127. Keshavarzian A, Iber FL. Gastrointestinal involvement in insulin-requiring diabetes mellitus. *J Clin Gastroenterol* 1987; **9**: 685–92.

128. Thomas PK, Tomlinson DR. Diabetic and hypoglycemic neuropathy. In Dyck PJ, Thomas PK (eds), *Peripheral Neuropathy*. Saunders: Philadelphia, PA, 1993: 1219.

129. Di Giulio AM, Tenconi B, La Croix R, Mantegazza P, Cattabeni F, Gorio A. Denervation and hyperinnervation in the nervous system of diabetic animals. I. The autonomic neuronal dystrophy of the gut. *J Neurosci Res* 1989; **24**: 355–61.
130. Schmidt RE, Plurad DA, Plurad SB, Cogswell BE *et al*. Ultrastructural and immunohistochemical characterization of autonomic neuropathy in genetically diabetic Chinese hamsters. *Lab Invest* 1989; **61**: 77–92.
131. Yagihashi S, Sima AA. Diabetic autonomic neuropathy. The distribution of structural changes in sympathetic nerves of the BB rat. *Am J Pathol* 1985; **121**: 138–47.
132. Abbate SL, Atkinson MB, Breuer AC. Amount and speed of fast axonal transport in diabetes. *Diabetes* 1991; **40**: 111–17.
133. Belai A, Burnstock G. Acrylamide-induced neuropathic changes in rat enteric nerves: similarities with effects of streptozotocin-diabetes. *J Autonom Nerv Syst* 1996; **58**: 56–62.
134. Iversen J, Miles DW. Evidence for a feedback inhibition of insulin on insulin secretion in the isolated, perfused canine pancreas. *Diabetes* 1971; **20**: 1–9.
135. Belai A, Milner P, Aberdeen J, Burnstock G. Selective damage to sensorimotor perivascular nerves in the mesenteric vessels of diabetic rats. *Diabetes* 1996; **45**: 139–43.
136. Schmidt RE, Plurad SB. Ultrastructural and biochemical characterization of autonomic neuropathy in rats with chronic streptozotocin diabetes. *J Neuropathol Exp Neurol* 1986; **45**: 525–44.
137. Schmidt RE, Plurad SB, Olack BJ, Scharp DW. The effect of pancreatic islet transplantation and insulin therapy on experimental diabetic autonomic neuropathy. *Diabetes* 1983; **32**: 532–40.
138. Schmidt RE, Plurad SB, Coleman BD, Williamson JR, Tilton RG. Effects of sorbinil, dietary myoinositol supplementation, and insulin on resolution of neuroaxonal dystrophy in mesenteric nerves of streptozocin-induced diabetic rats. *Diabetes* 1991; **40**: 574–82.
139. Kamijo M, Cherian PV, Sima AA. The preventive effect of aldose reductase inhibition on diabetic optic neuropathy in the BB/W-rat. *Diabetologia* 1993; **36**: 893–8.
140. Schmidt RE, Plurad SB, Sherman WR, Williamson JR, Tilton RG. Effects of aldose reductase inhibitor sorbinil on neuroaxonal dystrophy and levels of myoinositol and sorbitol in sympathetic autonomic ganglia of streptozocin-induced diabetic rats. *Diabetes* 1989; **38**: 569–79.
141. Sima AA, Prashar A, Zhang WX, Chakrabarti S, Greene DA. Preventive effect of long-term aldose reductase inhibition (ponalrestat) on nerve conduction and sural nerve structure in the spontaneously diabetic Bio-Breeding rat. *J Clin Invest* 1990; **85**: 1410–20.
142. Stearns SB, Benzo CA. A longitudinal and comparative study of some structural and hormonal alterations in the endocrine pancreas of spontaneously diabetic and streptozotocin-induced diabetic mice. *Acta Anat (Basel)* 1983; **115**: 193–203.
143. Low PA, Schmelzer JD, Ward KK, Yao JK. Experimental chronic hypoxic neuropathy: relevance to diabetic neuropathy. *Am J Physiol* 1986; **250**: E94–9.
144. Tuck RR, Schmelzer JD, Low PA. Endoneurial blood flow and oxygen tension in the sciatic nerves of rats with experimental diabetic neuropathy. *Brain* 1984; **107**: 935–50.
145. Van Buren T, Kasbergen CM, Gispen WH, De Wildt DJ. Presynaptic deficit of sympathetic nerves: a cause for disturbed sciatic nerve blood flow responsiveness in diabetic rats. *Eur J Pharmacol* 1996; **296**: 277–83.
146. Westerman R, Widdop R, Low A, Hannaford J *et al*. Non-invasive tests of neurovascular function: reduced axon reflex responses in diabetes mellitus of man and streptozotocin-induced diabetes of the rat. *Diabetes Res Clin Pract* 1988; **5**: 49–54.
147. Tribollet E, Raufaste D, Maffrand JP. Binding of the non-peptide vasopressin V-1a receptor antagonist Sr-49059 in the rat brain: an *in vitro* and *in vivo* autoradiographic study. *Neuroendocrinology* 1999; **69**: 113–20.

148. Schmidt RE, Plurad SB, Olack BJ, Scharp DW. The effect of pancreatic islet transplantation and insulin therapy on neuroaxonal dystrophy in sympathetic autonomic ganglia of chronic streptozocin-diabetic rats. *Brain Res* 1989; **497**: 393–8.

149. Belai A, Lincoln J, Milner P, Burnstock G. Differential effect of streptozotocin-induced diabetes on the innervation of the ileum and distal colon. *Gastroenterology* 1991; **100**: 1024–32.

150. Lincoln J, Bokor JT, Crowe R, Griffith SG, Haven AJ, Burnstock G. Myenteric plexus in streptozotocin-treated rats. Neurochemical and histochemical evidence for diabetic neuropathy in the gut. *Gastroenterology* 1984; **86**: 654–61.

151. Belai A, Facer P, Bishop A, Polak JM, Burnstock G. Effect of streptozotocin-diabetes on the level of VIP mRNA in myenteric neurones. *NeuroReport* 1993; **4**: 291–4.

152. Belai A, Burnstock G. Changes in adrenergic and peptidergic nerves in the submucous plexus of streptozocindiabetic rat ileum. *Gastroenterology* 1990; **98**: 1427–36.

153. Belai A, Lincoln J, Milner P, Crowe R *et al.* Enteric nerves in diabetic rats: increase in vasoactive intestinal polypeptide but not substance P. *Gastroenterology* 1985; **89**: 967–76.

154. Eaker EY, Sallustio JE, Marchand SD, Sahu A *et al.* Differential increase in neuropeptide Y-like levels and myenteric neuronal staining in diabetic rat intestine. *Regul Pept* 1996; **61**: 77–84.

155. Belai A, Lincoln J, Burnstock G. Lack of release of vasoactive intestinal polypeptide and calcitonin gene-related peptide during electrical stimulation of enteric nerves in streptozotocin-diabetic rats. *Gastroenterology* 1987; **93**: 1034–40.

156. Loesch A, Belai A, Lincoln J, Burnstock G. Enteric nerves in diabetic rats: electron microscopic evidence for neuropathy of vasoactive intestinal polypeptide-containing fibres. *Acta Neuropathol (Berl)* 1986; **70**: 161–8.

157. Belai A, Burnstock G. Selective damage of intrinsic calcitonin gene-related peptide-like immunoreactive enteric nerve fibers in streptozotocin-induced diabetic rats. *Gastroenterology* 1987; **92**: 730–34.

158. Soediono P, Belai A, Burnstock G. Prevention of neuropathy in the pyloric sphincter of streptozotocin-diabetic rats by gangliosides. *Gastroenterology* 1993; **104**: 1072–82.

159. Maeda CY, Fernandes TG, Timm HB, Irigoyen MC. Autonomic dysfunction in short-term experimental diabetes. *Hypertension* 1995; **26**: 1100–104.

160. Van Buren T, Schiereck P, De Ruiter GJ, Gispen WH, De Wildt DJ. Vagal efferent control of electrical properties of the heart in experimental diabetes. *Acta Diabetol* 1998; **35**: 19–25.

161. Anderson LC, Garrett JR, Thulin A, Proctor GB. Effects of streptozocin-induced diabetes on sympathetic and parasympathetic stimulation of parotid salivary gland function in rats. *Diabetes* 1989; **38**: 1381–9.

162. Belai A, Lefebvre RA, Burnstock G. Motor activity and neurotransmitter release in the gastric fundus of streptozotocin-diabetic rats. *Eur J Pharmacol* 1991; **194**: 225–34.

163. Medori R, Jenich H, Autilio-Gambetti L, Gambetti P. Experimental diabetic neuropathy: similar changes of slow axonal transport and axonal size in different animal models. *J Neurosci* 1988; **8**: 1814–21.

164. Wuarin-Bierman L, Zahnd GR, Kaufmann F, Burcklen L, Adler J. Hyperalgesia in spontaneous and experimental animal models of diabetic neuropathy. *Diabetologia* 1987; **30**: 653–8.

165. Kim HC, Im DH, Jhoo WK, Kim C, Wie MB. A low dose of streptozotocin prevents kainic acid-induced seizures and lethal effects in the rat. *Clin Exp Pharmacol Physiol* 1997; **24**: 503–505.

166. Al Deeb S, Al Moutaery K, Arshaduddin M, Biary N, Tariq M. Attenuation of acrylamide-induced neurotoxicity in diabetic rats. *Neurotoxicol Teratol* 2000; **22**: 247–53.

167. Kappelle AC, Biessels G, Bravenboer B *et al.* Beneficial effect of the Ca^{2+} antagonist, nimodipine, on existing diabetic neuropathy in the BB/Wor rat. *Br J Pharmacol* 1994; **111**: 887–93.

168. Cherian PV, Kamijo M, Angelides KJ, Sima AA. Nodal $Na^{(+)}$-channel displacement is associated with nerve-conduction slowing in the chronically diabetic BB/W rat: prevention by aldose reductase inhibition. *J Diabetes Complications* 1996; **10**: 192–200.

169. Sima AA, Zhang WX, Cherian PV, Chakrabarti S. Impaired visual evoked potential and primary axonopathy of the optic nerve in the diabetic BB/W-rat. *Diabetologia* 1992; **35**: 602–607.

170. Brismar T. Neuropathy-functional abnormalities in the BB rat. *Metabolism* 1983; **32**: 112–17.

171. Mohseni S, Hildebrand C. Neuropathy in diabetic BB/Wor rats treated with insulin implants. *Acta Neuropathol (Berl)* 1998; **96**: 144–50.

172. Sima AA, Zhang WX, Greene DA. Diabetic and hypoglycemic neuropathy—a comparison in the BB rat. *Diabetes Res Clin Pract* 1989; **6**: 279–96.

173. Paro M, Prosdocimi M, Zhang WX, Sutherland G, Sima AA. Autonomic neuropathy in BB rats and alterations in bladder function. *Diabetes* 1989; **38**: 1023–30.

174. Addicks K, Boy C, Rosen P. Sympathetic autonomic neuropathy in the heart of the spontaneous diabetic BB rat. *Anat Anz* 1993; **175**: 253–7.

175. Yagihashi S, Sima AA. Neuroaxonal and dendritic dystrophy in diabetic autonomic neuropathy. Classification and topographic distribution in the BB-rat. *J Neuropathol Exp Neurol* 1986; **45**: 545–65.

176. Yagihashi S, Sima AA. Diabetic autonomic neuropathy in the BB rat. Ultrastructural and morphometric changes in sympathetic nerves. *Diabetes* 1985; **34**: 558–64.

177. Gillis RA, Quest JA, Pagani FD, Norman WP. Control centers in the central nervous system for regulating gastrointestinal motility. Schultz SG, Wood JD, Rauner BB (eds), *The Gastrointestinal System, Motility and Circulation, Section 6, part 1.* American Physiological Society: Bethesda, MD, 1989; **1**: 621.

178. Pagani FD, Norman WP, Kasbekar DK, Gillis RA. Localization of sites within dorsal motor nucleus of vagus that affect gastric motility. *Am J Physiol* 1985; **249**: G73–84.

179. Hurley-Gius KM, Neafsey EJ. The medial frontal cortex and gastric motility: microstimulation results and their possible significance for the overall pattern of organization of rat frontal and parietal cortex. *Brain Res* 1986; **365**: 241–8.

180. Cannon WB. The movements of the intestine studied by means of Roentgen rays. *Am J Physiol* 1902; **6**: 251.

181. Wolf S, Wolff HG. *Human Gastric Function.* Oxford University Press: New York, 1943.

182. Bueno L. Assessment of CNS control of gastrointestinal motility. In Gaginella TS (ed.), *Handbook of Methods in Gastrointestinal Pharmacology.* CRC Press: Boca Raton, FC, 1996: 297–330.

183. Spencer SE, Talman WT. Modulation of gastric and arterial pressure by nucleus tractus solitarius in rat. *Am J Physiol* 1986; **250**: R996–1002.

184. Higgins GA, Hoffman GE, Wray S, Schwaber JS. Distribution of neurotensin-immunoreactivity within baroreceptive portions of the nucleus of the tractus solitarius and the dorsal vagal nucleus of the rat. *J Comp Neurol* 1984; **226**: 155–64.

185. Monnikes H, Lauer G, Bauer C, Tebbe J *et al.* Pathways of Fos expression in locus ceruleus, dorsal vagal complex, and PVN in response to intestinal lipid. *Am J Physiol* 1997; **273**: R2059–71.

186. Shapiro RE, Miselis RR. The central organization of the vagus nerve innervating the stomach of the rat. *J Comp Neurol* 1985; **238**: 473–88.

187. Rogers RC, McCann MJ. Intramedullary connections of the gastric region in the solitary nucleus: a biocytin histochemical tracing study in the rat. *J Autonom Nerv Syst* 1993; **42**: 119–130.

188. Fraser KA, Raizada E, Davison JS. Oral–pharyngeal–esophageal and gastric cues contribute to meal-induced c-fos expression. *Am J Physiol* 1995; **268**: R223–30.

189. Yuan CS, Barber WD. Area postrema: gastric vagal input from proximal stomach and interactions with nucleus tractus solitarius in cat. *Brain Res Bull* 1993; **30**: 119–25.

190. Nagano, T, Sato M, Mori Y, Du Y *et al.* Regional distribution of messenger RNA encoding the insulin-like growth factor type 2 receptor in the rat lower brainstem. *Brain Res Mol Brain Res* 1995; **32**: 14–24.

191. Carpenter DO, Briggs DB. Insulin excites neurons of the area postrema and causes emesis. *Neurosci Lett* 1986; **68**: 85–9.

192. van Houten M, Posner BI. Specific binding and internalization of blood-borne [^{125}I]-iodoinsulin by neurons of the rat area postrema. *Endocrinology* 1981; **109**: 853–9.

193. Hay M, McKenzie H, Lindsley K *et al.* Heterogeneity of metabotropic glutamate receptors in autonomic cell groups of the medulla oblongata of the rat [in process citation]. *J Comp Neurol* 1999; **403**: 486–501.

194. Hewlett WA, Trivedi BL, Zhang ZJ, *et al.* Characterization of (*S*)-des-4-amino-3-[^{125}I]iodozacopride ([^{125}I]DAIZAC), a selective high-affinity radioligand for 5-hydroxy-tryptamine3 receptors. *J Pharmacol Exp Ther* 1999; **288**: 221–31.

195. Baude A, Shigemoto R. Cellular and subcellular distribution of substance P receptor immunoreactivity in the dorsal vagal complex of the rat and cat: a light and electron microscope study (in process citation). *J Comp Neurol* 1998; **402**: 181–96.

196. Migita K, Hori N, Manako J, Saito R *et al.* Effects of arginine–vasopressin on neuronal interaction from the area postrema to the nucleus tractus solitarii in rat brain slices. *Neurosci Lett* 1998; **256**: 45–8.

197. Lowes VL, Sun K, Li Z, Ferguson AV. Vasopressin actions on area postrema neurons *in vitro. Am J Physiol* 1995; **269**: R463–8.

198. Gerstberger R, Fahrenholz F. Autoradiographic localization of V1 vasopressin binding sites in rat brain and kidney. *Eur J Pharmacol* 1989; **167**: 105–16.

199. Ruggiero DA, Regunathan S, Wang H, Milner TA, Reis DJ. Immunocytochemical localization of an imidazoline receptor protein in the central nervous system. *Brain Res* 1998; **780**: 270–93.

200. Lione LA, Nutt DJ, Hudson AL. Characterisation and localisation of [3H]2-(2-benzo-furanyl)-2-imidazoline binding in rat brain: a selective ligand for imidazoline I$_2$ receptors. *Eur J Pharmacol* 1998; **353**: 123–35.

201. Fitzsimons JT. Angiotensin, thirst, and sodium appetite. *Physiol Rev* 1998; **78**: 583–686.

202. Sirett NE, McLean AS, Bray JJ, Hubbard JI. Distribution of angiotensin II receptors in rat brain. *Brain Res* 1977; **122**: 299–312.

203. Göke R, Larsen PJ, Mikkelsen JD, Sheikh SP. Distribution of GLP-1 binding sites in the rat brain: evidence that exendin-4 is a ligand of brain GLP-1 binding sites. *Eur J Neurosci* 1995; **7**: 2294–300.

204. Orskov C, Poulsen SS, Moller M, Holst JJ. Glucagon-like peptide I receptors in the subfornical organ and the area postrema are accessible to circulating glucagon-like peptide I. *Diabetes* 1996; **45**: 832–5.

205. Larsen PJ, Tang-Christensen M, Jessop DS. Central administration of glucagon-like peptide-1 activates hypothalamic neuroendocrine neurons in the rat. *Endocrinology* 1997; **138**: 4445–55.

206. Larsen PJ, Kristensen P. The neuropeptide Y (Y4) receptor is highly expressed in neurones of the rat dorsal vagal complex. *Brain Res Mol Brain Res* 1997; **48**: 1–6.
207. Whitcomb DC, Puccio AM, Vigna SR, Taylor IL. Hoffman GE. Distribution of pancreatic polypeptide receptors in the rat brain. *Brain Res* 1997; **760**: 137–49.
208. Trinh T, van Dumont Y, Quirion R. High levels of specific neuropeptide Y/pancreatic polypeptide receptors in the rat hypothalamus and brainstem. *Eur J Pharmacol* 1996; **318**: R1–3.
209. Zajac JM, Gully D, Maffrand JP. [3H]-SR 27897B: a selective probe for autoradiographic labelling of CCK-A receptors in the brain. *J Recept Signal Transduct Res* 1996; **16**: 93–113.
210. Sun K, Ferguson AV. Cholecystokinin activates area postrema neurons in rat brain slices. *Am J Physiol* 1997; **272**: R1625–30.
211. Hashimoto H, Nogi H, Mori K et al. Distribution of the mRNA for a pituitary adenylate cyclase-activating polypeptide receptor in the rat brain: an *insitu* hybridization study. *J Comp Neurol* 1996; **371**: 567–77.
212. Herman JP, Dolgas CM, Rucker D, Langub MC Jr. Localization of natriuretic peptide-activated guanylate cyclase mRNAs in the rat brain. *J Comp Neurol* 1996; **369**: 165–87.
213. Yoshikawa T, Yoshida N, Hosoki K. Involvement of dopamine D3 receptors in the area postrema in *R*(+)-7-OH-DPAT-induced emesis in the ferret. *Eur J Pharmacol* 1996; **301**: 143–9.
214. Williams LM, Hannah LT, Hastings MH, Maywood ES. Melatonin receptors in the rat brain and pituitary. *J Pineal Res* 1995; **19**: 173–7.
215. Weaver DR, Deeds JD, Lee K, Segre GV. Localization of parathyroid hormone-related peptide (PTHrP) and PTH/PTHrP receptor mRNAs in rat brain. *Brain Res Mol Brain Res* 1995; **28**: 296–310.
216. Lei ZM, Rao CV, Kornyei JL, Licht P, Hiatt ES. Novel expression of human chorionic gonadotropin/luteinizing hormone receptor gene in brain. *Endocrinology* 1993; **132**: 2262–70.
217. Loup F, Tribollet E, Dubois-Dauphin M, Pizzolato G, Dreifuss JJ. Localization of oxytocin binding sites in the human brainstem and upper spinal cord: an autoradiographic study. *Brain Res* 1989; **500**: 223–30.
218. Wiedermann CJ, Sertl K, Zipser B, Hill JM, Pert CB. Vasoactive intestinal peptide receptors in rat spleen and brain: a shared communication network. *Peptides* 1988; **9**: 21–28.
219. Martin JL, Dietl MM, Hof PR, Palacios JM, Magistretti PJ. Autoradiographic mapping of [mono[125I]iodo-Tyr10, MetO17] vasoactive intestinal peptide binding sites in the rat brain. *Neuroscience* 1987; **23**: 539–65.
220. Shaffer MM, Moody TW. Autoradiographic visualization of CNS receptors for vasoactive intestinal peptide. *Peptides* 1986; **7**: 283–8.
221. Beleslin DB, Krstic SK. Further studies on nicotine-induced emesis: nicotinic mediation in area postrema. *Physiol Behav* 1987; **39**: 681–6.
222. Patel YC, Baquiran G, Srikant CB, Posner BI. Quantitative *in vivo* autoradiographic localization of [125I-Tyr11]somatostatin-14- and [Leu8,D-Trp22-125I-Tyr25]somatostatin-28-binding sites in rat brain. *Endocrinology* 1986; **119**: 2262–9.
223. Paakkari I, Karppanen H, Paakkari P. Site and mode of action of clonidine in the central nervous system. *Acta Med Scand* 1976; **602**: 106–9.
224. King BF, Jones MV, Ewart WR. Immunohistochemical localisation of a gastrin-releasing peptide-like material in area postrema, nucleus of the solitary tract and vagal motor nucleus in the brainstem of rat. *J Auton Nerv Syst* 1989; **28**: 97–104.

225. Hilton JM, Chai SY, Sexton PM. *In vitro* autoradiographic localization of the calcitonin receptor isoforms, C1a and C1b, in rat brain. *Neuroscience* 1995; **69**: 1223–37.

226. Morgan DG, Kulkarni RN, Hurley JD *et al*. Inhibition of glucose stimulated insulin secretion by neuropeptide Y is mediated via the Y1 receptor and inhibition of adenylyl cyclase in RIN 5AH rat insulinoma cells. *Diabetologia* 1998; **41**: 1482–91.

227. Riediger T, Rauch M, Jurat G, Schmid HA. Central nervous targets for pancreatic amylin. *Pflugers Arch* 1999; **437**: R142.

228. Kapas L, Obal F Jr, Farkas I *et al*. Cholecystokinin promotes sleep and reduces food intake in diabetic rats. *Physiol Behav* 1991; **50**: 417–20.

229. Chernausek SD, Attie KM, Cara JF, Rosenfeld RG, Frane J. Growth hormone therapy of Turner syndrome: the impact of age of estrogen replacement on final height. Genentech, Inc., Collaborative Study Group. *J Clin Endocrinol Metab* 2000; **85**: 2439–45.

230. Edmonds BK, Edwards GL. Dorsomedial hindbrain participation in glucoprivic feeding response to 2DG but not 2DG-induced hyperglycemia or activation of the HPA axis [in process citation]. *Brain Res* 1998; **801**: 21–8.

231. Herr RR, Jahnke JK, Argoudelis AD. The structure of streptozotocin. *J Am Chem Soc* 1967; **89**: 4808–9.

232. Schnedl WJ, Ferber S, Johnson JH, Newgard CB. STZ transport and cytotoxicity. Specific enhancement in GLUT2- expressing cells. *Diabetes* 1994; **43**: 1326–33.

233. Wang Z, Gleichmann H. GLUT2 in pancreatic islets: crucial target molecule in diabetes induced with multiple low doses of streptozotocin in mice. *Diabetes* 1998; **47**: 50–56.

234. Wang Z, Gleichmann H. Glucose transporter 2 expression: prevention of streptozotocin-induced reduction in β-cells with 5-thio-D-glucose. *Exp Clin Endocrinol Diabetes* 1995; **103**: 83–97.

235. Agarwal MK. Streptozotocin: mechanisms of action: proceedings of a workshop held on 21 June 1980, Washington, DC. *FEBS Lett* 1980; **120**: 1–3.

236. Leloup C, Arluison M, Lepetit N *et al*. Glucose transporter 2 (GLUT 2): expression in specific brain nuclei. *Brain Res* 1994; **638**: 221–6.

237. Tomlinson KC, Gardiner SM, Bennett T. Central effects of angiotensins I and II in conscious streptozotocin-treated rats. *Am J Physiol* 1990; **258**: R1147–56.

238. Young JK. A glial toxin reduces effects of gold thioglucose on the hypothalamus and area postrema. *Brain Res Bull* 1988; **20**: 97–104.

239. Powley TL, Prechtl JC. Gold thioglucose selectively damages dorsal vagal nuclei. *Brain Res* 1986; **367**: 192–200.

240. Brown DF, Floody OR. Gold thioglucose-induced brain lesions in hamsters. *Physiol Behav* 1987; **39**: 315–20.

241. Bird E, Cardone CC, Contreras RJ. Area postrema lesions disrupt food intake induced by cerebroventricular infusions of 5-thioglucose in the rat. *Brain Res* 1983; **270**: 193–6.

242. Caputo FA, Scallet AC. Postnatal MSG treatment attenuates angiotensin II (AII) induced drinking in rats. *Physiol Behav* 1995; **58**: 25–9.

243. Reddy VM, Meharg SS, Ritter S. Dose-related stimulation of feeding by systemic injections of monosodium glutamate. *Physiol Behav* 1986; **38**: 465–9.

244. Rogulja I, Harding JW, Ritter S. Reduction of ^{125}I-angiotensin II binding sites in rat brain following monosodium glutamate treatment. *Brain Res* 1987; **419**: 333–5.

245. Ritter S, Stone SL. Area postrema lesions block feeding induced by systemic injections of monosodium glutamate. *Physiol Behav* 1987; **41**: 21–4.

246. Printz H, Reiter S, Samadi N *et al*. Glp-1 release in man after lower large bowel resection or intrarectal glucose administration. *Digestion* 1998; **59**: 689–695.

247. Hoentjen F, Hopman WP, Jansen JB. Effect of circulating peptide YY on gall bladder motility in response to feeding in humans. Program and Abstracts, Digestive Disease Week, May 20–23, 2001, Atlanta, GA (abstr 65).

248. Gusev AA. [Cellular reaction of the area postrema of the medulla oblongata to experimental alloxan diabetes]. *Biull Eksp Biol Med* 1984; **98**: 753–5.
249. Arjune D, Bodnar RJ. Inhibition of deprivation-induced feeding by naloxone and cholecystokinin in rats: effects of central alloxan. *Brain Res Bull* 1990; **24**: 375–9.
250. Krolewski AS, Warram JH. Epidemiology of diabetes mellitus. In Marble A, Krall LP, Bradley RF, Christlieb AR, Soeldner JS (eds), *Joslin's Diabetes Mellitus*, 12th edn. Lea and Febiger: Philadelphia, 1985; 12–42.
251. Pipeleers D, Kiekens R, In't Veld P. Morphology of the pancreatic β-cell. In Ashcroft FM, Ashcroft SJH (eds), *Insulin: Molecular Biology to Pathology*. Oxford University Press: Oxford, 1992; 5–24.
252. Wahren J, Ekberg K, Johansson J *et al*. Role of C-peptide in human physiology. *Am J Physiol* 2000; **278**: E759–68.
253. Tatemoto K, Efendic S, Mutt V *et al*. Pancreastatin, a novel pancreatic peptide that inhibits insulin secretion. *Nature* 1986; **324**: 476–8.
254. Barkatullah SC, Curry WJ, Johnston CF, Hutton JC, Buchanan KD. Ontogenetic expression of chromogranin A and its derived peptides, WE-14 and pancreastatin, in the rat neuroendocrine system. *Histochem Cell Biol* 1997; **107**: 251–7.
255. Cooper GJS, Willis AC, Clark A, Turner RC *et al*. Purification and characterization of a peptide from amyloid-rich pancreases of type 2 diabetic patients. *Proc Natl Acad Sci USA* 1987; **84**: 8628–8632.
256. Saad MF, Knowler WC, Pettitt DJ, Nelson RG *et al*. Sequential changes in serum insulin concentration during development of non-insulin-dependent diabetes. *Lancet* 1989; **1**: 1356–59.
257. Koda JE, Fineman MS, Kolterman OG, Caro JF. 24 hour plasma amylin profiles are elevated in IGT subjects vs. normal controls. *Diabetes* 1995; **44**: 238A.
258. Gedulin B, Jodka C, Hoyt J, Young A. Evidence for amylin resistance for inhibition of gastric emptying in hyperamylinemic Fatty Zucker rats. Endocrine Society 81st Annual Meeting Program and Abstracts 1999; 217 (abstr P1-388).
259. Nauck MA, Heimesaat MM, Orskov C, Holst JJ *et al*. Preserved incretin activity of glucagon-like peptide 1 (7–36 amide) but not of synthetic human gastric inhibitory polypeptide in patients with type 2 diabetes mellitus. *J Clin Invest* 1993; **91**: 301–7.
260. Koda JE, Fineman M, Rink TJ, Dailey GE, Muchmore DB, Linarelli LG. Amylin concentrations and glucose control. *Lancet* 1992; **339**: 1179–1180.
261. Lorenzo A, Razzaboni B, Weir GC, Yankner BA. Pancreatic islet cell toxicity of amylin associated with type 2 diabetes mellitus. *Nature* 1994; **368**: 756–60.
262. MacGibbon GA, Cooper GJS, Dragunow M. Acute application of human amylin, unlike β-amyloid peptides, kills undifferentiated PC12 cells by apoptosis. *NeuroReport* 1997; **8**: 3945–9.
263. Young A, Denaro M. Roles of amylin in diabetes and in regulation of nutrient load. *Nutrition* 1998; **14**: 524–7.
264. Krowicki ZK, Nathan NA, Hornby PJ. Gastric motor and cardiovascular effects of insulin in dorsal vagal complex of the rat. *Am J Physiol* 1998; **275**: G964–72.
265. Gedulin BR, Young AA. Hypoglycemia overrides amylin-mediated regulation of gastric emptying in rats. *Diabetes* 1998; **47**: 93–7.
266. Kong MF, King P, Macdonald IA *et al*. Euglycaemic hyperinsulinaemia does not affect gastric emptying in type I and type II diabetes mellitus. *Diabetologia* 1999; **42**: 365–72.
267. Evangelista S, Santicioli P, Maggi CA. 2-Deoxy-D-glucose (2-DG)-induced increase in gastric acid secretion is impaired in capsaicin-pretreated rats. *Adv Exp Med Biol* 1991; **298**: 301–6.

268. Pennington AM, Corpe CP, Kellett GL. Rapid regulation of rat jejunal glucose transport by insulin in a luminally and vascularly perfused preparation. *J Physiol* 1994; **478**: 187–93.

269. Jamal H, Suda K, Bretherton-Watt D, Ghatei MA, Bloom SR. Molecular form of islet amyloid polypeptide (amylin) released from isolated rat islets of Langerhans. *Pancreas* 1993; **8**: 261–6.

270. Percy AJ, Trainor DA, Rittenhouse J, Phelps J, Koda JE. Development of sensitive immunoassays to detect amylin and amylin-like peptides in unextracted plasma. *Clin Chem* 1996; **42**: 576–85.

271. Dilts RP, Phelps J, Koda J, Beaumont K. Comparative distribution of amylin and calcitonin gene-related peptide (CGRP): immunoreactivities in the adult rat brain. *Soc Neurosci Abstr* 1995; **21**: 1116.

272. Young AA, Wang MW, Gedulin B, Rink TJ *et al.* Diabetogenic effects of salmon calcitonin are attributable to amylin-like activity. *Metabolism* 1995; **44**: 1581–9.

273. Kitamura K, Kangawa K, Kawamoto M *et al.* Adrenomedullin: a novel hypotensive peptide isolated from human pheochromocytoma. *Biochem Biophys Res Commun* 1993; **192**: 553–60.

274. Leighton B, Cooper GJS. Pancreatic amylin and calcitonin gene-related peptide cause resistance to insulin in skeletal muscle *in vitro*. *Nature* 1988; **335**: 632–5.

275. Young AA, Gedulin B, Wolfe-Lopez D, Greene HE *et al.* Amylin and insulin in rat soleus muscle: dose responses for cosecreted non-competitive antagonists. *Am J Physiol* 1992; **263**: E274–81.

276. Lupien JR, Young AA. No measurable effect of amylin on lipolysis in either white or brown isolated adipocytes from rats. *Diabet Nutr Metab* 1993; **6**: 13–18.

277. Young AA. Amylin and its effects on the Cori cycle. *Taking Control in Diabetes.* Synergy Medical Education: Surrey, UK, 1993; 15–21.

278. Dégano P, Silvestre RA, Salas M, Peiró E, Marco J. Amylin inhibits glucose-induced insulin secretion in a dose-dependent manner. Study in the perfused rat pancreas. *Regul Pept* 1993; **43**: 91–96.

279. Young AA, Vine W, Carlo P *et al.* Amylin stimulation of renin activity in rats: a possible link between insulin resistance and hypertension. *J Hypertension* 1994; **12**: S152.

280. Leighton B, Cooper GJS, Willis AC, Rothbard JB. Amylin inhibits glucose utilisation in the soleus muscle of the rat *in vitro*. *Diabetologia* 1988; **31**: 513A.

281. Young AA, Rink TJ, Vine W, Gedulin B. Amylin and syndrome-X. *Drug Dev Res* 1994; **32**: 90–99.

282. Young AA, Carlo P, Rink TJ, Wang M-W. 8-37hCGRP, an amylin receptor antagonist, enhances the insulin response and perturbs the glucose response to infused arginine in anesthetized rats. *Mol Cell Endocrinol* 1992; **84**: R1–5.

283. Young AA, Gedulin B, Gaeta LSL *et al.* Selective amylin antagonist suppresses rise in plasma lactate after intravenous glucose in the rat—evidence for a metabolic role of endogenous amylin. *FEBS Lett* 1994; **343**: 237–41.

284. Silvestre RA, Salas M, Rodriguez-Gallardo J, Garcia-Hermida O *et al.* Effect of (8–32) salmon calcitonin, an amylin antagonist, on insulin, glucagon and somatostatin release: study in the perfused pancreas of the rat. *Br J Pharmacol* 1996; **117**: 347–350.

285. Leaming R, Johnson A, Hook G, Hanley R, Baron A. Amylin modulates insulin secretion in humans. Studies with an amylin antagonist. *Diabetologia* 1995; **38**: A113.

286. Young A, Moore C, Herich J., Beaumont K. Neuroendocrine actions of amylin. In Poyner D, Marshall I, Brain SD (eds), *The CGRP Family: Calcitonin Gene-related Peptide (CGRP), Amylin, and Adrenomedullin*. Landes Bioscience; Georgetown, TX, 2000; 91–102.

287. Young AA, Gedulin B, Vine W, Percy A, Rink TJ. Gastric emptying is accelerated in diabetic BB rats and is slowed by subcutaneous injections of amylin. *Diabetologia.* 1995; **38**: 642–648.

288. Gedulin BR, Jodka CM, Green DL, Young AA. Comparison of 21 peptides on inhibition of gastric emptying in conscious rats. *Dig Dis Week* 1996: A–742.

289. Kong M, Stubbs T, King P *et al.* Effect of single doses of pramlintide on gastric emptying of two meals in type 1 diabetes [in German]. *Diabetes Stoffwechsel* 1998; **7**: 103–104.

290. Horowitz M, Edelbroek MA, Wishart JM, Straathof JW. Relationship between oral glucose tolerance and gastric emptying in normal healthy subjects. *Diabetologia* 1993; **36**: 857–62.

291. Brener W, Hendrix TR, McHugh PR. Regulation of the gastric emptying of glucose. *Gastroenterology* 1983; **85**: 76–82.

292. Young AA, Bogardus C, Stone K, Mott DM. Insulin response of components of whole-body and muscle carbohydrate metabolism in humans. *Am J Physiol* 1988; **254**: E231–6.

293. Thor P, Laskiewicz J, Konturek SJ, Creutzfeldt W. Role of GIP and insulin in glucose-induced changes in intestinal motility patterns. *Am J Physiol* 1987; **252**: G8–12.

294. Young AA, Gedulin BR, Rink TJ. Dose–responses for the slowing of gastric emptying in a rodent model by glucagon-like peptide (7–36) NH2, amylin, cholecystokinin, and other possible regulators of nutrient uptake. *Metabolism* 1996; **45**: 1–3.

295. Edwards GL, Gedulin BR, Jodka C, Dilts RP *et al.* Area postrema (AP)-lesions block the regulation of gastric emptying by amylin. *Neurogastroenterol Motil* 1998; **10**: 26.

296. Sexton PM, Paxinos G, Kenney MA, Wookey PJ, Beaumont K. *In vitro* autoradiographic localization of amylin binding sites in rat brain. *Neuroscience* 1994; **62**: 553–67.

297. Jodka C, Parkes D, Young A. Hypoglycemic override of inhibition of gastric emptying by exendin-4. *Diabetes* 2000; **49**: A285.

298. Young AA, Gedulin BR, Jodka C, Green D. Insulin-induced hypoglycemia reverses amylin-inhibition of gastric emptying in rats. *Diabetes* 1996; **45**: 187A.

299. Adachi A, Kobashi M, Funahashi M. Glucose-responsive neurons in the brainstem. *Obes Res* 1995; **3**: 735–40S.

300. Guidobono F, Coluzzi M, Pagani F, Pecile A, Netti C. Amylin given by central and peripheral routes inhibits gastric acid secretion. *Peptides* 1994; **15**: 699–702.

301. Gedulin BR, Lawler RL, Jodka CM, Grazzini ML, Young AA. Amylin inhibits pentagastrin-stimulated gastric acid secretion and protects against ethanol-induced gastric mucosal damage in rats. *Diabetologia* 1997; **40**: A299.

302. Jodka C, Gedulin B, Lawler R, Grazzini M, Young A. Amylin protects against ethanol-induced gastric mucosal damage and inhibits pentagastrin-stimulated gastric acid secretion in rats. *Diabetes* 1997; **46**: 365A.

303. Guidobono F, Pagani F, Ticozzi C, Sibilia V *et al.* Protection by amylin of gastric erosions induced by indomethacin or ethanol in rats. *Br J Pharmacol* 1997; **120**: 581–6.

304. Clementi G, Caruso A, Cutuli VMC, Prato A *et al.* Effect of amylin in various experimental models of gastric ulcer. *Eur J Pharmacol* 1997; **332**: 209–213.

305. Zanelli JM, Stracca-Gasser M, Gaines-Das RE, Guidobono F. The short term effect of peripherally administered brain-gut peptides on gastric acid secretion in rats. *Agents Actions* 1992; **35**: 122–9.

306. Holzer P, Lippe II, Raybould HE *et al.* Role of peptidergic sensory neurons in gastric mucosal blood flow and protection. *Ann NY Acad Sci* 1991; **632**: 272–82.

307. Tache Y, Raybould H, Wei JY. Central and peripheral actions of calcitonin gene-related peptide on gastric secretory and motor function. *Adv Exp Med Biol* 1991; **298**: 183–98.

308. Beglinger C, Born W, Hildebrand P *et al*. Calcitonin gene-related peptides I and II and calcitonin: distinct effects on gastric acid secretion in humans. *Gastroenterology* 1988; **95**: 958–65.

309. Lenz HJ, Brown MR. Intracerebroventricular administration of human calcitonin and human calcitonin gene-related peptide inhibits meal-stimulated gastric acid secretion in the dog. *Dig Dis Sci* 1987; **32**: 409–16.

310. Okimura Y, Chihara K, Abe H *et al*. Effect of intracerebroventricular administration of rat calcitonin gene-related peptide (CGRP), human calcitonin and [Asu1, 7]-eel calcitonin on gastric acid secretion in rats. *Endocrinol Jpn* 1986; **33**: 273–7.

311. Lenz HJ, Mortrud MT, Vale WW, Rivier JE, Brown MR. Calcitonin gene-related peptide acts within the central nervous system to inhibit gastric acid secretion. *Regul Pept* 1984; **9**: 271–7.

312. Guidobono F, Netti C, Pagani F *et al*. Effect of unmodified eel calcitonin on gastric acid secretion and gastric ulcers in the rat. *Farmaco* 1991; **46**: 555–63.

313. Doepfner W. Effects of synthetic salmon calcitonin on gastric secretion and ulcer formation in conscious cats and rats. In Goebell H, Hotz J (eds), *Effects of Calcitonin and Somatostatin on the Gastrointestinal Tract and Pancreas*. Demeter Verlag: Grafelfing, 1976: 60–70.

314. Tache Y. Inhibition of gastric acid secretion and ulcers by calcitonin gene-related peptide. *Ann N Y Acad Sci* 1992; **657**: 240–47.

315. Helton WS, Mulholland MM, Bunnett NW, Debas HT. Inhibition of gastric and pancreatic secretion in dogs by CGRP: role of somatostatin. *Am J Physiol* 1989; **256**: G715–20.

316. Okuma Y, Osumi Y. Central cholinergic descending pathway to the dorsal motor nucleus of the vagus in regulation of gastric functions. *Jpn J Pharmacol* 1986; **41**: 373–9.

317. Okuma Y, Osumi Y, Ishikawa T, Mitsuma T. Enhancement of gastric acid output and mucosal blood flow by tripeptide thyrotropin releasing hormone microinjected into the dorsal motor nucleus of the vagus in rats. *Jpn J Pharmacol* 1987; **43**: 173–8.

318. Tache Y, Stephens RL Jr, Ishikawa T. Central nervous system action of TRH to influence gastrointestinal function and ulceration. *Ann N Y Acad Sci* 1989; **553**: 269–85.

319. Zhang SX, Huang CG. [Stimulatory effect of vasoactive intestinal peptide microinjected into dorsal vagal complex on gastric acid secretion in rats]. *Sheng Li Hsueh Pao* 1993; **45**: 568–74.

320. Jonderko K, Konca A, Golab T, Jonderko G. Effect of calcitonin on gall-bladder volume in man. *J Gastroenterol Hepatol* 1989; **4**: 505–11.

321. Jonderko G, Jonderko K, Konca A, Golab T. [Effect of calcitonin on gallbladder volume between food intake and on its emptying after meals in humans]. *Pol Arch Med Wewn* 1989; **81**(1): 7–12.

322. Hashimoto T, Poston GJ, Greeley GH Jr, Thompson JC. Calcitonin gene-related peptide inhibits gallbladder contractility. *Surgery* 1988; **104**: 419–23.

323. Gedulin B, Lawler R, Jodka C, Young A. Amylin inhibits pentagastrin-stimulated gastric acid secretion: comparison with glucagon-like peptide-1 and exendin-4. *Diabetes* 1997; **40**: 188A.

324. Lutz TA, Geary N, Szabady MM, DelPrete E, Scharrer E. Amylin decreases meal size in rats. *Physiol Behav* 1995; **58**: 1197–202.

325. Morley JE, Morley PM, Flood JF. Anorectic effects of amylin in rats over the life span. *Pharmacol Biochem Behav* 1993; **44**: 577–80.

326. Bhavsar S, Watkins J, Young A. Synergy between amylin and cholecystokinin for inhibition of food intake in mice. *Physiol Behav* 1998; **64**: 557–61.

327. Lutz TA, Senn M, Althaus J, DelPrete E *et al*. Lesion of the area postrema nucleus of the solitary tract (AP/NTS) attenuates the anorectic effects of amylin and calcitonin gene-related peptide (CGRP) in rats. *Peptides* 1998; **19**: 309–17.

328. Lutz TA, Althaus J, Rossi R, Scharrer E. Anorectic effect of amylin is not transmitted by capsaicin-sensitive nerve fibers. *Am J Physiol* 1998; **274**: R1777–82.

329. Granqvist L, Permert J, Arnelo U *et al*. Effects of AC187, IAPP(8–37) and CGRP(8–37) on IAPP induced anorexia in rats. *Digestion* 1997; **58**: 55.

330. Rushing PA, Hagan MM, Seeley RJ *et al*. Inhibition of central amylin signaling increases food intake and body adiposity in rats. *Endocrinology* 2001; **142**: 5035.

331. Gebre-Medhin S, Mulder H, Pekny M *et al*. IAPP (amylin) null mutant mice; plasma levels of insulin and glucose, body weight and pain responses. *Diabetologia* 1997; **40**: A26.

332. Devine E, Young AA. Weight gain in male and female mice with amylin gene knockout. *Diabetes* 1998; **47**: A317.

333. Weyer C, Maggs DG, Young AA, Kolterman OG. Amylin replacement with pramlintide as an adjunct to insulin therapy in type 1 and type 2 diabetes mellitus: a physiological approach toward improved metabolic control. *Curr Pharm Des* 2001; **7**: 1353–73.

334. Samols E, Bonner-Weir S, Weir GC. Intra-islet insulin-glucagon-somatostatin relationships. *Clin Endocrinol Metab* 1986; **15**: 33–58.

335. Rothman DL, Magnusson I, Katz LD, Shulman RG, Shulman GI. Quantitation of hepatic glycogenolysis and gluconeogenesis in fasting humans with C-13 NMR. *Science* 1991; **254**: 573–6.

336. Unger RH, Orci L. The role of glucagon in the endogenous hyperglycemia of diabetes mellitus. *Ann Rev Med* 1997; **28**: 119–130.

337. Foster DW, McGarry JD. *The Regulation of Ketogenesis*. CIBA Foundation Symposia, Vol 87. Wiley: Chichester, 1982; 120–31.

338. Marliss EB, Nakhooda AF, Poussier P. Clinical forms and natural history of the diabetic syndrome and insulin and glucagon secretion in the BB rat. *Metabolism* 1983; **32**(suppl 1): 11–17.

339. Grill V, Herberg L. Glucose- and arginine-induced insulin and glucagon responses from the isolated perfused pancreas of the BB-Wistar diabetic rat. Evidence for selective impairment of glucose regulation. *Acta Endocrinol (Copenh)* 1983; **102**: 561–6.

340. Kanazawa M, Ikeda J, Sato J *et al*. Alteration of insulin and glucagon secretion from the perfused BB rat pancreas before and after the onset of diabetes. *Diabetes Res Clin Pract* 1988; **5**: 201–4.

341. Weir GC, Knowlton SD, Atkins RF, McKennan KX, Martin DB. Glucagon secretion from the perfused pancreas of streptozotocin-treated rats. *Diabetes* 1976; **25**: 275–82.

342. Goto Y, Berelowitz M, Frohman LA. Acute effects of alloxan- and streptozotocin-induced insulin deficiency on somatostatin and glucagon secretion by the perfused isolated rat pancreatico-duodenal preparation. *Diabetologia* 1981; **20**: 66–71.

343. Dunbar JC, Brown A. Glucagon secretion by dispersed alpha cell enriched islets from streptozotocin-treated hamsters in perifusion. *Horm Metab Res* 1984; **16**: 221–5.

344. Lykkelund C, Lund ED. Plasma glucagon responses to insulin-induced hypoglycaemia and arginine in normal and alloxan diabetic rats. *Scand J Clin Lab Invest* 1979; **39**: 151–7.

345. Giroix MH, Portha B, Kergoat M, Picon L. Glucagon secretion in rats with non-insulin-dependent diabetes: an *in vivo* and *in vitro* study. *Diabet Metab* 1984; **10**: 12–17.

346. Prosser PR, Karam JH. Diabetes mellitus following rodenticide ingestion in man. *J Am Med Assoc* 1978; **239**: 1148–50.

347. Raskin P, Fujita Y, Unger RH. Effect of insulin-glucose infusions on plasma glucagon levels in fasting diabetics and nondiabetics. *J Clin Invest* 1975; **56**: 1132–8.

348. Samols E, Bonner-Weir S, Weir GC. Intra-islet insulin–glucagon–somatostatin relationships. *Clin Endocrinol Metab* 1986; **15**: 33–58.

349. Filipponi P, Gregorio F, Cristallini S, Ferrandina C *et al*. Selective impairment of pancreatic A cell suppression by glucose during acute alloxan-induced insulinopenia: *in vitro* study on isolated perfused rat pancreas. *Endocrinology* 1986; **119**: 408–15.

350. Gotoh M, Okamura J, Monden M, Shima K. Glucagon secretory responses to insulin-induced hypoglycemia and arginine in streptozotocin-induced diabetic dogs. *Endocrinol Jpn* 1983; **30**: 443–50.

351. Nishikawa K, Ikeda H, Matsuo T. Abnormal glucagon secretion in Zucker fatty rats. *Horm Metab Res* 1981; **13**: 259–63.

352. Unger RH, Foster DW. Diabetes mellitus. In Wilson JD, Foster DW (eds), *Williams Textbook of Endocrinology*, 8th edn. W.B. Saunders: Philadelphia, PA, 1992: 1273–5.

353. Ishida K, Mizuno A, Sano T, Shi K, Shima K. Plasma glucagon responses to insulin-induced hypoglycemia and arginine in spontaneous non-insulin-dependent diabetes mellitus (NIDDM) rats, Otsuka Long Evans Tokushima Fatty (OLETF) strain. *Acta Endocrinol (Copenh)* 1993; **129**: 585–93.

354. Leahy JL, Weir GC. Unresponsiveness to glucose in a streptozocin model of diabetes. Inappropriate insulin and glucagon responses to a reduction of glucose concentration. *Diabetes* 1985; **34**: 653–9.

355. Young AA, Gedulin BR, Jodka C, Green D. Insulin-induced hypoglycemia reverses amylin-inhibition of gastric emptying in rats. *Diabetes* 1996; **45**: 187A.

356. Gedulin BR, Rink TJ, Young AA. Dose-response for glucagonostatic effect of amylin in rats. *Metabolism* 1997; **46**: 67–70.

357. Gedulin B, Jodka C, Percy A, Young A. Neutralizing antibody and the antagonist AC187 may inhibit glucagon secretion in rats. *Diabetes* 1997; **40**: 238A.

358. Silvestre RA, Rodriguez-Gallardo J, Jodka C *et al*. Selective amylin inhibition of the glucagon response to arginine is extrinsic to the pancreas. *Am J Physiol* 2001; **280**: E443–9.

359. Ohtomo Y, Bergman T, Johansson BL, Jornvall H, Wahren J. Differential effects of proinsulin C-peptide fragments on Na^+, K^+-ATPase activity of renal tubule segments. *Diabetologia* 1998; **41**: 287–91.

360. Forst T, De La Tour DD, Kunt T *et al*. Effects of proinsulin C-peptide on nitric oxide, microvascular blood flow and erythrocyte Na^+, K^+-ATPase activity in diabetes mellitus type I. *Clin Sci (Colch)* 2000; **98**: 283–90.

361. Johansson BL, Borg K, Fernqvist-Forbes E, Odergren T *et al*. C-peptide improves autonomic nerve function in IDDM patients. *Diabetologia* 1996; **39**: 687–95.

362. Johansson BL, Borg K, Fernqvist-Forbes E, Kernell A *et al*. Beneficial effects of C-peptide on incipient nephropathy and neuropathy in patients with type 1 diabetes mellitus. *Diabet Med* 2000; **17**: 181–9.

363. Johansson BL, Linde B, Wahren J. Effects of C-peptide on blood flow, capillary diffusion capacity and glucose utilization in the exercising forearm of type 1 (insulin-dependent) diabetic patients. *Diabetologia* 1992; **35**: 1151–8.

364. Walsh JH. Gastrointestinal hormones. In Johnson LR (ed.), *Physiology of the Gastrointestinal Tract*, 3rd edn. Raven: New York, 1994; **1**: 1–128.

365. Habener JF, inventor; The General Hospital Corporation, assignee. *Insulinotropic Hormone GLP-1 (7–36) and Uses Thereof*. US Patent 5,614,492, Mar 25 1997.

366. Mojsov S, Weir GC, Habener JF. Insulinotropin: glucagon-like peptide I (7–37) co-encoded in the glucagon gene is a potent stimulator of insulin release in the perfused rat pancreas. *J Clin Invest* 1987; **79**: 616–19.

367. Holst JJ, Orskov C, Nielsen OV, Schwartz TW. Truncated glucagon-like peptide I, an insulin-releasing hormone from the distal gut. *FEBS Lett* 1987; **211**: 169–74.

368. Weir GC, Mojsov S, Hendrick GK, Habener JF. Glucagon-like peptide I (7–37) actions on endocrine pancreas. *Diabetes* 1989; **38**: 338–42.

369. Göke R, Wagner B, Fehmann HC, Göke B. Glucose-dependency of the insulin stimulatory effect of glucagon-like peptide-1 (7–36) amide on the rat pancreas. *Res Exp Med (Berl)* 1993; **193**: 97–103.

370. Orskov C, Wettergren A, Holst JJ. Biological effects and metabolic rates of glucagon-like peptide-1 7–36 amide and glucagonlike peptide-1 7–37 in healthy subjects are indistinguishable. *Diabetes* 1993; **42**: 658–61.

371. Hansen L, Deacon CF, Orskov C, Holst JJ. Glucagon-like peptide-1-(7–36) amide is transformed to glucagon-like peptide-1-(9–36) amide by dipeptidyl peptidase IV in the capillaries supplying the L cells of the porcine intestine. *Endocrinology* 1999; **140**: 5356–63.

372. Knudsen LB, Pridal L. Glucagon-like peptide-1-(9–36) amide is a major metabolite of glucagon-like peptide-1-(7–36) amide after *in vivo* administration to dogs, and it acts as an antagonist on the pancreatic receptor. *Eur J Pharmacol* 1996; **318**: 429–35.

373. Wettergren A, Schjoldager B, Mortensen PE, Myhre J *et al*. Truncated GLP-1 (proglucagon 78–107 amide) inhibits gastric and pancreatic functions in man. *Dig Dis Sci* 1993; **38**: 665–73.

374. Dupre J, Behme MT, Hramiak IM *et al*. Glucagon-like peptide I reduces postprandial glycemic excursions in IDDM. *Diabetes* 1995; **44**: 626–30.

375. Willms B, Werner J, Holst JJ, Orskov C *et al*. Gastric emptying glucose responses, and insulin secretion after a liquid test meal: effects of exogenous glucagon-like peptide-1 (GLP-1)-(7–36) amide in type 2 (non-insulin-dependent) diabetic patients. *J Clin Endocrinol Metab* 1996; **81**: 327–32.

376. Dupre J, Behme MT, Hramiak IM, McDonald TJ. Subcutaneous glucagon-like peptide I combined with insulin normalizes postcibal glycemic excursions in IDDM. *Diabetes Care* 1997; **20**: 381–4.

377. Schirra J, Kuwert P, Wank U *et al*. Differential effects of subcutaneous GLP-1 on gastric emptying, antroduodenal motility, and pancreatic function in men. *Proc Assoc Am Physicians* 1997; **109**: 84–97.

378. Schirra J, Leicht P, Hildebrand P *et al*. Mechanisms of the antidiabetic action of subcutaneous glucagon-like peptide-1(7–36) amide in non-insulin-dependent diabetes mellitus. *J Endocrinol* 1998; **156**: 177–86.

379. Nauck MA, Niedereich-Holz U, Ettler R *et al*. Glucagon-like peptide 1 inhibition of gastric emptying outweighs its insulinotropic effects in healthy humans. *Am J Physiol* 1997; **273**: E981–8.

380. Vaag AA, Holst JJ, Volund A, BeckNielsen H. Gut incretin hormones in identical twins discordant for non-insulin-dependent diabetes mellitus (NIDDM)—Evidence for decreased glucagon-like peptide 1 secretion during oral glucose ingestion in NIDDM twins. *Eur J Endocrinol* 1996; **135**: 425–32.

381. Legakis IN, Tzioras C, Phenekos C. Decreased GLP-1 levels in type 2 diabetes. *Program and Abstracts, 82nd Annual Endocrine Meeting*, June 21–24, Toronto, Canada, 2000; 431.

382. Puente J, Molina LM, Márquez L *et al*. GLP-1 secretion in morbid obesity after vertical banded gastroplasty. *Diabetologia* 1999; **42**: A196.

383. Toft-Nielsen M-B, Damholt MB, Hilsted L *et al*. GLP-1 secretion is decreased in NIDDM patients compared to matched control subjects with normal glucose tolerance. *Diabetologia* 1999; **42**: A40.

384. Hopwood NJ, Hintz RL, Gertner JM *et al*. Growth response of children with non-growth-hormone deficiency and marked short stature during three years of growth hormone therapy. *J Pediat* 1993; **123**: 215–22.

385. Kreymann B, Yiangou Y, Kanse S, Williams G *et al*. Isolation and characterisation of GLP-1 7–36 amide from rat intestine. Elevated levels in diabetic rats. *FEBS Lett* 1988; **242**: 167–70.

386. Brubaker PL, So DC, Drucker DJ. Tissue-specific differences in the levels of pro-glucagon-derived peptides in streptozotocin-induced diabetes. *Endocrinology* 1989; **124**: 3003–9.

387. Roberge JN, Brubaker PL. Secretion of proglucagon-derived peptides in response to intestinal luminal nutrients. *Endocrinology*. 1991; **128**: 3169–74.

388. Plaisancie P, Bernard C, Chayvialle JA, Cuber JC. Regulation of glucagon-like peptide-1-(7–36) amide secretion by intestinal neurotransmitters and hormones in the isolated vascularly perfused rat colon. *Endocrinology* 1994; **135**: 2398–403.

389. Dell' Anna C, Lugari R, Dei Cas A *et al*. Gastric emptying and glucagon-like peptide 1 (7–36 amide) response to a solid test meal in type 1 diabetes. *Diabetologia* 1999; **42** (suppl 1): A197.

390. Schjoldager BT, Mortensen PE, Christiansen J, Orskov C, Holst JJ. GLP-1 (glucagon-like peptide 1) and truncated GLP-1 fragments of human proglucagon, inhibit gastric acid secretion in humans. *Dig Dis Sci* 1989; **34**: 703–8.

391. O'Halloran DJ, Nikou GC, Kreymann B, Ghatei MA, Bloom SR. Glucagon-like peptide-1 (7–36)-NH2: a physiological inhibitor of gastric acid secretion in man. *J Endocrinol* 1990; **126**: 169–73.

392. Wettergren A, Maina P, Boesby S, Holst JJ. Glucagon-like peptide-1 7–36 amide and peptide YY have additive inhibitory effect on gastric acid secretion in man. *Scand J Gastroenterol* 1997; **32**: 552–5.

393. Fung LC, Chisholm C, Greenberg GR. Glucagon-like peptide-1-(7–36) amide and peptide YY, mediate intraduodenal fat-induced inhibition of acid secretion in dogs. *Endocrinology* 1998; **139**: 189–94.

394. Wojdemann M, Wettergren A, Sternby B *et al*. Inhibition of human gastric lipase secretion by glucagon-like peptide-1. *Dig Dis Sci* 1998; **43**: 799–805.

395. Wettergren A, Wojdemann M, Holst JJ. Glucagon-like peptide-1 inhibits gastropancreatic function by inhibiting central parasympathetic outflow. *Am J Physiol* 1998; **38**: G984–92.

396. Lloyd KCK, Amirmoazzami S, Friedik F, Heynio A *et al*. Candidate canine enterogastrones: acid inhibition before and after vagotomy. *Am J Physiol* 1997; **35**: G1236–42.

397. Wettergren A, Wojdemann M, Meisner S, Stadil F, Holst JJ. The inhibitory effect of glucagon-like peptide-1 (GLP-1) 7–36 amide on gastric acid secretion in humans depends on an intact vagal innervation. *Gut* 1997; **40**: 597–601.

398. Imeryuz N, Yegen BC, Bozkurt A, Coskun T *et al*. Glucagon-like peptide-1 inhibits gastric emptying via vagal afferent-mediated central mechanisms. *Am J Physiol* 1997; **273**: G920–27.

399. Rossowski WJ, Cheng BL, Jiang NY, Coy DH. Examination of somatostatin involvement in the inhibitory action of GIP, GLP-1, amylin and adrenomedullin on gastric acid release using a new SRIF antagonist analogue. *Br J Pharmacol* 1998; **125**: 1081–87.

400. Lloyd KC, Amirmoazzami S, Friedik F, Heynio A *et al*. Candidate canine enterogastrones: acid inhibition before and after vagotomy. *Am J Physiol* 1997; **272**: G1236–42.

401. Gedulin BR, Lawler RL, Jodka CM, Young AA. Comparison of effects of amylin, glucagon-like peptide-1 and exendin-4 to inhibit pentagastrin-stimulated gastric acid secretion. *Diabetologia* 1997; **40**(suppl 1): A300.

402. Nauck MA, Bartels E, Orskov C, Ebert R, Creutzfeldt W. Lack of effect of synthetic human gastric inhibitory polypeptide and glucagon-like peptide 1 [7–36 amide] infused at near-physiological concentrations on pentagastrin-stimulated gastric acid secretion in normal human subjects. *Digestion* 1992; **52**: 214–21.
403. Turton MD, O'Shea D, Gunn I *et al*. A role for glucagon-like peptide-1 in the central regulation of feeding [see comments]. *Nature* 1996; **379**: 69–72.
404. Tang-Christensen M, Larsen PJ, Göke R *et al*. Central administration of GLP-1-(7–36) amide inhibits food and water intake in rats. *Am J Physiol* 1996; **271**: R848–56.
405. Navarro M, Rodriquez de Fonseca F, Alvarez E *et al*. Colocalization of glucagon-like peptide-1 (GLP-1) receptors, glucose transporter GLUT-2, and glucokinase mRNAs in rat hypothalamic cells: evidence for a role of GLP-1 receptor agonists as an inhibitory signal for food and water intake. *J Neurochem* 1996; **67**: 1982–91.
406. Rodriquez de Fonseca F, Navarro M, Alvarez E *et al*. Glucagon-like peptide-1 receptor agonist induce an inhibitory signal for food intake in obese Zucker rats. *Diabetologia* 1997; **40**: A267.
407. Furuse M, Matsumoto M, Mori R, Sugahara K *et al*. Influence of fasting and neuropeptide Y on the suppressive food intake induced by intracerebroventricular injection of glucagon-like peptide-1 in the neonatal chick. *Brain Res* 1997; **764**: 289–92.
408. Furuse M, Matsumoto M, Okumura J, Sugahara K, Hasegawa S. Intracerebroventricular injection of mammalian and chicken glucagon-like peptide-1 inhibits food intake of the neonatal chick. *Brain Res* 1997; **755**: 167–9.
409. Donahey JCK, vanDijk G, Woods SC, Seeley RJ. Intraventricular GLP-1 reduces short- but not long-term food intake or body weight in lean and obese rats. *Brain Res* 1998; **779**: 75–83.
410. Wang TL, Edwards GL, Baile CA. Glucagon-like peptide-1 (7–36) amide administered into the third cerebroventricle inhibits water intake in rats. *Proc Soc Exp Biol Med* 1998; **219**: 85–91.
411. Jensen P, Larsen P, Holst J, Madsen O. Taste aversion responsible for the glucagonoma induced anorexia. *Proce Endocr Soc* 1998: P1–453.
412. Thiele TE, Seeley RJ, D'Alessio D *et al*. Central infusion of glucagon-like peptide-1-(7–36) amide (GLP-1) receptor antagonist attenuates lithium chloride-induced c-Fos induction in rat brainstem. *Brain Res* 1998; **801**: 164–70.
413. Thiele TE, Van Dijk G, Campfield LA *et al*. Central infusion of GLP-1, but not leptin, produces conditioned taste aversions in rats. *Am J Physiol* 1997; **272**: R726–30.
414. Van Dijk G, Thiele TE. Glucagon-like peptide-1 and satiety. *Nature* 1997; **385**: 214.
415. Bhavsar S, Watkins J, Young A. Comparison of central and peripheral effects of exendin-4 and GLP-1 on food intake in rats. Program and Abstracts: 80th Annual Meeting of the Endocrine Society, June 24–27, 1998, New Orleans, LA, 1998; 433.
416. Scrocchi LA, Brown TJ, MaClusky N *et al*. Glucose intolerance but normal satiety in mice with a null mutation in the glucagon-like peptide I receptor gene. *Nature Med* 1996; **2**: 1254–8.
417. Scrocchi LA, Drucker DJ. Effects of aging and a high fat diet on body weight and glucose tolerance in glucagon-like peptide-1 receptor $(-/-)$ mice. *Endocrinology* 1998; **139**: 3127–32.
418. McMahon LR, Wellman PJ. Decreased intake of a liquid diet in nonfood-deprived rats following intra-PVN injections of GLP-1 (7–36) amide. *Pharmacol Biochem Behav* 1997; **58**: 673–7.
419. McMahon LR, Wellman PJ. PVN infusion of GLP-1-(7–36) amide suppresses feeding but does not induce aversion or alter locomotion in rats. *Am J Physiol* 1998; **43**: R23–9.

420. Tang-Christensen M, Vrang N, Larsen PJ. Glucagon-like peptide 1(7–36) amide's central inhibition of feeding and peripheral inhibition of drinking are abolished by neonatal monosodium glutamate treatment. *Diabetes* 1998; **47**: 530–37.

421. Flint A, Raben A, Astrup A, Holst JJ. Glucagon-like peptide 1 promotes satiety and suppresses energy intake in humans. *J Clin Invest* 1998; **101**: 515–20.

422. Flint A, Raben A, Ersboll AK, Holst JJ, Astrup A. The effect of physiological levels of glucagon-like peptide-1 on appetite, gastric emptying, energy and substrate metabolism in obesity. *Int J Obes Relat Metab Disord* 2001; **25**: 78–92.

423. Gutzwiller JP, Drewe J, Göke B *et al.* Glucagon-like peptide-1 promotes satiety and reduces food intake in patients with diabetes mellitus type 2. *Am J Physiol* 1999; **45**: R1541–4.

424. Gutzwiller JP, Göke B, Drewe J *et al.* Glucagon-like peptide-1: a potent regulator of food intake in humans. *Gut* 1999; **44**: 81–6.

425. Thiele TE, Seeley RJ, D'Alessio D *et al.* Central infusion of glucagon-like peptide-1-(7–36) amide (GLP-1) receptor antagonist attenuates lithium chloride-induced c-Fos induction in rat brainstem. *Brain Res* 1998; **801**: 164–70.

426. Larsen PJ, Fledelius C, Knudsen LB, Tang-Christensen M. Systemic administration of the long-acting GLP-1 derivative NN2211 induces lasting and reversible weight loss in both normal and obese rats. *Diabetes* 2001; **50**: 2530–39.

427. Rodriquez de Fonseca F, Navarro M, Alvarez E *et al.* Peripheral vs. central effects of glucagon-like peptide-1 receptor agonists on satiety and body weight loss in Zucker obese rats. *Metabolism* 2000; **49**: 709–17.

428. Siegel EG, Schulze A, Schmidt WE, Creutzfeldt W. Comparison of the effect of GIP and GLP-1 (7–36 amide) on insulin release from rat pancreatic islets. *Eur J Clin Invest* 1992; **22**: 154–7.

429. Zawalich WS, Zawalich KC, Rasmussen H. Influence of glucagon-like peptide-1 on β-cell responsiveness. *Regul Pept* 1993; **44**: 227–83.

430. Holz GG, Kuhtreiber WM, Habener JF. Pancreatic β-cells are rendered glucose-competent by the insulinotropic hormone glucagon-like peptide-1 (7–37). *Nature* 1993; **361**: 362–5.

431. Hargrove DM, Nardone NA, Persson LM *et al.* Comparison of the glucose dependency of glucagon-like peptide-1(7–37) and glyburide *in vitro* and *in vivo*. *Metabolism* 1996; **45**: 404–9.

432. Parkes D, Pittner R, Ackerman J, Watts L, Young A. Insulinotropic actions of exendin-4 and GLP-1 in isolated rat pancreatic islets. Programs and Abstracts: 80th Annual Meeting of the Endocrine Society, June 24–27, 1998, New Orleans, LA, 1998: 275.

433. Fridolf T, Ahren B. GLP-1 (7–36) amide stimulates insulin secretion in rat islets: studies on the mode of action. *Diabetes Res* 1991; **16**: 185–91.

434. Sreenan SK, Mittal AA, Dralyuk F, Pugh WL *et al.* Glucagon-like peptide-1 stimulates insulin secretion by a Ca^{2+}- independent mechanism in Zucker diabetic fatty rat islets of Langerhans. *Metabolism* 2000; **49**: 1579–87.

435. Fehmann HC, Göke R, Göke B. Cell and molecular biology of the incretin hormones glucagon-like peptide-I and glucose-dependent insulin releasing polypeptide. *Endocr Rev* 1995; **16**: 390–410.

436. Masiello P, Gjinovci A, Bombara M, Wollheim CB, Bergamini E. Effects of age, diet and obesity on insulin secretion from isolated perfused rat pancreas: response to glucose, arginine and glucagon-like peptide 1 (7–37). *Diabetes Nutr Metab* 1995; **8**: 346–52.

437. Gutniak MK, Guenifi A, Berggren LJ, Holst JJ *et al.* Glucagon-like peptide I enhances the insulinotropic effect of glibenclamide in NIDDM patients and in the perfused rat pancreas. *Diabetes Care* 1996; **19**: 857–63.

438. Malhotra R, Singh L, Eng J, Raufman JP. Exendin-4, a new peptide from *Heloderma suspectum* venom, potentiates cholecystokinin-induced amylase release from rat pancreatic acini. *Regul Pept* 1992; **41**: 149–56.

439. Dachicourt N, Serradas P, Bailbe D, Kergoat M *et al.* Glucagon-like peptide-1 (7–36)-amide confers glucose sensitivity to previously glucose-incompetent β-cells in diabetic rats: *in vivo* and *in vitro* studies. *J Endocrinol* 1997; **155**: 369–76.

440. Shen HQ, Roth MD, Peterson RG. The effect of glucose and glucagon-like peptide-1 stimulation on insulin release in the perfused pancreas in a non-insulin-dependent diabetes mellitus animal model. *Metab Clin Exp* 1998; **47**: 1042–7.

441. Parkes DG, Pittner R, Jodka C, Smith P, Young A. Insulinotropic actions of exendin-4 and glucagon-like peptide-1 *in vivo* and *in vitro*. *Metabolism* 2001; **50**: 583–9.

442. Kawai K, Suzuki S, Ohashi S, Mukai H *et al.* Effects of truncated glucagon-like peptide-1 on pancreatic hormone release in normal conscious dogs. *Acta Endocrinol (Copenh)* 1990; **123**: 661–7.

443. Ribel U, Hvidt M, Larsen MO, Rolin B *et al.* Glucose-lowering effect of the protracted GLP-1 derivative, NN2211, in the Betacell Reduced Minipig. *Diabetologia* 2000; **43**: A145.

444. Nauck MA, Wollschlager D, Werner J *et al.* Effects of subcutaneous glucagon-like peptide 1 (GLP-1 [7–36 amide]) in patients with NIDDM. *Diabetologia* 1996; **39**: 1546–53.

445. Porksen N, Grofte T, Nyholm B *et al.* Effects of GLP-1 on regularity, frequency, amplitude, and mass of coordinate pulsatile insulin secretion in healthy humans. *Diabetologia* 1997; **40**(suppl 1): A127.

446. Porksen N, Grofte T, Nyholm B *et al.* Glucagon-like peptide 1 increases mass but not frequency or orderliness of pulsatile insulin secretion. *Diabetes* 1998; **47**: 45–9.

447. Byrne MM, Gliem K, Wank U *et al.* Glucagon-like peptide 1 improves the ability of the β-cell to sense and respond to glucose in subjects with impaired glucose tolerance. *Diabetes* 1998; **47**: 1259–65.

448. Edwards CMB, Todd JF, Ghatei MA, Bloom SR. Subcutaneous glucagon-like peptide-I (7–36) amide is insulinotropic and can cause hypoglycaemia in fasted healthy subjects. *Clin Sci* 1998; **95**: 719–24.

449. Heimesaat MM, Behle K, Ritzel R, Schmiegel W, Nauck MA. Glucose-dependence of insulinotropic GLP-1 actions in the hypoglycaemic range: an *in vivo* study in healthy volunteers. *Diabetologia* 1999; **42**(suppl 1): A198.

450. Müller WA, Faloona GR, Aguilar-Parada E, Unger RH. Abnormal α-cell function in diabetes. Response to carbohydrate and protein ingestion. *N Engl J Med* 1970; **283**: 109–15.

451. Unger RH. Glucagon physiology and pathophysiology. *N Engl J Med* 1971; **285**: 443–9.

452. Creutzfeldt WOC, Orskov C, Kleine N, Holst JJ *et al.* Glucagonostatic actions and reduction of fasting hyperglycemia by exogenous glucagon-like peptide I (7–36) amide in type I diabetic patients. *Diabetes Care* 1996; **19**: 580–86.

453. Ritzel R, Orskov C, Holst JJ, Nauck MA. Pharmacokinetic, insulinotropic, and glucagonostatic properties of GLP-1 [7–36 amide] after subcutaneous injection in healthy volunteers. Dose–response relationships. *Diabetologia* 1995; **38**: 720–2.

454. Rodriguez-Gallardo J, Silvestre RA, Egido EM, Marco J. Insulin secretory pattern induced by exendin-4. Study in the perfused rat pancreas. *Diabetologia* 2000; **43**(suppl 1): A138.

455. Freyse EJ, Becher T, El-Hag O, Knospe S *et al.* Blood glucose lowering and glucagonostatic effects of glucagon-like peptide I in insulin-deprived diabetic dogs. *Diabetes* 1997; **46**: 824–8.

456. Suzuki S, Kawai K, Ohashi S, Mukai H *et al.* Reduced insulinotropic effects of gluca-gonlike peptide I-(7–36)-amide and gastric inhibitory polypeptide in isolated perfused diabetic rat pancreas. *Diabetes* 1990; **39**: 1320–25.

457. Jia X, Elliott R, Kwok YN, Pederson RA, McIntosh CH. Altered glucose dependence of glucagon-like peptide I (7–36)-induced insulin secretion from the Zucker (fa/fa) rat pancreas. *Diabetes* 1995; **44**: 495–500.

458. Drucker DJ. Glucagon-like peptide 2. *J Clin Endocrinol Metab* 2001; **86**: 1759–64.

459. Fischer KD, Dhanvantari S, Drucker DJ, Brubaker PL. Intestinal growth is associated with elevated levels of glucagon-like peptide 2 in diabetic rats. *Am J Physiol* 1997; **36**: E815–20.

460. Brubaker PL, Izzo A, Hill M, Drucker DJ. Intestinal function in mice with small bowel growth induced by glucagon-like peptide-2. *Am J Physiol* 1997; **35**: E1050–58.

461. Shibata C, Naito H, Jin XL *et al.* Effect of glucagon, glicentin, glucagon-like peptide-1 and -2 on interdigestive gastroduodenal motility in dogs with a vagally denervated gastric pouch. *Scand J Gastroenterol* 2001; **36**: 1049–55.

462. Wojdemann M, Wettergren A, Hartmann B, Holst JJ. Glucagon-like peptide-2 inhibits centrally induced antral motility in pigs. *Scand J Gastroenterol* 1998; **33**: 828–32.

463. Bozkurt A, Naslund E, Hellstrom PM. GLP-1 and GLP-2 act in synergy to inhibit fasting small bowel motility in the rat. Program and Abstracts, Digestive Diseases Week, May 21–24, 2000, San Diego, CA, 2000 A–630.

464. Tang-Christensen M, Larsen PJ, Thulesen J, Nielsen JR, Vrang N. [Glucagon-like pep-tide 2, a neurotransmitter with a newly discovered role in the regulation of food ingestion]. *Ugeskr Laeger* 2001; **163**: 287–91.

465. Barragan JM, Rodriguez RE, Blazquez E. Changes in arterial blood pressure and heart rate induced by glucagon-like peptide-1 (7–36) amide in rats. *Am J Physiol* 1994; **266**: E459–66.

466. Benito E, Blazquez E, Bosch MA. Glucagon-like peptide-1 (7–36)amide increases pulmonary surfactant secretion through a cyclic adenosine $3', 5'$-monophosphate-dependent protein kinase mechanism in rat type II pneumocytes. *Endocrinology* 1998; **139**: 2363–8.

467. Brubaker PL, Efendic S, Greenberg GR. Truncated and full-length glucagon-like peptide-1 (GLP-1) differentially stimulate intestinal somatostatin release. *Endocrine* 1997; **6**: 91–5.

468. Miki H, Namba M, Nishimura T *et al.* Glucagon-like peptide-1 (7–36) amide enhances insulin-stimulated glucose uptake and decreases intracellular cAMP content in isolated rat adipocytes. *Biochim Biophys Acta* 1996; **1312**: 132–6.

469. Schepp W, Dehne K, Riedel T, Schmidtler J *et al.* Oxyntomodulin: a cAMP-dependent stimulus of rat parietal cell function via the receptor for glucagon-like peptide-1 (7–36) NH$_2$. *Digestion* 1996; **57**: 398–405.

470. Schmidt WE, Siegel EG, Creutzfeldt W. Glucagon-like peptide-1 but not glucagon-like peptide-2 stimulates insulin release from isolated rat pancreatic islets. *Diabetologia* 1985; **28**: 704–7.

471. Flatt PR, Bailey CJ, Kwasowski P, Swanston-Flatt SK, Marks V. Abnormalities of GIP in spontaneous syndromes of obesity and diabetes in mice. *Diabetes* 1983; **32**: 433–5.

472. Schulz TB, Jorde R, Burhol PG. Fasting portal vein plasma levels of gastric inhibitory polypeptide (GIP) and extractable fasting GIP in the duodenal wall in rats treated with methylprednisolone or alloxan compared with normal controls. *Scand J Gastroenterol* 1982; **17**: 487–90.

473. Bailey CJ, Flatt PR, Kwasowski P, Adams M. Gastric inhibitory polypeptide and the entero-insular axis in streptozotocin diabetic mice. *Diabet Metab* 1986; **12**: 351–4.

474. Spannagel AW, Green GM, Guan D, Liddle RA et al. Purification and characterization of a luminal cholecystokinin-releasing factor from rat intestinal secretion. *Proc Natl Acad Sci USA* 1996; **93**: 4415–20.

475. Chandrasekar B, Korc M. Alteration of cholecystokinin-mediated phosphatidylinositol hydrolysis in pancreatic acini from insulin-deficient rats. Evidence for defective G protein activation. *Diabetes* 1991; **40**: 1282–91.

476. Takiguchi S, Takata Y, Funakoshi A et al. Disrupted cholecystokinin type-A receptor (CCKAR) gene in OLETF rats. *Gene* 1997; **197**: 169–75.

477. Miyasaka K, Kanai S, Ohta M, Kawanami T et al. Lack of satiety effect of cholecystokinin (CCK) in a new rat model not expressing the CCK-A receptor gene. *Neurosci Lett* 1994; **180**: 143–6.

478. Moran TH, Katz LF, Plata-Salaman CR, Schwartz GJ. Disordered food intake and obesity in rats lacking cholecystokinin A receptors. *Am J Physiol* 1998; **274**: R618–25.

479. Funakoshi A, Miyasaka K, Kanai S et al. Pancreatic endocrine dysfunction in rats not expressing the cholecystokinin-A receptor. *Pancreas* 1996; **12**: 230–36.

480. Jimi A, Kojiro M, Miyasaka K, Kono A, Funakoshi A. Apoptosis in the pancreas of genetically diabetic rats with a disrupted cholecystokinin (CCK-A) receptor gene. *Pancreas* 1997; **14**: 109–12.

481. Parmar NS, Tariq M, Ageel AM. Proglumide, a cholecystokinin receptor antagonist, exacerbates alloxan-induced diabetes mellitus in Swiss mice. *J Pharm Pharmacol* 1987; **39**: 1028–30.

482. El-Salhy M, Zachrisson S, Spangeus A. Abnormalities of small intestinal endocrine cells in non-obese diabetic mice. *J Diabetes Complications* 1998; **12**: 215–23.

483. El-Salhy M, Spangeus A. Neuropeptide contents in the duodenum of non-obese diabetic mice. *Acta Diabetol* 1998; **35**: 9–12.

484. Flatt PR, Bailey CJ, Conlon JM. Somatostatin, gastrin-releasing peptide and gastrin in the stomach of rats with streptozotocin-induced diabetes and insulinoma. *J Nutr* 1991; **121**: 1414–17.

485. Haraguchi Y, Sakamoto A, Yoshida T, Tanaka K. Plasma GRP-like immunoreactivity in healthy and diseased subjects. *Gastroenterol Jpn* 1988; **23**: 247–50.

486. Tallroth G, Ryding E, Ekman R, Agardh CD. The response of regulatory peptides to moderate hypoglycaemia of short duration in type 1 (insulin-dependent) diabetes mellitus and in normal man. *Diabetes Res* 1992; **20**: 73–85.

487. Ballmann M, Conlon JM. Changes in the somatostatin, substance P and vasoactive intestinal polypeptide content of the gastrointestinal tract following streptozotocin-induced diabetes in the rat. *Diabetologia* 1985; **28**: 355–8.

488. Kazumi T, Utsumi M, Yoshino G et al. Somatostatin concentration responds to arginine in portal plasma: effects of fasting, streptozotocin diabetes, and insulin administration in diabetic rats. *Diabetes* 1980; **29**: 71–3.

489. Nwokolo CU, Debnam ES, Booth JD et al. Neuroendocrine changes in rat stomach during experimental diabetes mellitus. *Dig Dis Sci* 1992; **37**: 751–6.

490. Patel YC, Wheatley T, Zingg HH. Increased blood somatostatin concentration in streptozotocin diabetic rats. *Life Sci* 1980; **27**: 1563–70.

491. Tomita T, Sasaki S, Doull V, Bunag R, Kimmel JR. Pancreatic hormones in streptozotocin-diabetic rats. *Int J Pancreatol* 1986; **1**: 265–78.

492. Chiba T, Kadowaki S, Taminato T et al. Concentration and secretion of gastric somatostatin in streptozotocin-diabetic rats. *Diabetes* 1981; **30**: 188–91.

493. Karakida T, Sakai M, Ito S, Yamada Y, Homma S. Changes of substance P and somatostatin contents in the gastrointestinal tract of streptozotocin diabetic rats. *Neurosci Lett* 1991; **129**: 173–6.

494. Lee W, Wakasugi H, Ibayashi H. Comparison of somatostatin distribution in pancreatic duct ligated rats and streptozotocin diabetic rats. *Gastroenterol Jpn* 1983; **18**: 453–8.

495. Deville de Periere D, Hillaire-Buys D, Gross R, Puech R, Arancibia S. Increases in concentrations of somatostatin- and insulin-like immunoreactivities in submandibular salivary gland of diabetic rats: effect of insulin treatment. *Acta Endocrinol (Copenh)* 1989; **120**: 790–94.

496. Kadowaki S, Taminato T, Chiba T *et al.* Somatostatin release from the isolated, perfused diabetic rat pancreas: inverse relationship between pancreatic somatostatin and insulin. *Diabetes* 1980; **29**: 960–63.

497. Kazumi T, Utsumi M, Yoshino G *et al.* Increase of pancreatic somatostatin concentration in early phases of streptozotocin diabetes in rats. *Endocrinol Jpn* 1980; **27**: 23–6.

498. Makino H, Kanatsuka A, Matsushima Y, Yamamoto M, Kumagai A. Effect of streptozotocin administration on somatostatin content of pancreas and hypothalamus in rats. *Endocrinol Jpn* 1977; **24**: 295–9.

499. Patel YC, Cameron DP, Bankier A *et al.* Changes in somatostatin concentration in pancreas and other tissues of streptozotocin diabetic rats. *Endocrinology* 1978; **103**: 917–23.

500. Tabata M, Shima K, Tanaka R *et al.* Changes in somatostatin release from perfused pancreas of streptozotocin-induced diabetic rats. *Endocrinol Jpn* 1981; **28**: 101–9.

501. Schauder P, McIntosh C, Herberg L *et al.* Increased somatostatin secretion from pancreatic islets of streptozotocin-diabetic rats in response to glucose. *Mol Cell Endocrinol* 1980; **20**: 243–50.

502. Zerbib A, Ribes G, Gross R, Puech R, Loubatieres-Mariani MM. Hypersensitivity to arginine of both B and D pancreatic cells in adult streptozotocin-diabetic rats. *Acta Endocrinol (Copenh)* 1989; **121**: 345–9.

503. Trimble ER, Gerber PP, Renold AE. Abnormalities of pancreatic somatostatin secretion corrected by *in vivo* insulin treatment of streptozotocin-diabetic rats. *Diabetes* 1981; **30**: 865–7.

504. Patel YC, Wheatley T, Malaisse-Lagae F, Orci L. Elevated portal and peripheral blood concentration of immunoreactive somatostatin in spontaneously diabetic (BBL) Wistar rats: suppression with insulin. *Diabetes* 1980; **29**: 757–61.

505. Chiba T, Taminato T, Kadowaki S *et al.* Reversal of increased gastric somatostatin in streptozotocin-diabetic rats by whole pancreas transplantation. *Diabetes* 1981; **30**: 724–7.

506. Seno M, Tsuda K, Kitano N *et al.* Degradation and conversion of somatostatin in normal and diabetic rats *in vivo* and *in vitro*. *Can J Physiol Pharmacol* 1988; **66**: 55–60.

507. Papaccio G, Mezzogiorno V. Morphological aspects of glucagon and somatostatin islet cells in diabetic Bio-Breeding and low-dose streptozocin-treated Wistar rats. *Pancreas* 1989; **4**: 289–94.

508. Verhaeghe J, Peeters TL, Vandeputte M, Rombauts W *et al.* Maternal and fetal endocrine pancreas in the spontaneously diabetic BB rat. *Biol Neonate* 1989; **55**: 298–308.

509. Patel YC, Ruggere D, Malaisse-Lagae F, Orci L. Alterations in somatostatin and other islet cell functions in the spontaneously diabetic BB Wistar rat: biochemical and morphological characterization. *Metabolism* 1983; **32**: 18–25.

510. Seemayer TA, Colle E, Tannenbaum GS, Oligny LL *et al.* Spontaneous diabetes mellitus syndrome in the rat. III. Pancreatic alterations in aglycosuric and untreated diabetic BB Wistar-derived rats. *Metabolism* 1983; **32**: 26–32.

511. Pederson RA, Curtis SB, Chisholm CB, Gaba NR *et al*. Insulin secretion and islet endocrine cell content at onset and during the early stages of diabetes in the BB rat: effect of the level of glycemic control. *Can J Physiol Pharmacol* 1991; **69**: 1230–36.

512. Boden G, Naji A, Barker CF, June V, Matschinsky FM. Effect of spontaneous diabetes on hormone release in BB/Phi rats: comparison between the isolated perfused pancreas/stomach/duodenum/spleen and the isolated perfused pancreas. *Endocrinology* 1983; **112**: 1777–81.

513. Kurose T, Tsuda K, Ishida H *et al*. Glucagon, insulin and somatostatin secretion in response to sympathetic neural activation in streptozotocin-induced diabetic rats. A study with the isolated perfused rat pancreas *in vitro*. *Diabetologia* 1992; **35**: 1035–41.

514. Srikant CB, Patel YC. Somatostatin receptors on rat pancreatic acinar cells. Pharmacological and structural characterization and demonstration of downregulation in streptozotocin diabetes. *J Biol Chem* 1986; **261**: 7690–96.

515. Curtis SB, Buchan AM, Pederson RA, Brown JC. Insulin response of cultured islets from diabetic and non-diabetic BB rats. *Metabolism* 1992; **41**: 1047–52.

516. Spangeus A, Kand M, El-Salhy M. Gastrointestinal endocrine cells in an animal model for human type 2 diabetes. *Dig Dis Sci* 1999; **44**: 979–85.

517. El-Salhy M. Neuroendocrine peptides of the gastrointestinal tract of an animal model of human type 2 diabetes mellitus. *Acta Diabetol* 1998; **35**: 194–98.

518. El-Salhy M. Neuroendocrine peptides in stomach and colon of an animal model for human diabetes type I. *J Diabetes Complications* 1999; **13**: 170–73.

519. Allen JM, Fitzpatrick ML, Yeats JC, Darcy K *et al*. Effects of peptide YY and neuropeptide Y on gastric emptying in man. *Digestion* 1984; **30**: 255–62.

520. Savage AP, Adrian TE, Carolan G, Chatterjee VK, Bloom SR. Effects of peptide YY (PYY) on mouth to caecum intestinal transit time and on the rate of gastric emptying in healthy volunteers. *Gut* 1987; **28**: 166–70.

521. Pappas TN, Debas HT, Chang AM, Taylor IL. Peptide YY release by fatty acids is sufficient to inhibit gastric emptying in dogs. *Gastroenterology* 1986; **91**: 1386–9.

522. Hanefeld M, Fischer S, Schulze J *et al*. Therapeutic potentials of acarbose as first-line drug in NIDDM insufficiently treated with diet alone. *Diabetes Care* 1991; **14**: 732–7.

523. Young AA, Gedulin B, Srivastava V, Jodka C, Nikoulina S. Peptide YY(3–36) inhibits gastric emptying via a neuroendocrine pathway that includes the *area postrema*. *Diabetes* 2002 (submitted).

524. Wettergren A, Petersen H, Orskov C, Christiansen J *et al*. Glucagon-like peptide-1 7–36 amide and peptide YY from the L-cell of the ileal mucosa are potent inhibitors of vagally induced gastric acid secretion in man. *Scand J Gastroenterol* 1994; **29**: 501–5.

525. Layer P, Holst JJ, Grandt D, Goebell H. Ileal release of glucagon-like peptide-1 (GLP-1). Association with inhibition of gastric acid secretion in humans. *Dig Dis Sci* 1995; **40**: 1074–82.

526. Fung LC, Chisholm C, Greenberg GR. Glucagon-like peptide-1-(7–36) amide and peptide YY mediate intraduodenal fat-induced inhibition of acid secretion in dogs. *Endocrinology* 1998; **139**: 189–94.

527. Hoentjen F, Hopman WP, Maas MI, Jansen JB. Role of circulating peptide YY in the inhibition of gastric acid secretion by dietary fat in humans. *Scand J Gastroenterol* 2000; **35**: 166–71.

528. Adrian TE, Savage AP, Sagor GR *et al*. Effect of peptide YY on gastric, pancreatic, and biliary function in humans. *Gastroenterology* 1985; **89**: 494–9.

529. Greeley GH Jr, Guo YS, Gomez G, Lluis F *et al*. Inhibition of gastric acid secretion by peptide YY is independent of gastric somatostatin release in the rat. *Proc Soc Exp Biol Med* 1988; **189**: 325–8.

530. Pironi L, Stanghellini V, Miglioli M *et al.* Fat-induced ileal brake in humans: a dose-dependent phenomenon correlated to the plasma levels of peptide YY. *Gastroenterology* 1993; **105**: 733–9.

531. Clave P, Lluis F, Thompson JC, Greeley GH Jr. Peptide YY inhibits gastric acid secretion stimulated by the autonomic nervous system. *Biol Signals* 1992; **1**: 40–45.

532. Nikoulina S, Gedulin B, Smith P, Young A. Effect of PYY(3–36) on gastric acid secretion and gastroprotection in rats. American Diabetes Association 62nd Annual Meeting and Scientific Sessions, San Francisco, CA, (submitted).

533. Sheikh SP. Neuropeptide Y and peptide YY: major modulators of gastrointestinal blood flow and function. *Am J Physiol* 1991; **261**: G701–15.

534. Adrian TE, Sagor GR, Savage AP, Bacarese-Hamilton AJ *et al.* Peptide YY kinetics and effects on blood pressure and circulating pancreatic and gastrointestinal hormones and metabolites in man. *J Clin Endocrinol Metab* 1986; **63**: 803–7.

535. Szecowka J, Tatemoto K, Rajamaki G, Efendic S. Effects of PYY and PP on endocrine pancreas. *Acta Physiol Scand* 1983; **119**: 123–6.

3

Oesophageal Function

André J. P. M. Smout

Introduction

In comparison with other parts of the gastrointestinal tract, the human oesophagus is a relatively simple organ with relatively simple functions. Despite this simplicity, disordered oesophageal function is not uncommon. It can be anticipated that the prevalence of disordered oesophageal function is higher in patients with diabetes mellitus, since autonomic neuropathy as well as hyperglycaemia have been shown to impair gastrointestinal function. In this chapter the available information on disordered oesophageal functions (abnormal motility and transit, reflux and abnormal perception) are reviewed. First, normal oesophageal functions and the techniques to study these are summarised. The prevalence and

Gastrointestinal Function in Diabetes Mellitus. Edited by Michael Horowitz and Melvin Samsom
© 2004 John Wiley & Sons, Ltd   ISBN: 0-471-89916-X

pathophysiology of disordered function is then reviewed. Thereafter, clinical manifestations, diagnosis and treatment are discussed.

Normal oesophageal function and methods of investigation

Oesophageal motor function

The human oesophagus is a muscular tube that connects the pharyngeal cavity to the stomach. At its proximal end there is a 2–3 cm long sphincter composed of striated muscle (upper oesophageal sphincter; UOS); at its distal end there is a 3–4 cm long sphincter composed of smooth muscle (lower oesophageal sphincter; LOS). The most important functions of the human oesophagus and its sphincters are to propel swallowed food boluses to the stomach and to prevent gastro-oesophageal and oesophagopharyngeal reflux. The former function is accomplished by swallow-induced peristalsis in the oesophageal body and timely opening of the UOS and LOS, the latter by high-pressure zones at the oesophagogastric and oesophagopharyngeal junctions. Oesophageal motor functions can be evaluated by a number of techniques.

Radiographic techniques allow an assessment of the movements of the pharyngeal and UOS muscles during swallowing, to visualise the peristaltic activity in the oesophageal body and oesophageal emptying. Substantial disadvantages are the requirements for exposure to relatively high levels of irradiation and the difficulties in quantifying the phenomena observed.

Scintigraphic measurement of oesophageal transit of radioactively labelled solid or liquid boluses allows accurate and quantitative assessment of oesophageal transit at acceptable radiation exposure levels. However, this technique is not widely used and has not been standardised.

The most frequently used technique for investigation of oesophageal contractile activity and LOS function is *manometry*. This technique is available in many centres and has been standardised to a great extent. Manometry can also be used to study the function of the UOS, but this necessitates expertise that is not available in most clinical laboratories.

Oesophageal manometry is usually performed with perfused catheters. A minimum of three recording orifices is required for assessment of peristalsis, but many laboratories now use catheters with 6 or more channels, often with side holes spaced at 3 cm or 5 cm intervals. A low-compliance perfusion system [1] should be used in order to be able to record oesophageal pressures with adequate fidelity. Alternatively, oesophageal manometry can be performed using a catheter that includes miniature 'solid-state' pressure transducers. The fragility of these catheters and their high price limit their widespread application in routine diagnostic tests.

Both types of manometry (perfused and non-perfused) suffer from the disadvantage that considerable axial displacement of the pressure sensors may occur

as a result of respiratory movements and swallowing. For this reason it is not feasible to position a single side hole in the LOS for prolonged periods of time. To
overcome this problem, a manometric catheter equipped with a perfused 5–6 cm
long membrane, the so-called Dent sleeve, has been developed [2]. The sleeve
device measures the highest pressure exerted at any point of its length, thus
allowing continuous measurement of LOS pressure despite axial movements.

Following a swallow, the human oesophagus exhibits a circular contraction
that is propagated in an aboral direction. This phenomenon is called primary
peristalsis (Figure 3.1, left panel). The propagation velocity is 2 cm/s in the
proximal part and 3 cm/s in the distal part of the oesophageal body. The amplitude of the peristaltic wave recorded is 30–120 mmHg in the proximal part
and 50–180 mmHg in the distal part. In healthy subjects more than 80% of the
contractions following a 'wet' swallow (5 ml water) are propagated. Up to 20%
of the pressure waves recorded after a wet swallow are simultaneous or do not
propagate from the UOS to the LOS; the latter phenomenon is categorised as
incomplete peristalsis [3]. Occasionally a wet swallow is not followed by any
motor response in the oesophageal body (so-called 'failed peristalsis').

When the oesophagus is distended by a food bolus that was not cleared
by primary peristalsis or an episode of gastro-oesophageal reflux, secondary
peristaltic waves may occur in the absence of swallowing. The term 'tertiary
peristalsis' is sometimes used to denote spontaneous, i.e. not swallow-induced,
simultaneous, contractile activity. Manometrically, the LOS is a high-pressure
zone. When a manometric catheter without a sleeve sensor is used, this zone
can be identified by withdrawing the catheter in a stepwise, or continuous,
fashion from the stomach into the oesophagus. The normal LOS pressure is
7.5–20 mmHg; this decreases to a value equal or close to intragastric pressure

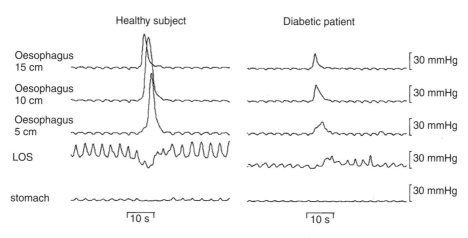

Figure 3.1 Disordered oesophageal peristalsis, as measured with intraluminal manometry,
in a patient with diabetes and severe autonomic neuropathy (right), in comparison with
normal peristalsis in a healthy subject (left)

with swallowing. The competence of the antireflux barrier is now recognised to be dependent on the crural diaphragm surrounding the LOS, as well as the LOS.

The LOS relaxes not only following a swallow, but also spontaneously. In healthy subjects these so-called 'transient LOS relaxations' (TLOSRs) occur at a rate of 1–5 per hour [4]. Their duration is longer than that of the swallow-associated relaxations. Distension of the proximal stomach is the most important stimulus for induction of TLOSR [5]. TLOSRs constitute the major mechanism responsible for gastro-oesophageal reflux in health and in the majority of patients with gastro-oesophageal reflux disease [6].

The process of oesophageal peristalsis and relaxation of UOS and LOS is neuronally controlled. A swallowing centre in the brain stem signals to the dorsal motor nucleus of the vagus nerve. Most of the afferent information required for oesophageal peristalsis is relayed through vagal fibres.

Oesophageal sensory function

An additional function of the oesophagus is perception. Most of the efferent information from the oesophagus uses vagal pathways. Whereas the passage of liquid and solid food boluses through the oesophagus, and even acid gastro-oesophageal reflux, are usually not perceived, the likelihood of perception is greater under pathological circumstances, e.g. when transit of food through the oesophagus is impaired, the hold-up may give rise to the sensation of dysphagia; when excessive gastro-oesophageal reflux has led to oesophagitis, acid reflux usually causes the sensation of heartburn. However, the relationship between oesophageal perception and stimulation is highly variable, e.g. patients with severe oesophagitis may deny any oesophageal symptom, while others with an endoscopically normal oesophagus may suffer from severe reflux symptoms.

The sensitivity of the oesophagus can be tested by applying mechanical (usually balloon distension), electrical (using electrodes mounted on a catheter) or chemical (infusion of hydrochloric acid) stimuli. The latter stimulus was used widely in the past, as a test for gastro-oesophageal reflux disease (Bernstein test) [7].

In recent years attempts were made to measure a physiological (objective) signal in addition to the sensation score (subjective) reported by the patient. The technique of evoked potential recording measures the cerebral potentials that are generated in response to electrical or mechanical stimulation of the oesophagus. These potentials are recorded from electrodes placed on the scalp. Repeated stimulation and an averaging technique are required to distinguish the response to the stimulus from the background electrical activity. The typical oesophageal evoked potential is multiphasic, with peak latencies of 100–500 ms [8]. It has been shown that the amplitude of the evoked potential correlates with the intensity of the oesophageal sensation (usually retrosternal pain).

Prevalence of abnormal oesophageal function in diabetes

The earliest reports on abnormal oesophageal function in diabetes date from the late 1960s. In 1967, using cineradiographic techniques, Mandelstam and Lieber observed in diabetics with evidence of neuropathy reduced or absent primary peristaltic waves, an increased prevalence of tertiary contractions and delayed oesophageal emptying [9]. Some years later, manometric evidence of a reduced amplitude of both pharyngeal and oesophageal contractions and a reduced LOS pressure in diabetics was reported by the same group [10].

While it is clear that oesophageal dysfunction occurs frequently in diabetes mellitus, there is considerable variation in the reported prevalence between different studies.

Oesophageal transit

Numerous studies have shown that oesophageal transit, as measured with radionuclide techniques, is slower in patients with diabetes than in age- and sex-matched healthy controls [11–29] oesophageal transit appears to be delayed in 40–60% of patients with long-standing diabetes (Figure 3.2, Table 3.1). The relationship between oesophageal transit and the rate of gastric emptying appears to be poor [26].

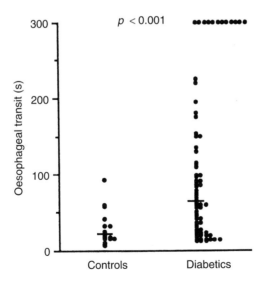

Figure 3.2 Oesophageal transit of a radioactively labelled solid bolus in 25 healthy subjects (controls) and 87 diabetic patients (67 type 1, 20 type 2). The horizontal lines represent median values. From Horowitz *et al.* [14], with permission

Table 3.1   Prevalence of delayed oesophageal transit in patients with diabetes

Authors [ref.]	Year	Type	n	Prevalence %	CVAN-related
Channer et al. [24]	1985	1	34	56	+
Westin et al. [18]	1986	1	40	33	?
Vannini et al. [19]	1989	1	29	45	+
Horowitz et al. [14]	1990	1 + 2	87	48	+
Tsai et al. [29]	1995	2	15	93	?
Annese et al. [23]	1999	2	35	46	−

CVAN, cardiovascular autonomic neuropathy.

Contractile activity of the oesophageal body

Although information relating to the prevalence of manometric abnormalities of the oesophagus is limited, the available data indicate that these are evident in approximately 50% of patients with diabetes [11,14,17,23,24,30] (Table 3.2).

A variety of oesophageal motor abnormalities has been demonstrated in patients with diabetes mellitus (Table 3.3). These include a decreased amplitude [10,11,30,31] and number [30,32,33] of peristaltic contractions (Figure 3.1), and an increased incidence of simultaneous [12,17,34] and non-propagated [10] contractions, as well as abnormal wave forms [17,30,32]. The latter include repetitive and multipeaked contractions [32]. An increased incidence of spontaneous, i.e. non-swallow-related, contractions was observed in one study [30]. Interestingly, an increased amplitude of peristaltic contractions has also been observed in patients with diabetes mellitus [30,31].

A recent study, combining oesophageal manometry and radionuclide measurement of oesophageal transit has shown that retarded oesophageal transit

Table 3.2   Prevalence of abnormal oesophageal motility in patients with diabetes, as studied with manometry

Authors [ref.]	Year	Type	n	Prevalence %	CVAN-related
Oesophageal body					
Vela and Balart [38]	1970	?	25	96	?
Stewart et al. [34]	1976	1+2	26	62	+
Murray et al. [11]	1987	?	20	35	+
Keshavarzian et al. [17]	1987	?	15	80	?
Sundkvist et al. [21]	1989	?	13	55	?
Annese et al. [23]	1999	2	35	48	−
Lower oesophageal sphincter					
Vela and Balart [38]	1970	?	25	92	?
Murray et al. [11]	1987	?	20	15	?

CVAN, cardiovascular autonomic neuropathy.

Table 3.3 Types of oesophageal motor abnormalities in patients with diabetes, as studied with manometry

Oesophageal body
Decreased peristaltic amplitude [11,10,30,31]
Decreased incidence of peristaltic contractions [30,32,33,34]
Increased peristaltic amplitude [17,31]
Increased incidence of simultaneous pressure waves [12,17,34]
Increased incidence of non-transmitted pressure waves [10]
Abnormal wave forms [17,30,32]
Lower oesophageal sphincter
Decreased LOS pressure [10,11,34,38,39]

usually reflects either peristaltic failure or focal low-amplitude waves and that the level of the bolus hold-up coincides with the level of peristaltic failure [35].

In the only published study relating to upper oesophageal function in diabetes, radiological evidence of disordered pharyngeal function was found in 14 of 18 patients (78%) with swallowing complaints [36].

Gastro-oesophageal reflux and LOS function

The available information indicates that the prevalence of gastro-oesophageal reflux disease is higher in diabetes. Murray and co-workers studied 20 diabetic patients (14 type 1, six type 2), of whom nine (45%) were found to have excessive gastro-oesophageal acid reflux, as assessed by 24 h oesophageal pH monitoring [5].

In a larger study of 50 type 1 diabetic patients without symptoms or history of gastro-oesophageal disease, abnormal gastro-oesophageal reflux, defined as a percentage of time with esophageal pH < 4 exceeding 3.5%, was detected in 14 patients (28%) [37].

In accordance with the increased prevalence of gastro-oesophageal reflux disease in diabetes, the LOS has been found to be hypotensive in diabetics [10,11,34,38,39]. In only one study was no significant difference in LOS pressure between diabetes and health observed [11]. The prevalence of LOS hypotension in diabetes is difficult to estimate, since the two studies that reported on the prevalence of this abnormality yielded highly discrepant results (Table 3.2). The impact of diabetes mellitus on the incidence of transient LOS relaxations appears not to have been reported.

Whereas gastro-oesophageal reflux, as measured by pH monitoring, is more prevalent in diabetics than in controls, there is no evidence that oesophagitis is more common in diabetics than in those without the disease. Formal studies of the prevalence of oesophagitis in diabetics appear not to have been carried out.

Oesophageal perception

There is little information about the perception of oesophageal stimuli in patients with diabetes. Rathmann and co-workers used the cortical evoked potential recording technique in a study of 10 patients with type 1 diabetes using electrical stimulation of the oesophagus (32 cm from the incisors) at an intensity just above the perception threshold. All control subjects exhibited regular evoked potentials, whereas in six of the 10 diabetic patients there was no evoked potential and in these patients the perception thresholds were significantly elevated [40]. In the four patients in whom the perception threshold was normal, evoked potentials of normal configuration, but decreased amplitude were recorded.

Somewhat contrasting findings were made in another evoked potential study. Two patients with type 1 diabetes and evidence of autonomic neuropathy were studied using cortical evoked responses following oesophageal balloon and electrical stimulation [41]. Both patients had symptomatic gastroparesis and abnormal gastroduodenal motility. In both patients normal evoked potential responses were recorded, even though one patient could not feel the electrical stimulation. The evoked potential peaks occurred after an abnormally long latency [42]. The authors concluded that afferent vagal pathways are affected in severe diabetes [42]. Kamath and colleagues applied electrical stimuli to the oesophagus in six diabetic patients and 14 control subjects. In addition to cortical evoked potentials, they also measured heart rate variability. Whereas reproducible evoked potentials were recorded in all healthy subjects, in all patients the response to electrical stimulation of the oesophagus was erratic and non-reproducible [43]. However, during electrical stimulation there was a similar decrease in the ratio of the low-frequency to the high-frequency component in the heart rate power spectra in the diabetic patients compound to the healthy volunteers, indicative of increased efferent vagal output to the heart. The authors interpreted their observations as suggestive of an intact subcortical reflex circuitry in patients with diabetes [43]. However, this conclusion may not be correct if the vagal centres and vagal efferent fibres that innervate the heart are not affected by diabetic neuropathy to the same extent as the vagal centres and pathways involved in oesophageal motility and perception.

The evoked potential studies summarized above suggest that, in patients with diabetes, there is an impaired perception of oesophageal stimuli as a consequence of visceral afferent neuropathy. Despite this, there is an increased overall prevalence of oesophageal symptoms in diabetics. This suggests that an even higher prevalence of oesophageal symptoms would be found if impaired perception were not present.

Pathophysiology

Our understanding of the pathophysiology of disordered oesophageal function in diabetes is still far from complete. Since the reported manometric abnormalities are indicative of disorganisation of contractile patterns, rather than abnormal smooth muscle *per se*, it is generally assumed that the contractile apparatus of the oesophagus is normal in diabetes and that disordered oesophageal function reflects neuronal abnormalities [30,32].

Autonomic neuropathy is considered to play a pivotal role in the pathophysiology but, as will be discussed, the available information suggests that oesophageal dysfunction is not closely related to autonomic neuropathy.

Autonomic neuropathy

Abnormal oesophageal motility in diabetes has been traditionally attributed to autonomic neuropathy [10–12,14,30,34,44]. If so, the question arises as to whether neuropathic changes in the intramural oesophageal plexuses, the extrinsic neuronal pathways or in the motor centres in the central nervous system are primarily at fault. There is indirect evidence that the myenteric plexuses of the oesophagus and lower oesophageal sphincter are not severely affected in diabetes.

Stewart and co-workers observed that 2.5 mg bethanechol given subcutaneously to 29 diabetics, with and without evidence of autonomic neuropathy, increased lower oesophageal pressure more than in controls, but the final pressures were comparable in the two groups [34]. In contrast, in achalasia and Chagas' disease, which are characterized by degeneration of post-ganglionic nerves of the myenteric plexus, there is a pronounced hypersensitivity to cholinergic agents such as bethanechol. Thus, the absence of an exaggerated oesophageal motor response to cholinergic drugs supports the concept that the myenteric plexus is normal in patients with diabetes.

In a study focusing on the phenomenon of multipeaked peristaltic waves in diabetics with autonomic neuropathy, the pharmacological responses to edrophonium and atropine were found to suggest a possible increased cholinergic tone as the basis of this abnormality [32].

In contrast, there is unequivocal evidence of damage to the extrinsic nerve supply to the oesophagus in diabetes mellitus. The results of examination of the oesophagus in 20 patients who died from diabetes disclosed histologic abnormalities in 18 of them [45], particularly demyelination in the vagus and Schwann cell loss in the parasympathetic fibres arising from the oesophagus [46].

Zhao and co-workers investigated the occurrence of IgG or IgM deposits in the microvasculature of certain organs of diabetics, using routine autopsy materials [47]. In the oesophagus and/or tongue of diabetics, IgG was frequently deposited in the microvasculature. In total, IgG deposits were found in 13 of 16 diabetics, in either the oesophagus or the tongue, but in only 3 of 16 controls. These observations suggest that deposition of immunoglobulins is a component of diabetic microangiopathy, but its relationship to autonomic neuropathy remains speculative [47].

Several studies have shown that abnormal oesophageal motility is more frequent in diabetic patients who have evidence of peripheral or autonomic neuropathy than in those without [11–14,17,19,20,24,25,48,49]. In one of the largest studies that focused on the relationship between neuropathy and disordered oesophageal function, 50 consecutive insulin-requiring diabetics were stratified into three groups: (a) patients without peripheral neuropathy ($n = 18$); (b) patients with peripheral neuropathy but no autonomic neuropathy ($n = 20$); and (c) patients with both peripheral and autonomic neuropathy ($n = 12$). Radionuclide oesophageal emptying was found to be abnormal in 55%, 70% and 83% of patients in groups A, B and C, respectively [17].

An association between gastro-oesophageal reflux and the severity of autonomic neuropathy could not be demonstrated in one study [11]. In another study, the presence of abnormal gastro-oesophageal reflux in diabetic patients was associated with autonomic neuropathy. Pathological reflux was present in 38.7% of diabetic patients with abnormal cardiovascular tests, whereas only 10.5% of diabetic patients without signs of autonomic neuropathy had pathological reflux [50].

It must be emphasised, however, that although several studies have provided evidence for the existence of a relationship between disordered oesophageal function and diabetic autonomic neuropathy, this relationship is relatively weak [13,14,17,27,37,49]. By no means can evaluation of autonomic function be used to predict the presence or absence of abnormal oesophageal motility.

It should be noted that in all of the studies on this subject the evidence for the presence of autonomic neuropathy was derived from cardiovascular reflex tests, usually based on the criteria described by Ewing and Clarke [51]. It is conceivable that there is not a close concordance between the extent and severity of autonomic neuropathy in the gastrointestinal tract and the severity of cardiovascular neuropathy. A practical and validated test for gastrointestinal autonomic neuropathy in humans has not yet been described (Chapter 9).

Glycaemic control

Several studies have shown that the gastrointestinal motor responses to various stimuli are impaired during acute hyperglycaemia in both healthy subjects and diabetic patients [52–54]. The potential effect of hyperglycaemia on oesophageal function has only recently received attention.

De Boer and co-workers investigated the effect of acute hyperglycaemia on oesophageal motility and LOS pressure in seven healthy volunteers, during euglycaemia and during hyperglycaemia [55]. At 90 min, motility was stimulated with edrophonium chloride (0.08 mg/kg intravenously). Plasma levels of pancreatic polypeptide (PP) were used as an indirect measure of vagal cholinergic tone. During hyperglycaemia the LOS pressure decreased significantly from 20.1 ± 1.6 to 10.7 ± 0.6 mmHg. As expected, plasma PP levels were also significantly decreased during hyperglycaemia. Edrophonium increased LOS pressure and PP levels in both experiments. However, after edrophonium stimulation, LOS pressure and PP levels remained significantly reduced during hyperglycaemia compared with euglycaemia. During hyperglycaemia an increase in peristaltic wave duration and a decrease in peristaltic velocity were observed in the distal part of the oesophagus. It was concluded that acute hyperglycaemia reduces LOS pressure and impairs oesophageal motility under both basal and edrophonium-stimulated conditions, suggesting impaired vagal cholinergic activity during hyperglycaemia.

Hyperglycaemia may also affect the perception of sensations arising from the oesophagus, as well as other regions of the gut. Rayner and colleagues examined the effects of hyperglycaemia on cortical potentials evoked by oesophageal distension in 16 healthy volunteers [56]. A series of 50 distensions was performed at both a lower volume (producing definite sensation) and a higher volume (producing unpleasant sensation), at blood glucose concentrations of 5 and 13 mmol/l, while cortical potentials were recorded from a scalp electrode. During euglycaemia, peak amplitudes were greater at the higher than at the lower balloon volume. At the lower balloon volume, the peak amplitudes were greater during hyperglycaemia than euglycaemia, while there was no effect of the blood glucose concentration on evoked potential amplitude at the higher balloon volume. The observed increase in amplitude of the cortical response to moderate oesophageal distension during hyperglycaemia suggests that either afferent signal conduction or central processing of afferent information from the oesophagus is enhanced during hyperglycaemia.

Psychological factors

There is little information about the relationships between psychological factors and oesophageal function in diabetes. In a study in 30 patients with type 1 or type 2 diabetes mellitus, oesophageal motor abnormalities, neuropathy and psychiatric illness were independently determined [25]. Fifteen patients (50%) were found to have oesophageal contraction abnormalities. The prevalence of depression, dysthymia or generalized anxiety disorder was substantially greater in those with contraction abnormalities (87%) when compared to 21% in patients with normal manometric patterns. Log-linear analysis confirmed that this association was independent of neuropathy effects [25]. Thus, it appears that some of the oesophageal neuromuscular dysfunction observed in diabetics may be associated with psychiatric disorders. This observation seems to provide an additional explanation for the discrepant relationship of motility disturbances to neuropathy noted in prior reports [25].

Clinical manifestations

In contrast to the relatively simple function of the oesophagus, the symptoms of oesophageal dysfunction are surprisingly diverse. The most common symptom is heartburn, defined as a short-lived burning sensation behind the sternum or in the epigastric region. Heartburn is rather specific for gastro-oesophageal reflux, but its sensitivity as an indicator of this disease is low. Occasionally, heartburn is reported by patients who do not have any reflux, such as in achalasia, suggesting that some patients perceive abnormal oesophageal motility as heartburn. Another common symptom of gastro-oesophageal reflux disease is regurgitation, and the combination of heartburn and regurgitation of acid material is highly specific for reflux disease. Belching is a non-specific oesophageal symptom. It may occur in reflux disease, in aerophagia and with gastric motor disorders. The most characteristic symptom of impaired oesophageal transit is dysphagia. It should be recognised that dysphagia is caused more often by mechanical obstruction (tumour, peptic stenosis) than by disordered motility of the oesophageal body or LOS. The site of the hold-up of the food passage that the patient perceives is notoriously imprecise, e.g. patients with achalasia may point to the upper end of sternum when indicating the site of delayed transit in the distal oesophagus. Dysphagia (i.e. oesophageal dysphagia) must be distinguished from swallowing problems (oropharyngeal dysphagia). The latter is a symptom of obstructive or motor disorders of the pharynx or UES. Chest pain, retrosternally located in the midline, can be a symptom of reflux and of an oesophageal motor disorder. The pain may be indistinguishable from that in angina pectoris or myocardial infarction and may radiate to the jaws, shoulders and arms.

There is considerable disagreement in the literature as to the prevalence of symptoms of oesophageal dysfunction in diabetes mellitus. Some publications indicate that patients with diabetes mellitus usually do not complain about oesophageal symptoms, even when severe oesophageal dysfunction is present. For example, in a manometric and radiographic study of 14 diabetics with manifestations of gastroenteropathy, 12 of whom had abnormal oesophageal motility, only three had symptoms referable to the oesophagus [9,10]. In another series, only six of 50 patients with type 1 diabetes and one of 31 type 2 diabetics complained of dysphagia. In yet another study, none of the 40 type 1 diabetics reported oesophageal symptoms. However, in other studies a high prevalence of oesophageal symptoms in diabetics has been documented. For example, 27% of 137 unselected diabetics attending an outpatient clinic admitted to having dysphagia when specifically asked for [44]. Russell *et al.* reported

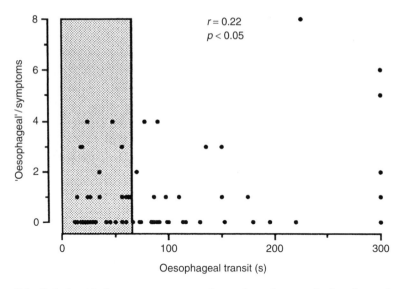

Figure 3.3   Relationship between symptoms of oesophageal motor dysfunction and oesophageal transit of a solid bolus in the same 87 randomly selected diabetics as in Figure 3.2. Courtesy of M. Horowitz

that dysphagia occurred in 42% of a cohort of insulin-dependent diabetics who had other gastrointestinal symptoms, such as nausea, vomiting and diarrhoea, which were assumed to reflect diabetic gastroenteropathy [12]. In a study of 30 patients with type 1 or type 2 diabetes mellitus, Clouse and co-workers found oesophageal symptoms such as dysphagia and heartburn in 12 [31]. In yet another study, heartburn was reported in 40 of 50 unselected patients with diabetes mellitus [30].

Several studies have addressed the relationship between delayed oesophageal transit, abnormal oesophageal motility and oesophageal symptoms (Figure 3.3). In these studies this relationship was usually found to be poor [14,30,31,37,57,58]. The poor association between oesophageal dysfunction and symptoms in patients with diabetes may reflect impaired perception of oesophageal stimuli caused by neuropathic abnormalities in afferent pathways. The development of symptoms and signs of gastro-oesophageal reflux disease in diabetics may in part be counteracted by a decrease in gastric acid secretion [59].

Diagnostic testing

Given the fact that oesophageal dysfunction is common in diabetes, and that the predictive value of oesophageal symptoms in these patients is rather poor, one may argue that oesophageal function tests should be carried out in all patients with diabetes. However, the treatment of oesophageal motor disorders is usually not very successful and treatment of asymptomatic patients is often not indicated.

Therefore, routine testing for oesophageal motor disorders in diabetics without symptoms thereof cannot be recommended. However, when oesophageal motility tests are considered, e.g. in a patient with oesophageal symptoms, endoscopy should always be carried out first to exclude organic abnormalities, particularly obstruction (tumour, peptic stenosis) and oesophageal candidiasis. The latter occurs more frequently in diabetics than in the general population and treatment with fungicidal agents usually results in rapid symptom relief.

The discussion about routine testing is more complex in the case of gastro-oesophageal reflux disease. As discussed, oesophageal acid exposure is increased in about 40% of diabetics and it is known that the absence of reflux symptoms does not exclude the presence of severe oesophagitis and/or Barrett's metaplasia. Due to impaired oesophageal perception, the proportion of asymptomatic patients with reflux disease may be higher in the presence of diabetes than when diabetes is absent. It might, therefore, be argued that a screening upper gastrointestinal endoscopy should be performed in diabetic patients, even when no oesophageal or gastric symptoms are reported. However, more cost-effective and realistic approach may be to perform endoscopy in diabetics with other risk factors for reflux disease, in particular severe obesity.

The tests of oesophageal function that combine sufficient specificity and sensitivity and clinical applicability are oesophageal manometry, 24 hour pH-monitoring and measurement of oesophageal transit by means of radiographic or scintigraphic techniques.

The question has arisen to what extent oesophageal motor abnormalities can be used as a marker of gastrointestinal involvement in diabetes. A possible answer to this question is provided by a study of Keshavarzian and Iber [60]. They evaluated the frequency, extent and clinical significance of gastrointestinal complications in 75 consecutive, male, insulin-requiring diabetics (46 with neuropathy); 19% of the 75 patients and 30% of those with neuropathy had one or more GI symptoms. Oesophageal, gastric, gall bladder and small intestinal functions were studied in 30 patients using radionuclide oesophageal and gastric emptying, postprandial gallbladder emptying, and intestinal transit of lactulose. The patients were divided into three groups: 10 patients without neuropathy; 10 patients with peripheral neuropathy; and 10 patients with autonomic and peripheral neuropathy; 25 patients (83%) had abnormalities of at least one gastrointestinal organ, and 57% had abnormalities of two. In 19 of the 25 patients (76%) with gastrointestinal involvement and eight of nine (89%) symptomatic diabetics, oesophageal emptying was delayed. There was a higher prevalence of retinopathy, neuropathy and autonomic dysfunction in symptomatic when compared to asymptomatic diabetics, who also had more widespread and more severe gastrointestinal involvement than asymptomatic diabetics. Therefore, the results of this study indicate that, in diabetics, delayed oesophageal transit, especially in symptomatic diabetics, could serve as a marker of more widespread gastrointestinal involvement.

Treatment

Since upper gastrointestinal symptoms correlate poorly with objective abnormalities of gastrointestinal motor function in diabetes, the symptomatic benefit that could be expected from correction of these motor abnormalities is questionable. Only a few studies have investigated the effect of drug treatment on impaired oesophageal function in diabetes mellitus.

Domperidone did not increase oesophageal emptying of a solid bolus in 12 insulin-dependent diabetic patients after either acute or chronic administration [16]. In a study in 20 type 1 diabetics, a single dose of cisapride (20 mg) increased oesophageal emptying as well as both solid and liquid gastric emptying. The response to cisapride was most marked in patients with the greatest delay in oesophageal emptying. However, after administration of cisapride for 4 weeks, gastric emptying of solid and liquid meal components was still accelerated, but oesophageal emptying was not significantly different from placebo [61].

De Caestecker and co-workers studied 19 diabetic patients with autonomic neuropathy in a double-blind cross-over study of cisapride, metoclopramide and placebo [62]. Symptoms were evaluated from diary cards and from assessments undertaken at the end of each 8 week treatment period. Measurements of oesophageal transit, gastric emptying and whole gut transit were made before treatment began and at the end of each treatment period. Three patients dropped out early in the study, and the results from 16 patients were analysed. The severity of autonomic neuropathy, as assessed by cardiovascular reflex tests, correlated with delayed oesophageal transit and prolonged gastric emptying, but abnormal oesophageal transit and gastric emptying were often unrelated to the presence of upper gastrointestinal symptoms. Neither cisapride nor metoclopramide had a significant effect on oesophageal transit, gastric emptying or whole-gut transit, nor was any significant effect on symptoms identified.

Recently, cisapride has been withdrawn from the market in many countries because of reports of cardiac arrhythmias caused by prolongation of the Q–T interval (discussed further in Chapter 4). These restrictions obviously limit the use of cisapride for gastrointestinal manifestations of diabetes.

A recent study from Taiwan suggests that a 2 week oral treatment with erythromycin might be beneficial in non-insulin-dependent patients with delayed oesophageal transit. A significant reduction of mean oesophageal transit time was found [29]. In addition, the rates of gastric emptying and fasting blood glucose levels were improved. However, the study was not placebo-controlled and an order effect cannot be excluded, rendering the conclusions drawn by the authors insufficiently well-founded.

In a study by Fabiani and co-workers, the influence of tolrestat, an aldosereductase inhibitor, on both oesophageal and gallbladder motility was investigated in 66 type 2 diabetic patients with asymptomatic diabetic neuropathy [63].

The patients were randomly assigned to receive tolrestat 200 mg once daily (33 patients) or were left without specific treatment (33 patients) for 12 months. Efficacy and safety evaluation were done at 4.5 and 12 months by persons blinded to the patient's treatment regimen. Scintigraphic evaluation of oesophageal motility showed significant changes in transit time for tolrestat at 12 months. In addition, the vibration perception threshold at two sites of the dominant leg improved in the tolrestat group and remained unchanged or slightly deteriorated in the control group. Tendon reflexes and blood pressure fall after standing were also improved in the tolrestat group. Thus, the authors concluded that one year's treatment with tolrestat significantly improves oesophageal motility and vibration perception in type 2 diabetic patients with asymptomatic diabetic neuropathy [63]. Tolrestat can cause hepatic necrosis and is not available for clinical use.

Prognosis

Little or nothing is known about the prognosis of disordered oesophageal function in diabetes. Long-term follow-up studies are lacking. However, there is evidence that disordered oesophageal function in a diabetic patient is not indicative of a particularly poor prognosis. In a recent study, 86 patients (66 type 1, 20 type 2) were followed up who, between 1984 and 1989, underwent assessment of oesophageal transit (by scintigraphy), gastrointestinal symptoms (by questionnaire), autonomic nerve function (by cardiovascular reflex tests) and glycaemic control (by HbAlc and blood glucose concentrations during gastric emptying measurement) [64]. At follow-up in 1998, 62 patients were known to be alive, 21 had died, and three were lost to follow-up. In the group who had died, the duration of diabetes had been longer, the score for autonomic neuropathy higher and oesophageal transit slower than in those patients who were still alive. After adjustment for the effects of other factors that showed a relationship with the risk of dying, there was no significant relationship between either gastric emptying or oesophageal transit and death. In this relatively large cohort of outpatients with diabetes, there was no evidence that delayed oesophageal transit or gastroparesis was associated with a poor prognosis.

Summary

Disordered oesophageal function clearly is more common in diabetics than in healthy control subjects. Delayed oesophageal transit caused by ineffective oesophageal peristalsis and increased gastro-oesophageal reflux can be found in at least 30% of the patients. The chance of abnormal oesophageal function increases with increasing severity of autonomic neuropathy, but the correlation is not particularly strong. There is no solid evidence for the existence of a correlation between the presence of oesophageal dysfunction and the type of diabetes.

It is unclear whether the prevalence of oesophageal symptoms in patients with diabetes parallels that of abnormal oesophageal function. In clinical practice, oesophageal motor disorders should probably not be actively searched when the patient has no oesophageal symptoms, but upper gastrointestinal endoscopy should be carried out more liberally in diabetics than in non-diabetic patients.

References

1. Arndorfer RC, Stef JJ, Dodds WJ, Linehan JH, Hogan WJ. Improved infusion system for intraluminal esophageal manometry. *Gastroenterology* 1977; **73**: 23–7.
2. Dent J, Chir B. A new technique for continuous sphincter pressure measurement. *Gastroenterology* 1976; **71**: 263–7.
3. Spechler SJ, Castell DO. Classification of oesophageal motility abnormalities. *Gut* 2001; **49**: 145–51.
4. Mittal RK, McCallum RW. Characteristics and frequency of transient relaxations of the lower esophageal sphincter in patients with reflux esophagitis. *Gastroenterology* 1988; **95**: 593–9.
5. Holloway RH, Kocyan P, Dent J. Provocation of transient lower esophageal sphincter relaxations by meals in patients with symptomatic gastroesophageal reflux. *Dig Dis Sci* 1991; **36**: 1034–9.
6. Dent J, Holloway RH, Toouli J, Dodds WJ. Mechanisms of lower oesophageal sphincter incompetence in patients with symptomatic gastrooesophageal reflux. *Gut* 1988; **29**: 1020–28.
7. Bernstein LM, Baker L. A clinical test for esophagitis. *Gastroenterology* 1958; **34**: 760–81.
8. Smout AJPM, DeVore MS, Castell DO. Cerebral potentials evoked by esophageal distension in humans. *Am J Physiol* 1990; **259**: G955–9.
9. Mandelstam P, Lieber A. Esophageal dysfunction in diabetic neuropathy gastroenteropathy—clinical and roentgenological manifestations. *J Am Med Assoc* 1967; **210**: 582–6.
10. Mandelstam P, Siegel CI, Lieber A, Siegel M. The swallowing disorder in patients with diabetic neuropathy–gastroenteropathy. *Gastroenterology* 1969; **56**: 1–12.
11. Murray FE, Lombard MG, Ashe J *et al.* Esophageal function in diabetes mellitus with special reference to acid studies and relationship to peripheral neuropathy. *Am J Gastroenterol* 1987; **82**: 840–43.
12. Russell RO, Gannan R, Coatsworth J *et al.* Relationship among esophageal dysfunction, diabetic gastroenteropathy and peripheral neuropathy. *Dig Dis Sci* 1983; **28**: 289–93.
13. Steffey DL, Wahl RL, Shapiro B. Diabetic oesophagoparesis: assessment by solid phase radionuclide scintigraphy. *Nucl Med Commun* 1986; **7**: 165–71.
14. Horowitz M, Maddox AF, Wishart JM, Harding PE *et al.* Relationships between oesophageal transit and solid and liquid gastric emptying in diabetes mellitus. *Eur J Nucl Med* 1991; **18**: 229–34.
15. Channer KS, Jackson PC, O'Brien I *et al.* Oesophageal function in diabetes mellitus and its association with autonomic neuropathy. *Diabet Med* 1985; **2**: 378–82.
16. Maddern GJ, Horowitz M, Jamieson GG. The effect of domperidone on oesophageal emptying in diabetic autonomic neuropathy. *Br J Clin Pharmacol* 1985; **19**: 441–4.
17. Keshavarzian A, Iber FL, Nasrallah S. Radionuclide oesophageal emptying and manometric studies in diabetes mellitus. *Am J Gastroenterol* 1987; **82**: 625–31.
18. Westin L, Lilja B, Sundkvist G. Oesophagus scintigraphy in patients with diabetes mellitus. *Scand J Gastroenterol* 1986; **21**: 1200–1204.

19. Vannini P, Ciavarella A, Corbelli C *et al*. Oesophageal transit time and cardiovascular autonomic neuropathy in type 1 (insulin-dependent) diabetes mellitus. *Diabetes Res* 1989; **11**: 21–5.

20. Horowitz M, Harding PE, Maddox A *et al*. Gastric and oesophageal emptying in insulin-dependent diabetes mellitus. *J Gastroenterol Hepatol* 1986; **1**: 97–113.

21. Sundkvist G, Hilarp B, Lilja B, Ekberg O. Esophageal motor function evaluated by scintigraphy, video-radiography and manometry in diabetic patients. *Acta Radiol* 1989; **30**: 17–19.

22. Jermendy G, Fornet B, Koltai MZ *et al*. Correlation between oesophageal motility and cardiovascular autonomic dysfunction in diabetic patients without gastrointestinal symptoms of autonomic neuropathy. *Diabetes Res* 1991; **16**: 193–7.

23. Annese V, Bassotti G, Caruso N *et al*. Gastrointestinal motor dysfunction, symptoms, and neuropathy in non-insulin-dependent (type 2) diabetes mellitus. *J Clin Gastroenterol* 1999; **29**: 171–7.

24. Channer KS, Jackson PC, O'Brien I *et al*. Oesophageal function in diabetes mellitus and its association with autonomic neuropathy. *Diabet Med* 1985; **2**: 378–82.

25. Clouse RE, Lustman PJ, Reidel WL. Correlation of esophageal motility abnormalities with neuropsychiatric status in diabetics. *Gastroenterology* 1986; **90**: 1146–54.

26. Horowitz M, Maddox AF, Wishart JM, Harding PE, *et al*. Relationships between oesophageal transit and solid and liquid gastric emptying in diabetes mellitus. *Eur J Nucl Med* 1991; **18**: 229–34.

27. Jermendy G, Fornet B, Koltai MZ, Pogatsa G. Correlation between oesophageal dysmotility and cardiovascular autonomic dysfunction in diabetic patients without gastrointestinal symptoms of autonomic neuropathy. *Diabetes Res* 1991; **16**: 193–7.

28. Karayalcin B, Karayalcin U, Aburano T *et al*. Esophageal clearance scintigraphy in diabetic patients—a preliminary study. *Ann Nucl Med* 1992; **6**: 89–93.

29. Kao CH, Wang SJ, Pang DY. Effects of oral erythromycin on upper gastrointestinal motility in patients with non-insulin-dependent diabetes mellitus. *Nucl Med Commun* 1995; **16**: 790–93.

30. Hollis JB, Castell DO, Braddom RL. Esophageal function in diabetes mellitus and its relation to peripheral neuropathy. *Gastroenterology* 1977; **73**: 1098–1102.

31. Clouse RE, Lustman PJ, Reidel WL. Correlation of oesophageal motility abnormalities with neuropsychiatric status in diabetes. *Gastroenterology* 1986; **90**: 1146–54.

32. Loo FD, Dodds WJ, Soergel KH *et al*. Multipeaked oesophageal peristaltic pressure waves in patients with diabetic neuropathy. *Gastroenterology* 1985; **88**: 485–91.

33. Silber W. Diabetes and oesophageal dysfunction. *Br Med J* 1969; **3**: 688–90.

34. Stewart IM, Hosking DJ, Preston BJ, Atkinson M. Oesophageal motor changes in diabetes mellitus. *Thorax* 1976; **31**: 278–83.

35. Holloway RH, Tippett MD, Horowitz M, Maddox AF *et al*. Relationship between esophageal motility and transit in patients with type I diabetes mellitus. *Am J Gastroenterol* 1999; **94**: 3150–57.

36. Borgstrom PS, Olsson R, Sundkvist G, Ekberg O. Pharyngeal and oesophageal function in patients with diabetes mellitus and swallowing complaints. *Br J Radiol* 1988; **61**: 817–21.

37. Horowitz M, Harding PE, Maddox AF *et al*. Gastric and oesophageal emptying in patients with type 2 (non-insulin-dependent) diabetes mellitus. *Diabetologia* 1989; **32**: 151–9.

38. Vela AR, Balart LA. Esophageal motor manifestations in diabetes mellitus. *Am J Surg* 1970; **119**: 21–6.

39. Horgan JH, Doyle JS. A comparative study of oesophageal motility in diabetics with neuropathy. *Chest* 1971; **60**: 170–74.

40. Rathmann W, Enck P, Frieling T, Gries FA. Visceral afferent neuropathy in diabetic gastroparesis. *Diabetes Care* 1991; **14**: 1086–9.

41. Tougas G, Hunt RH, Fitzpatrick D, Upton AR. Evidence of impaired afferent vagal function in patients with diabetic gastroparesis. *Pacing Clin Electrophysiol* 1992; **15**: 1597–602.

42. Rydberg L, Ruth M, Lundell L. Does oesophageal motor function improve with time after successful antireflux surgery? Results of a prospective, randomised clinical study. *Gut* 1997; **41**: 82–6.

43. Kamath MV, Tougas G, Fitzpatrick D *et al*. Assessment of the visceral afferent and autonomic pathways in response to esophageal stimulation in control subjects and in patients with diabetes. *Clin Invest Med* 1998; **21**: 100–113.

44. Feldman M, Schiller LR. Disorders of gastrointestinal motility associated with diabetes mellitus. *Ann Intern Med* 1983; **98**: 378–84.

45. Smith B. Neuropathology of the oesophagus in diabetes mellitus. *J Neurol Neurosurg Psychol* 1974; **37**: 1151–54.

46. Kristensson K, Nordborg C, Olsson Y *et al*. Changes in the vagus nerve in diabetes mellitus. *Acta Pathol Microbiol Scand* 1971; **79**: 684–5.

47. Zhao JB, Mikata A, Azuma K. Immunoglobulin deposits in diabetic microangiopathy. Observations in autopsy materials. *Acta Pathol Jpn* 1990; **40**: 729–734.

48. Horowitz M, Harding PE, Maddox AF *et al*. Gastric and oesophageal emptying in patients with type 2 (non-insulin-dependent) diabetes mellitus. *Diabetologia* 1989; **32**: 151–9.

49. Frusciante V, Modoni S, Bonazza A *et al*. Scintigraphic oesophageal clearance in diabetics: clinical usefulness. *Nucl Med Commun* 1988; **9**: 955–64.

50. Lluch I, Ascaso JF, Mora F *et al*. Gastroesophageal reflux in diabetes mellitus. *Am J Gastroenterol* 1999; **94**: 919–24.

51. Ewing DJ, Clarke BF. Diagnosis and management of diabetic autonomic neuropathy. *Br Med J* 1982; **285**: 916–8.

52. Bjornsson ES, Urbanavicius V, Eliasson B, Attvall S *et al*. Effects of hyperglycemia on interdigestive gastrointestinal motility in humans. *Scand J Gastroenterol* 1994; **29**: 1096–104.

53. Hebbard GS, Samsom M, Sun WM, Dent J, Horowitz M. Hyperglycemia affects proximal gastric motor and sensory function during small intestinal triglyceride infusion. *Am J Physiol* 1996; **271**: G814–19.

54. Fraser R, Horowitz M, Dent J. Hyperglycaemia stimulates pyloric motility in normal subjects. *Gut* 1991; **32**: 475–8.

55. De Boer SY, Masclee AA, Lam WF, Lamers CB. Effect of acute hyperglycemia on esophageal motility and lower esophageal sphincter pressure in humans. *Gastroenterology* 1992; **103**: 775–80.

56. Rayner CK, Smout AJPM, Sun WM *et al*. Effects of hyperglycemia on cortical response to esophageal distension in normal subjects. *Dig Dis Sci* 1999; **44**: 279–85.

57. Grishaw EK, Ott DJ, Frederick MG, Gelfand DW, Chen MY. Functional abnormalities of the esophagus: a prospective analysis of radiographic findings relative to age and symptoms. *Am J Roentgenol* 2000; **1996**: 719–23.

58. Huppe D, Tegenthoff M, Faig J *et al*. Esophageal dysfunction in diabetes mellitus: is there a relation to clinical manifestation of neuropathy? *Clin Invest* 1992; **70**: 740–47.

59. Hosking DJ, Moody F, Stewart IM, Atkinson M. Vagal impairment of gastric secretion in diabetic autonomic neuropathy. *Br Med J* 1975; **2**: 588–93.

60. Keshavarzian A, Iber FL. Gastrointestinal involvement in insulin-requiring diabetes mellitus. *J Clin Gastroenterol* 1987; **9**: 685–92.

61. Horowitz M, Harding PE, Maddox AF *et al*. Effect of cisapride on gastric and oesophageal emptying in insulin-dependent diabetes mellitus. *Gastroenterology* 1987; **92**: 1899–907.

62. De Caestecker JS, Ewing DJ, Tothill P, Clarke BF, Heading RC. Evaluation of oral cisapride and metoclopramide in diabetic autonomic neuropathy: an eight-week double-blind crossover study. *Aliment Pharmacol Ther* 1989; **3**: 69–81.

63. Fabiani F, De Vincentis N, Staffilano A. Effect of Tolrestat on oesophageal transit time and cholecystic motility in type 2 diabetic patients with asymptomatic diabetic neuropathy. *Diabetes Metab* 1995; **21**: 360–64.

64. Kong MF, Horowitz M, Jones KL, Wishart JM, Harding PE. Natural history of diabetic gastroparesis. *Diabetes Care* 1999; **22**: 503–7.

4

Gastric Function

Michael Horowitz, Karen L. Jones, Louis M. A. Akkermans and Melvin Samsom

Introduction
Gastric motility in diabetes
Management of gastroparesis associated with gastrointestinal symptoms
Gastric secretion in diabetes
Gastric blood supply in diabetes
Acknowledgements
References

Introduction

The focus of this chapter relates to the effects of diabetes on gastric motor function. Abnormally delayed gastric emptying, or gastroparesis, was once considered to be a rare sequela of diabetes mellitus, occurring occasionally in patients who had long-standing diabetes complicated by symptomatic autonomic neuropathy, and inevitably associated with both intractable upper gastrointestinal symptoms and a poor prognosis [1]. Consequent upon the development of a number of techniques to quantify gastric motility, particularly radioisotopic measurement of gastric emptying, and the rapid expansion of knowledge relating to both normal and disordered gastric motor function in humans over the last ~ 20 years, it is now recognised that these concepts are incorrect.

The functions of the stomach are, of course, not limited to the storage and processing of food. Diabetes may be associated with impaired gastric mucosal function, potentially resulting in abnormal gastric acid secretion and gastritis,

Gastrointestinal Function in Diabetes Mellitus. Edited by Michael Horowitz and Melvin Samsom
© 2004 John Wiley & Sons, Ltd ISBN: 0-471-89916-X

although this subject has received substantially less attention, and is of lesser clinical relevance, than disordered gastric motility.

For convenience, gastric motor and mucosal function in diabetes are dealt with separately; for completeness there is also a brief discussion of the potential effects of diabetes on the vascular supply to the stomach.

Gastric motility in diabetes

Delayed gastric emptying represents a frequent, and clinically important, complication of diabetes mellitus.

Prevalence

I believe that this syndrome gastroparesis diabeticorum ... is more frequently overlooked than diagnosed (Kassander, 1958).

Gastric motility in patients with diabetes mellitus has usually been quantified by measurement of gastric emptying. Delayed gastric emptying in diabetes was first reported by Boas in 1925 [2], with subsequent radiological studies by Ferroir in 1937 [3]. The latter noted: 'X-ray examination showed that in diabetics ... the stomach motor responses are weaker than normal: contractions are slow,

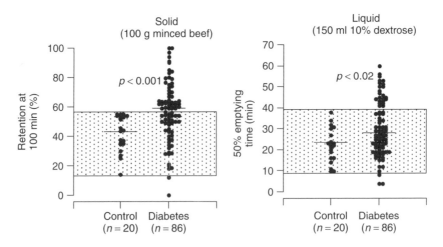

Figure 4.1 Gastric emptying of a mixed solid (100 g minced beef) and liquid (150 ml 10% dextrose) meal in 20 normal subjects and 86 unselected outpatients with diabetes (66 type 1, 20 type 2). For solid the amount remaining in the stomach at 100 min after completion of the meal, and for liquid the 50% gastric emptying time are shown. Gastric emptying of the minced beef is greater than the upper limit of the normal range in 57% of the patients and that of dextrose in 34%. Horizontal lines represent median values. From Jones *et al.* [31], with permission

lack vigour and die out quickly' [3,4]. Rundles and his colleagues, who in 1945 provided the first detailed description of the association between delayed gastric emptying and diabetes, reported that gastric emptying of barium was abnormally slow in five of 35 patients with clinical evidence of peripheral neuropathy [1,5]. In a seminal monograph, published in 1958, Kassander named the condition 'gastroparesis diabeticorum', referring to abnormal retention of liquid barium detected radiologically in asymptomatic patients [6].

Cross-sectional studies, in most cases using radionuclide techniques to measure gastric emptying, have established that gastric emptying of solid, or nutrient liquid, meals is abnormally slow in some 30–50% of outpatients with long-standing type 1 [7–20] or type 2 [20–26] diabetes (Figures 4.1 and 4.2). Early studies, using insensitive barium contrast techniques to quantify gastric emptying, clearly underestimated the prevalence substantially [1,27]. The reported prevalence of delayed gastric emptying is highest when gastric emptying of

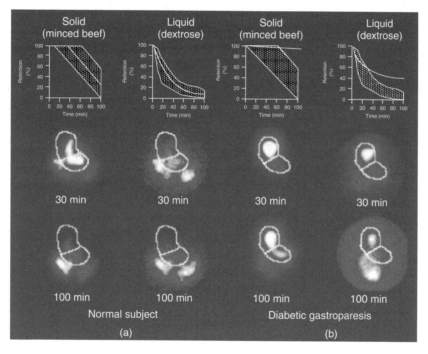

Figure 4.2 Gastric emptying curves, derived from the intragastric retention of isotope between 0 (time of meal completion) and 100 min, and scintigraphic images showing the abdominal distribution of radioactivity at 30 and 100 min following a meal of 100 g minced beef labelled with ^{99m}Tc sulphur colloid and 150 ml 10% dextrose labelled with ^{67}Ga-EDTA in (a) a healthy volunteer and (b) a patient with long-standing type 1 diabetes. The normal range for gastric emptying (mean ± 2 SD) is shown in the shaded areas. Scintigraphic images illustrate total, proximal and distal stomach regions of interest. There is a marked delay of solid and liquid emptying in the type 1 patient; the mean blood glucose concentration during the gastric emptying measurement was 11 mmol/l

both solid and nutrient-containing liquids (or semi-solids) are measured, either simultaneously or on separate occasions [17,28,29], as there is a relatively poor correlation between gastric emptying of solids and liquids in diabetes [28–30]. The latter may reflect differences in the gastroduodenal mechanisms which control gastric emptying of different meal components (to be discussed). While it has been suggested that evaluation of gastric emptying of solids may be more sensitive than that of liquids or semi-solids in the diagnosis of delayed gastric emptying in diabetes [30], this concept is based primarily on studies in which gastric emptying of low rather than high-nutrient liquids has been measured.

It should be recognised that in many cases the magnitude of the delay in gastric emptying of solids or liquids is relatively modest (i.e. gastric emptying rates are just outside the upper limit of a normal range) (Figure 4.1), and it can be argued that a distinction should be made between 'gastroparesis', as opposed to 'delayed gastric emptying'. This would imply that the diagnosis of gastroparesis should be restricted to those patients in whom emptying is grossly delayed [e.g. emptying rates outside mean ± 3 standard derivations (SD) of a control range]. It is self-evident that the diagnosis of 'gastroparesis' is also critically dependent on the definition of the 'normal range', for which there is a lack of consistency between studies, e.g. mean ± 2 SD [28,31], or mean ± 1.5 SD—in this chapter the term 'gastroparesis' should be inferred to indicate emptying rates which are $\geq$ mean ± 2 SD [32]. Not surprisingly, intragastric meal distribution is also frequently abnormal in outpatients with diabetes, with increased retention of food in both the proximal and distal stomach [31,33]. The former may potentially be important in the aetiology of gastro-oesophageal reflux [34], which appears to occur more frequently in patients with diabetes [35] (as discussed in Chapter 3). The prevalence of delayed gastric emptying in patients with 'brittle' type 1 diabetes is probably comparable to that which exists in patients with long-standing type 1 or type 2 diabetes [36]. It is now recognised that delayed gastric emptying also occurs frequently (perhaps about 30%) in children and adolescents with type 1 diabetes [37–39]. In contrast to some animal models of diabetes [40,41] (discussed in Chapter 2), gastric emptying is accelerated in only a minority ($\sim 5\%$) of patients with type 1 diabetes [9,13,28,42–45]. However, there is evidence, albeit inconsistent [46], that gastric emptying in patients with 'early' type 2 diabetes, particularly that of nutrient liquids, is not infrequently abnormally rapid [29,47–50]; it has been suggested that this may predispose to the development of type 2 diabetes by leading to higher postprandial blood glucose concentrations [47]. Further studies are required to explore this issue—in a study evaluating gastric emptying of a solid (pancake) meal in 'early' type 2 patients, differences from control subjects were modest [48]. No studies have evaluated the prevalence of disordered gastric emptying in patients with recently diagnosed type 1 diabetes, or in older people with type 2 diabetes. The prevalence of delayed emptying in ketoacidosis is also not known, although characteristic symptoms of nausea, abdominal discomfort and vomiting are often attributed to gastric stasis, and acute gastric dilatation is a recognised, albeit rare, complication [51]. Gastric emptying has hitherto not been evaluated in the rare cases where diabetes is a component of a mitochondrial disease, although pseudo-obstruction is a recognised complication of the so-called MELAS syndrome (myoencephalopathy, lactic acidosis, stroke-like episodes). In evaluating the information presented above, it should be recognised that there are no true population-based studies of gastric emptying in diabetes (this may prove feasible with the advent of carbon breath tests [12,19]), and no studies have been performed during euglycaemia (as will be discussed, the prevalence of delayed emptying is presumably less during euglycaemia than during hyperglycaemia). Moreover, there has hitherto only been one long-term, longitudinal study to evaluate the natural history of gastric emptying in diabetes [52]; in a cohort of 20 patients (16 type 1, four type 2) there was minimal change in gastric emptying of either solid (minced beef) or liquid (10% glucose) despite a deterioration in cardiovascular autonomic function, over a mean follow-up of about 12 years (Figure 4.3). While this suggests that gastric emptying is usually relatively stable over time, in this study there was a concomitant improvement in glycaemic control, presumably reflecting the increased therapeutic efforts directed at the normalisation of blood glucose levels in patients with diabetes subsequent to the DCCT [53] and UKPDS [54] studies. As will be discussed, the improvement in glycaemic control would favour faster gastric emptying and may 'balance' the deterioration in autonomic nerve function. Hence, additional studies are required to explore the associations of delayed gastric emptying with other diabetic complications and chronic glycaemic control.

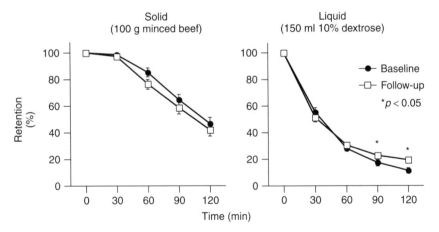

Figure 4.3   Gastric emptying of a mixed solid (100 g minced beef) and liquid (150 ml 10% dextrose) meal at baseline and follow-up (12.3 ± 0.7 years) in 20 outpatients with diabetes (16 type 1, four type 2). There is no change in gastric emptying of solid and a marginal slowing of liquid emptying at follow-up. Data are mean ± SEM. *$p < 0.05$ baseline vs. follow-up by ANOVA. From Jones *et al.* [52], with permission

Although it is recognised that disordered gastroduodenal contractile activity, as assessed by manometry, occurs frequently in diabetes [55,56], there have been no population-based studies. It is, however, reasonable to assume that the prevalence of abnormal motility will be even higher than that of disordered gastric emptying—in a series of 84 type 1 and type 2 patients referred for evaluation of upper gastrointestinal symptoms (such as nausea, vomiting and abdominal bloating), abnormal antral motility was evident in 83% [55].

Diabetic gastroparesis is often associated with motor dysfunction in other areas of the gut, e.g. oesophageal transit is delayed in some 50% of patients with long-standing diabetes [8]. However, there is a relatively poor relationship between transit in different regions [56], e.g. measurement of oesophageal transit cannot be used to predict the rate of gastric emptying.

Physiology of gastric emptying

Gastric emptying involves storage of ingested food, mixing with gastric secretions, grinding of solid food into particles 1–2 mm in diameter, and the regulated delivery of chyme into the small intestine at a rate designed to optimise digestion and absorption (Figure 4.4). Understanding of the mechanical factors by which the stomach moves its contents into the small intestine is still limited [57,58].

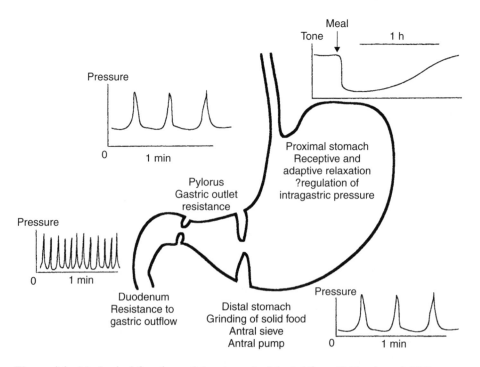

Figure 4.4   Mechanical functions of the stomach. Adapted from Hebbard *et al.* [57]

This situation reflects, at least in part, the technical difficulties associated with the investigation of human gastric motility; an optimal strategy to evaluate gastric mechanics dictates that a number of factors—gastric muscular contractions in different regions of the stomach and proximal small intestine, gastroduodenal pressure gradients and transpyloric flow—are measured, ideally simultaneously [58]. While most attention has focused on the frequency and amplitude of contractions, it is now recognised that the spatiotemporal organisation of muscular activity is an important determinant of the movement of luminal content; there are also fundamental differences in the mechanical impact of contractions which result in occlusion of the lumen, when compared to those that do not, on luminal flow [57].

Recent studies have confirmed observations, initially made by Cannon (1911) in animals, that transpyloric flow is predominantly pulsatile, rather than continuous. Thus, most liquefied chyme is propelled into the duodenum as a series of small gushes; the characteristics of individual flow pulses (both duration and volume) vary considerably, so that forward, interrupted and reverse flow may all occur [59,60]. A short episode of duodenogastric reflux often precedes pyloric closure [61]. Contrary to the previous suggestion that one motor region could exert the dominant role, patterns of transpyloric flow are dependent on the integration of motor activity in the proximal stomach, antrum, pylorus and proximal small intestine [58]. The stomach is capable of considerable compensation before the overall rate of emptying, as opposed to the characteristics of individual flow pulses, is modified substantially [59].

Gastric motility is controlled by a number of neural networks that are located in the gastric wall, prevertebral ganglia, spinal cord and brain. The stomach, like other parts of the gastrointestinal tract, is innervated by extrinsic nerves—the sympathetic and parasympathetic parts of the autonomic nervous system and sensory nerves that project to the spinal cord (splanchnic and sacral efferents) and brain stem (vagal efferents). Gastric motility is controlled predominantly by the vagus nerve—vagal efferents project to the nucleus tractus solitarius, where they form synapses with interneurones that project to the dorsal motor nucleus of the vagus and to higher brain centres. From the dorsal motor nucleus of the vagus there are efferent projections to the stomach, which modulate the activity of muscle cells through activation of either inhibitory or excitatory motor neurones. This circuit has been called a 'vago-vagal' reflex [62].

The enteric nervous system (ENS), also termed the 'brain of the gut' since it is able to function without input from the central nervous system, is located within the gastric wall and consists of the myenteric (or Auerbach) plexus, which is between the circular and longitudinal layers, and the submucosal (or Meissner) plexus, located beneath the mucosa. The enteric nervous system contains sensory neurones, interneurones and motor neurones which are closely integrated. The principal excitatory neurotransmitters are acetylcholine and substance P, and the major inhibitory neurotransmitters are vasoactive intestinal peptide and nitric oxide [57]. Thus, the enteric nervous system consists of local circuitries for the performance of integrative functions independent of extrinsic innervation.

The proximal region of the stomach is primarily concerned with storage of ingested food. During swallowing, there is a vagally-mediated, transient 'receptive' relaxation, which is followed by a more prolonged relaxation, known as 'accommodation', so that an increase in gastric volume is not usually associated with a substantial rise in intragastric pressure [63]. The accommodation response may be triggered by mechanoreceptors in both the proximal stomach and the antrum. The contractions of the distal stomach are controlled by electrical signals ('slow waves'), generated by a pacemaker region located on the greater curvature, which discharges at a rate of about 3/min [57]. The generation of slow waves within the gastric wall is dependent on the so-called interstitial cells of Cajal, which are interspersed in the circular and longitudinal muscle layers [64]. The interstitial cells of Cajal are also required for effective neurotransmission. Slow waves are continuous rhythmic changes in the membrane potential which, *per se*, do not initiate contractions, i.e. contractile activity of the distal stomach is always associated with gastric slow waves, but slow waves persist in the absence of gastric contractile activity. Accordingly, other neurohumoral factors determine whether a slow wave induces gastric contractile activity.

As first described by Code and Marlett in 1975 [65], fasting antral motility is cyclical and has been termed the 'migrating motor complex' (or MMC). The latter consists of three phases, which have a cycle time of about 100 min: phase 1, motor quiescence (about 40 min); phase 2, irregular contractions (about 50 min); and phase 3, regular, high-amplitude contractions at the maximal rate (i.e. the frequency of the gastric pacemaker) of 3/min for 5–10 min. During late phase 2 (and phase 3), indigestible residues, dead cells, secretions and bacteria are emptied from the stomach into the small intestine—not surprisingly, the MMC has been referred to as the 'gastrointestinal housekeeper' [65]. About 80% of phase 3 episodes originate in the antrum and the remainder in the small intestine. Recent studies indicate that large particles are sometimes emptied from the stomach without phase 3 activity.

Meal ingestion disrupts the MMC and causes distinct changes in gastric motility, characterised by initial relaxation and a subsequent increase in tonic activity of the proximal stomach, irregular contractile activity in the antrum and an increase in tonic and phasic pyloric pressures. Antral contractions play the major role in grinding digestible solid food into small particles, generally < 2 mm in size; ingestion of a solid meal induces strong antral contractions. Postprandial patterns of intraluminal pressure in the distal stomach are very complex [66]. While pyloric contractile activity is regulated by the gastric slow wave, the muscle of the pylorus is specialised and its control mechanisms differ from those of the antrum. Phasic and tonic pyloric contractions occur over a narrow zone (~ 2 mm), either in isolation or in temporal association with antral contractions, and probably play a major role in the regulation of gastric emptying by acting as a brake [58], i.e. transpyloric flow can only occur when the pylorus is open.

The mechanical determinants of individual transpyloric flow episodes are poorly defined. Flow could reflect a local increase in the antroduodenal pressure difference due to peristaltic antral contractions, or be associated with a 'common-cavity' pressure difference between the distal antrum and proximal duodenum during periods of relative antral quiescence [67]. Recent studies suggest that the latter mechanism (so-called 'pressure', as opposed to 'peristaltic', pump) may be of primary importance [67], so that substantial transpyloric flow may occur in the absence of antral peristalsis [68]. Duodenal contractions may potentially facilitate or retard gastric emptying; patterns of duodenal motility are complex, with substantial regional variations [69].

Overall patterns of gastric emptying are critically dependent on the physical and chemical composition of a meal, so that there are substantial differences between solids, semi-solids, nutrient liquids and non-nutrient liquids [70]. The emptying of digestible solids is characterised by an initial lag phase (usually 20–40 min in duration) before emptying commences, when solids are ground into small particles and redistributed from the proximal into the distal stomach [71], followed by an emptying phase that approximates a linear pattern, at least for the majority of emptying. After the lag phase the overall emptying rates of solid, semi-solid and high-nutrient liquid meals are comparable. In contrast, non-nutrient liquids empty from the stomach in a mono-exponential pattern; emptying is influenced by both posture and intragastric volume. The major factor regulating gastric emptying of nutrients (liquids and 'liquefied' solids) is feedback inhibition, triggered by receptors that are distributed throughout the small intestine [72]; as a result of this inhibition, nutrient-containing liquids usually empty from the stomach at an overall rate of about 2 kcal/min, after an initial emptying phase that may be somewhat faster [73]. These small intestinal receptors also respond to pH, osmolality and distension, as well as nutrient content. Triglycerides must be digested to fatty acids in order to slow emptying. The extent of small intestinal feedback is dependent on both the length and region of small intestine that has been exposed [72]. Small intestinal sensing probably involves both neural and hormonal mechanisms—the interaction of nutrients with the small intestine triggers the release of a number of hormones that may slow gastric emptying, including cholecystokinin, glucagon-like peptide-1, amylin and peptide YY. Caeco-ileal reflux of short-chain fatty acids may also potentially contribute to the regulation of gastric emptying [74].

A number of studies have evaluated the motor correlates of small intestinal feedback. Infusion of nutrients directly into the small intestine slows gastric emptying, and this is associated with suppression of antral pressure waves, the stimulation of pressure waves localised to the pylorus, and proximal stomach relaxation [63,70]. In general, provided that small intestinal feedback is intact, the elimination of individual motor components does not prevent the slowing of emptying by nutrients.

While the differential emptying rates of solids, nutrient and non-nutrient liquids when ingested alone is well established, there is much less information about the interaction between different meal components. When liquids and solids are consumed together, liquids empty preferentially ($\sim$80% before the solid starts to empty) (see Figure 4.3) and the presence of a solid meal results in an overall slowing of a simultaneously ingested liquid [71,75,76]. Therefore, while it is clear that the stomach can, to some extent, regulate the emptying of liquids and solids separately, the mechanisms by which this is accomplished remain poorly defined. Extracellular fat has a much lower density than water and is liquid at body temperature. The pattern of gastric emptying of fat, and its effects on emptying of other meal components are, therefore, dependent on posture—in the left lateral posture oil accumulates in the stomach and empties early, which markedly delays emptying of a nutrient liquid [77]. Gastric emptying is also influenced by patterns of previous nutrient intake. In healthy young and older subjects, supplementation of the diet with glucose is associated with acceleration of gastric emptying of glucose [78,79], while short-term starvation slows gastric emptying [80] presumably as a result of changes in the sensitivity of small intestinal receptors.

Pathophysiology of disordered gastric emptying in diabetes

The pathogenesis of disordered gastric emptying in diabetes is now recognised to be multifactorial; those factors which appear to be dominant, autonomic neuropathy and glycaemic control, are closely related, e.g. both acute [81] and chronic [82] changes in the blood glucose concentration may affect autonomic function.

Autonomic and enteric neuropathy

Putative similarities in the symptoms experienced by patients following surgical vagotomy and those with long-standing diabetes led to the initial assumption that disordered gastric motility in diabetes reflected irreversible vagal damage [1]. As there is a lack of tests to assess gastrointestinal autonomic function directly (discussed in Chapter 9), evaluation of cardiovascular autonomic function has usually been employed as a surrogate marker of the function of the abdominal vagus. It is well recognised that there is a high prevalence of cardiovascular autonomic neuropathy in diabetes which is, not infrequently, evident at the time of diagnosis [83]. While the prevalence of disordered gastric emptying/gastric motility is clearly higher in patients with cardiovascular autonomic neuropathy than in those without [12,16,28,61,84–86], the correlation between disordered motility and either abnormal cardiovascular autonomic function (parasympathetic or sympathetic) or peripheral nerve function is relatively weak [12,16–18,28,42,85]. This may be interpreted as evidence for selective autonomic impairment of the gastrointestinal tract [87]; however, it is more likely that other factors, such as hyperglycaemia, are important [88]. Moreover, as discussed, in a recent longitudinal study, progression in cardiovascular autonomic dysfunction was not associated with slowing of gastric emptying [52].

As discussed in Chapter 2, in animal models of diabetes a number of morphological changes are evident in the autonomic nerves supplying the gut and the myenteric plexus, including a reduction in the number of myelinated axons in the vagosympathetic trunk and neurons in the dorsal root ganglia, abnormalities in neurotransmitters (including metenkephalin, serotonin, substance P, neuropeptide-Y, vasoactive intestinal peptide and calcitonin gene-related peptide), as well as a reduced number of interstitial cells of Cajal in the fundus and antrum [89–92]. In contrast, there is hitherto little evidence of a fixed pathological process in the neural tissue of humans with diabetes; while two studies reported a reduction in the number of axons (myelinated and unmyelinated) in the vagus [93,94], the most comprehensive study, in which the myenteric plexus was evaluated by silver staining, showed no abnormalities [95]. Data relating to enteric innervation in human diabetes is even more limited. However, in a recent case report of a type 1 patient with gastroparesis, there was a marked decrease in the number of interstitial cells of Cajal in a jejunal biopsy taken at the time of performing a jejunostomy [96], consistent with observations in diabetic mice [90]. Nitric oxide (NO) is a key transmitter in the regulation of gastrointestinal motor function [97]. In some rodent models of diabetes (streptozotocin-induced and non-obese diabetic mice), there is a marked reduction in NO-synthase expression in gastric myenteric neurons [98] (Chapter 2), which is associated with delayed gastric emptying. The latter is normalised by administration of insulin or the cGMP-specific phosphodiesterase sildenafil, which acts as an NO donor [99]. Accordingly, in rodent models of diabetes abnormally slow gastric emptying may reflect reversible downregulation of neuronal nitric oxidase synthase (nNOS) expression. It has been suggested that this has implications for the treatment of diabetic gastroparesis in humans [99], particularly as there is evidence of a reduced number of nNOS neurons in human diabetic gastroparesis [96]. However, it should be recognised that the effects of NO on gastric emptying appear to differ between animals and humans, e.g. in healthy humans NO donors slow [100], while inhibition accelerates [101], gastric emptying. Hence, while formal studies are required, it may be anticipated that drugs such as sildenafil will slow, rather than accelerate, gastric emptying in patients with diabetes and potentially exacerbate gastroparesis. Further evaluation of the impact of diabetes mellitus on the enteric nervous system in humans is required.

Blood glucose concentration

While a clear-cut association between disordered gastrointestinal function in diabetes mellitus and the presence of autonomic neuropathy remains to be established, it is now recognised that acute changes in the blood glucose concentration have a substantial, and reversible, effect on gastric (as well as oesophageal, intestinal, gallbladder and anorectal) motility, in both healthy subjects and patients with diabetes [17,39,102–112]. Indeed, it was suggested some 20 years ago that diabetic gastroparesis may be the result of poor glycaemic control *per se* [102]. Marked hyperglycaemia (blood glucose concentration ∼ 15 mmol/l) affects motility in every region of the gastrointestinal tract [103].

Although some cross-sectional studies have, perhaps not surprisingly, failed to demonstrate any relationship between the rate of gastric emptying and the blood glucose concentration immediately preceding the gastric emptying measurement in type 1 patients [12,16,43], the use of glucose clamp techniques has established unequivocally that in both type 1 patients and healthy subjects, acute hyperglycaemia (blood glucose 16–20 mmol/l) slows gastric emptying of both solids and nutrient liquids significantly, when compared to euglycaemia (blood glucose 5–8 mmol/l) [107–109]. Cross-sectional studies suggest that hyperglycaemia also slows gastric emptying in type 2 patients, and there seems little reason to suggest that this would not be the case [21,46]. As discussed in Chapter 2, an effect of hyperglycaemia on gastric emptying of liquids is also evident in rodents [99,113]. While the magnitude of the effect of acute hyperglycaemia on gastric emptying in humans appears to be substantial, and hyperglycaemia slows gastric emptying in type 1 patients who have cardiovascular autonomic neuropathy [109,110], further studies are indicated to quantify the magnitude of the effect of hyperglycaemia, as well as the 'dose–response', more precisely. Moreover, it remains to be established whether the response to hyperglycaemia is dependent on the rate of gastric emptying during euglycaemia, previous (long-term) glycaemic control and/or autonomic nerve function.

In healthy subjects [114] and patients with uncomplicated type 1 diabetes [115], gastric emptying is accelerated markedly during hypoglycaemia (blood glucose ∼ 2.5 mmol/l) (Figure 4.5); this response is likely to be important in the counterregulation of hypoglycaemia. It is not known whether the magnitude of the effect of hypoglycaemia on gastric emptying is influenced by gastroparesis and/or autonomic neuropathy.

Recent studies have established that changes in the blood glucose concentration within the normal postprandial range also influence gastric emptying and motility [104–106]; emptying of solids and nutrient-containing liquids is slower at a blood glucose of 8 mmol/l than at 4 mmol/l in both healthy subjects and patients with type 1 diabetes (Figure 4.6) [104]. Accordingly, it is not surprising that a modest improvement in glycaemic control (postprandial blood glucose of 15.4 ± 2.2 mmol/l vs. 11.7 ± 1.7 mmol/l) had no significant effect on gastric emptying in a small cohort of patients with type 2 diabetes [116]. The concept that the risk of gastroparesis is influenced by chronic glycaemic control independent of acute glycaemia (analogous to the situation with diabetic microvascular

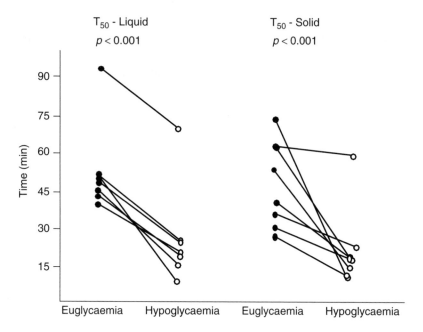

Figure 4.5 Effect of hypoglycaemia (blood glucose ~ 1.9 mmol/l) on gastric emptying [50% emptying time (T_{50})] of a mixed solid (egg, beef and vegetables) and liquid (water) meal in patients with uncomplicated type 1 diabetes mellitus. Gastric emptying of solids and liquids is accelerated markedly during hypoglycaemia. Adapted from Schvarcz *et al.* [115]

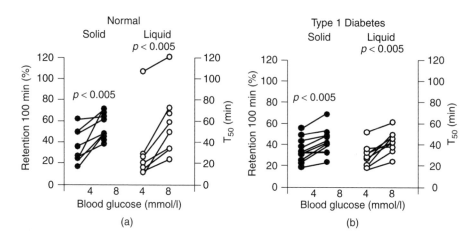

Figure 4.6 Effect of physiological changes in the blood glucose concentration (4 vs. 8 mmol/l) on gastric emptying (solid retention at 100 min and 50% emptying time for liquid) of a meal containing solid (egg omelet, 380 kcal) and liquid (lemonade, 70 kcal) components in (a) normal subjects and (b) patients with uncomplicated type 1 diabetes mellitus. Gastric emptying of solid and liquid is slower at a blood glucose of 8 mmol/l than 4 mmol/l. Adapted from Schvarcz *et al.* [104]

complications [53,54]) is supported by uncontrolled observations of improvement in gastric emptying after pancreatic transplantation [82,117], but requires formal evaluation.

There is relatively little information about potential mechanisms mediating the effects of the blood glucose concentration on gut motor function. Animal studies have demonstrated the presence of glucose-responsive neurons in the central nervous system, which may modify vagal efferent activity [118,119]. The various subtypes of central glucose-sensing neurons respond to physiological, as well as pathological, changes in extracellular glucose [120]. In healthy subjects the secretion of pancreatic polypeptide, which is under vagal cholinergic control, is diminished during acute hyperglycaemia, indicative of a reversible impairment of vagal efferent function [121,122], but such an effect has, hitherto, not been demonstrated in patients with diabetes mellitus [104]. The observed reduction in the heart rate response to standing during acute hyperglycaemia in healthy volunteers is also indicative of transient impairment of vagal parasympathetic function [81]; the concept that the inhibitory effect of hyperglycaemia on gastric emptying is mediated in part by impaired vagal activity is also supported by animal studies [113]. Neurons responsive to glucose have also been identified in the rat small intestine [123] and presumably exist in humans. Insulin, released in response to oral or intravenous glucose in healthy subjects and type 2 diabetes, does not appear to play a major role, as indicated by studies of the effects of euglycaemic hyperinsulinaemia [124,125]. Prostaglandins may be involved in the induction of abnormal gastric electrical rhythms (to be discussed) by hyperglycaemia [124]. Further studies are indicated to define the neural, humoral and cellular mechanisms by which systemic glucose affects gastrointestinal motility.

Other factors

A number of other (poorly defined) factors may affect gastric motility in diabetes. The prevalence of disordered motility is weakly associated with the duration of known diabetes [28,38,125]; this may be attributable to an increased prevalence of autonomic neuropathy. The prevalence of gastroparesis appears to be higher in females than males, for uncertain reasons [126]; this is also the case in patients with functional dyspepsia [127]. There is no apparent effect of body weight on gastric emptying in diabetes; reports relating to the effects of obesity on gastric emptying in otherwise healthy subjects are inconsistent; anorexia nervosa is known to be associated with delayed gastric emptying [70]. A number of electrolyte abnormalities (e.g. hyper- and hypokalaemia) may affect gastric motility [70]. Abnormalities in the secretion of gastrointestinal hormones, apart from insulin, have been reported in patients with diabetic gastroparesis; e.g. plasma motilin and gastrin levels are often increased [128,129], but their significance is uncertain. There is evidence that the elevation of plasma motilin may respond to insulin therapy [130] and be compensatory to a reduction in fasting antral motility [128]. *Helicobacter pylori* infection does not appear to affect gastric emptying or upper gastrointestinal symptoms in diabetes [11,131]; a study suggesting that eradication therapy may be associated with slowing of gastric emptying [132] requires confirmation. In type 1 patients there is no relationship between the rate of gastric emptying and the presence of parietal cell antibodies [17]. There is limited evidence that myopathic abnormalities may contribute to delayed gastric emptying; in one report, gastric smooth muscle degeneration and eosinophilic inclusion bodies were evident in a small number of patients with intractable gastroparesis [133]. The response to prokinetic drugs (to be discussed) argues against the concept of a primary disturbance of smooth muscle in most cases.

Gastroduodenal motor dysfunctions—effect of blood glucose

Abnormally slow stomach emptying can potentially be considered to result from defective mechanical breakdown of food, ineffective propulsion of intragastric content, and/or an abnormally high resistance to emptying. In view of the incomplete understanding of the mechanisms that underlie normal gastric emptying, it is not surprising that the motor dysfunctions responsible for disordered gastric emptying in diabetes are poorly characterised. An improved understanding may allow therapy designed to accelerate gastric emptying to be targeted more effectively. It is important to recognise that most studies in patients with diabetes have been performed either without blood glucose monitoring or during hyperglycaemia, in symptomatic patients with type 1 diabetes who were assumed to have gastroparesis [134–137]. An additional limitation is that usually only the function of only one or two components (most often the antrum) in an integrated system has been assessed. Nevertheless, it is clear that disordered fasting and postprandial motility occur frequently during 'euglycaemia' (i.e. blood glucose ~ 4–10 mmol/l), that the motor abnormalities are heterogeneous, and that the organisation of gastric contractile activity is frequently impaired [56,138–141].

Proximal gastric function is abnormal in many patients, with impairment of gastric relaxation induced by a meal [139,140,142,143]. There is, however, evidence that proximal gastric compliance or 'distensibility', as assessed by gastric balloon distension, may be greater [139]. Antral motility has usually been evaluated as an 'index' that takes into account the amplitude and frequency of pressure waves, but provides no information about their organisation [55,135]. Both fasting (reduced phase III activity) [56] and postprandial antral hypomotility [56,135] occur frequently in patients with long standing diabetes (Figure 4.7). In many patients there is a postprandial reduction in the number of antral waves that are temporally associated with duodenal waves, which may be a major factor contributing to slow gastric emptying [56,61,141]; in others there is the absence of a transition from a fasting to a fed motor pattern. An increase in both fasting and postprandial antral width, as assessed by ultrasound,

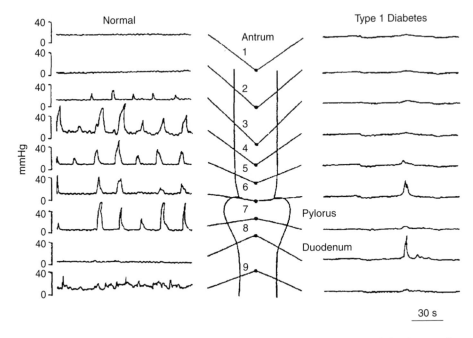

Figure 4.7   Manometric recording of pressures in the antrum, pylorus and duodenum after ingestion of a solid (minced beef) meal in a normal volunteer (left panel) and a type 1 patient with gastroparesis (right panel). In the normal volunteer there are a number of antral pressure waves. In the patient there is marked antral hypomotility. The spacing of the side-holes on the manometric catheter is shown

has been demonstrated [142] and may potentially account for disordered proximal gastric function. Increased pyloric motility does not appear to be a major factor contributing to gastroparesis, at least during euglycaemia [141]. A study that reported increased tonic pyloric activity in a cohort of diabetics with symptoms of nausea and vomiting [136] used a suboptimal technique to evaluate pyloric motility, and blood glucose concentrations were not monitored. Abnormal proximal small intestinal motor function also occurs frequently in patients with diabetes, but has been poorly characterised [144,145].

In most patients, the activity of the gastric pacemaker is normal during euglycaemia [146]; reports of an increased prevalence of gastric arrhythmias, particularly tachygastria, as assessed by cutaneous electrogastrography [26,84,134], may be indicative of an effect of acute hyperglycaemia [84,124,146] as well as inconsistencies in patient selection. There does not appear to be a significant relationship between the rate of gastric emptying and gastric myoelectrical activity in diabetes [26,147].

As discussed, acute elevations in the blood glucose concentration, even within the normal postprandial range, effect gastric emptying [103]. In both healthy subjects and type 1 patients, acute hyperglycaemia (blood glucose $\sim$ 15 mmol/l)

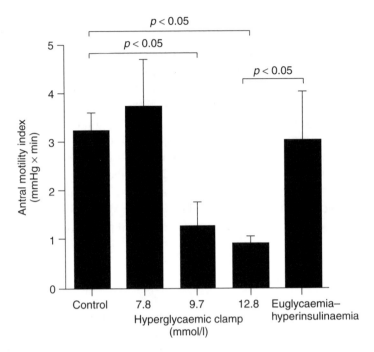

Figure 4.8   Dose-dependent effect of acute hyperglycaemia on postprandial antral motility in six healthy subjects. The antral motility index is less than the control value during hyperglycaemic clamping at both 9.7 mmol/l and 12.8 mmol/l; in contrast, hyperinsulinaemia *per se* had no effect on antral motility. From Hasler *et al.* [124], with permission

induces a motor pattern associated with retardation of gastric emptying (and comparable to that induced by small intestinal nutrients), characterised by relaxation of the proximal stomach [148,149], inhibition of antral pressure waves in both the fasted [150] and fed [124] (Figure 4.8) states (particularly propagated antral pressure waves [110]), stimulation of pressure waves localised to the pylorus [151] (the 'pylorospasm' that has been reported in patients with diabetes [136] is likely to be due to hyperglycaemia) and induction of gastric tachyarrhythmias [124,146]. The reduced number of propagated antral pressure waves during hyperglycaemia is associated with less frequent episodes of anterograde pyloric flow [61]. The threshold for an effect of hyperglycaemia on motility may differ between different regions of the stomach and in the fasted, as compared to the postprandial, state [123,150,152].

Clinical features

Disordered gastric motility in diabetes mellitus may, at least theoretically, be associated with upper gastrointestinal symptoms, changes in oral drug absorption and alterations in glycaemic control. Gastric bezoar is a rare, but well recognised, complication of disordered gastric motility in diabetes [153], which may occur as a result of a reduction in antral phase 3 activity.

Recent studies suggest that the rate of gastric emptying is a significant factor in postprandial hypotension. The latter, which may lead to syncope and falls, is an important clinical problem, particularly in the elderly and patients with autonomic dysfunction (usually diabetes mellitus), occurring more frequently than orthostatic hypotension [154]. In type 2 patients the magnitude of the fall in blood pressure after a glucose drink is related to the rate of gastric emptying [155]. Moreover, slowing of gastric emptying (and the rate of small intestinal glucose absorption), by the addition of guar gum to the glucose attenuates the fall in blood pressure [156]. These observations suggest that therapies which slow the rate of carbohydrate entry into the small intestine and/or carbohydrate absorption may be effective in the treatment of postprandial hypotension in diabetes.

Gastrointestinal symptoms

As discussed in Chapter 1, there is a paucity of information about the prevalence, determinants, or importance of gastrointestinal symptoms in patients with diabetes mellitus, and the significance of this problem remains controversial. As was the case with sexual dysfunction some years ago, clinicians may not inquire specifically about gastrointestinal symptoms. A major limitation is that there are few population-based studies and a number of reports relate to patients recruited from tertiary referral centres, with an inherent high probability of selection bias. In evaluating studies relating to gastrointestinal symptoms in diabetes, it should also be recognised that there is a high prevalence of gastrointestinal symptoms in the community, particularly those associated with functional dyspepsia and the irritable bowel syndrome, which are known to be related to both demographic and psychological variables [157]. Studies relating to gastrointestinal symptoms in diabetes should, therefore, ideally take into account a number of factors, including age, sex, body weight, psychological/psychiatric status and use of drugs (including alcohol and nicotine), as well as 'diabetes-specific' variables, including the type and duration of diabetes, acute and chronic glycaemic control, diabetic micro- and macrovascular complications, autonomic nerve function and usage of oral hypoglycaemic medications. Although validated measures to evaluate gastrointestinal symptoms exist for a number of diseases [157], until the recent development of the Diabetes Bowel Symptom Questionnaire [158,159], no 'diabetes-specific' validated questionnaire was available. Cross-sectional studies are inherently associated with substantial limitations; at present, as is the case with gastric motility, there is limited information about the natural history of gastrointestinal symptoms in diabetes, i.e. the number of patients who have persistent, as opposed to transient or relapsing symptoms, as well as the determinants of symptom turnover [52,160]. Community studies in non-diabetics have established that there is substantial fluctuation in the reporting of gastrointestinal symptoms [157]. A recent longitudinal study in predominantly type 2 patients indicates that there is a significant fluctuation in both upper and lower gastrointestinal symptoms over a 3 year period, with a relatively constant prevalence [160]. This information has important implications for the management of gastrointestinal symptoms in diabetes. The majority of community studies relating to gastrointestinal symptoms in diabetes have, unsurprisingly, related to type 2, rather than type 1, diabetes.

Despite these caveats, it is clear that the prevalence of upper gastrointestinal symptoms is high in both type 1 and 2 diabetes [158,160–167] and probably exceeds that in the general population, especially in women [158,161,165]. For example, in a study of 110 outpatients with long-standing type 1 diabetes, Schvarcz *et al.* [161] reported that the prevalence of postprandial fullness was 19%, compared to 8.5% in control subjects (Chapter 1). In a recent study from Australia that focused on type 2 diabetes, all upper and lower gastrointestinal symptoms evaluated were more common in community-dwelling people with diabetes than in controls [158]. In a US study of 483 patients with type 2 diabetes, 50% reported one or more upper gastrointestinal symptoms, compared with 38% in matched controls [165]; similar observations have been made in Sweden [162]. As discussed in Chapter 1, the impact of gastrointestinal symptoms, as opposed to other aspects of diabetes, on 'health-related quality of life' amongst patients with diabetes is poorly documented. The available studies support an association between impairments in both quality of life [117,166–169] and psychological function [166,170] with gastrointestinal symptoms, independent of other diabetic complications, but additional studies are required.

Potential determinants of gastrointestinal symptoms in diabetes include disordered motility, glycaemic control, psychological and demographic variables, autonomic neuropathy, visceral hypersensitivity, disordered gastric myoelectrical activity, use of medications, and *H. pylori* infection.

It has been assumed that upper gastrointestinal symptoms are a direct result of delayed gastric emptying [6]; this concept, while intuitively appealing, is overly simplistic. In particular, the relationship between upper gastrointestinal symptoms and the rate of gastric emptying appears to be relatively weak (Figure 4.9) [9,12,28,46,56]; some patients with marked delay in gastric emptying may have few, or no, upper gastrointestinal symptoms (Figure 4.9). As will be discussed, there is also a relatively poor relationship between the effects of prokinetic drugs on symptoms and gastric emptying. Moreover, many patients experience symptoms in the fasted, as well as postprandial, states. The relationship between symptoms and gastric emptying does not appear to be substantially stronger when symptoms are evaluated postprandially, rather than while fasting [171], neither do patterns of intragastric meal distribution appear to predict symptoms [31]. These observations are not altogether surprising, e.g. patients with pyloric stenosis may exhibit few, or no, symptoms. It should, however, be

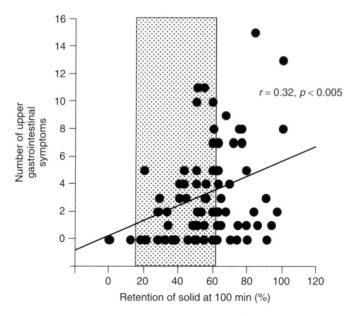

Figure 4.9   The relationship between upper gastrointestinal symptoms (maximum total score of 27) and gastric emptying (retention at 100 min) of the solid (100 g minced beef) component of a mixed solid/liquid meal in 86 outpatients with diabetes mellitus (66 type 1, 20 type 2). The normal range for gastric emptying is shown in the shaded area. There is a statistically significant, but weak, relationship. From Jones *et al.* [31], with permission

recognised that in most studies symptoms were not evaluated using validated measures and that total symptom scores, rather than the severity of individual symptoms, were quantified. In highly selected patients with functional dyspepsia, there is evidence of a close association between certain symptoms (such as postprandial fullness) and delayed gastric emptying of solids, when these symptoms are severe enough to influence daily activities [127]. This may also be the case in diabetes mellitus; in a recent study, the perception of fullness/abdominal bloating (but not nausea or vomiting) was predictive of delay in solid emptying [126]. While it is clear that additional studies are required to evaluate the association between symptoms and gastric emptying, it is appropriate to regard delay in gastric emptying more as a marker of gastroduodenal motor abnormality than a direct cause of symptoms, the aetiology of which is likely to be multifactorial. For example, there is evidence in patients with diabetes that symptoms may reflect visceral hypersensitivity, as is the case in patients with functional dyspepsia [140,149]. Studies in relatively small cohorts indicate that, during euglycaemia, the perception of gastric distension is increased in type 1 patients with [140] and without [149] gastrointestinal symptoms when compared with healthy subjects. Impaired gastric accommodation [44,141,143] and disordered antral motility, as well as gastric electrical activity [172], may also be potentially important in the aetiology of symptoms. Symptoms may also reflect disordered oesophageal, small intestinal or colonic motility, as well as psychiatric abnormality [173]. Uraemia may contribute to nausea and also affect gut motility [70].

Acute changes in the blood glucose concentration have been shown to affect the perception of sensations arising from the stomach and duodenum, although this issue has been studied less comprehensively than the effect of hypergly-caemia on gastric motility [103]. For example, in normal subjects, the per-ceptions of nausea and fullness produced by proximal gastric or duodenal distension, or small intestinal nutrient infusion [103,148,174], are more intense during hyperglycaemia (blood glucose 11–15 mmol/l) when compared to eugly-caemia. In healthy subjects, the amplitude of cortical evoked potentials elicited by oesophageal distension is increased during hyperglycaemia, providing an objective measure of increased perception [175]. Elevations in the blood glu-cose concentration that are within the normal postprandial range also affect the perception of gastroduodenal stimuli [105,174]. There is evidence that the blood glucose concentration also affects perception in diabetes mellitus, e.g. in patients with type 1 and type 2 diabetes the perception of postprandial fullness is related to the blood glucose concentration [103,171]. As discussed in Chapter 1, a role for hyperglycaemia in the aetiology of gastrointestinal symptoms is also sup-ported by cross-sectional, epidemiological studies [158,161]. The mechanism(s) by which hyperglycaemia affects gut perception/symptoms is unknown.

While 'lower' gastrointestinal symptoms, such as diarrhoea and faecal incon-tinence, are increased by the use of metformin (and presumably α-galactosidase inhibitors, such as acarbose), chronic use of oral hypoglycaemic medication is not clearly associated with an increased prevalence of upper gastrointestinal symptoms [159]. In considering other factors, H. pylori infection is probably not associated with upper gastrointestinal symptoms in diabetes in the absence of peptic ulceration (discussed on p. 156) [131,176,177], although there are no controlled studies of the effects of H. pylori eradication in this group—it is also possible that H. pylori may be more difficult to eradicate in patients with diabetes. Psychological disorders occur frequently in diabetes and may be associated with abnormal motility [173]; moreover, both psychological distress and impaired well-being are associated with poor glycaemic control [170,178]. Further studies are required to evaluate these issues.

Oral drug absorption

Gastric emptying is potentially an important determinant of oral drug absorption; most orally administered drugs (including alcohol) are absorbed more slowly from the stomach than from the small intestine because the latter has a much greater surface area [179,180]. Thus, delayed gastric emptying (particularly that of tablets or capsules, which are not degraded easily in the stomach) and a reduc-tion in antral phase 3 activity, may potentially lead to fluctuations in the serum

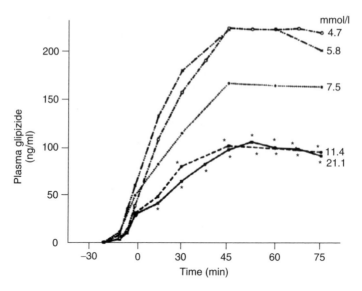

Figure 4.10 Absorption of the oral sulphonylurea, glipizide (5 mg p.o.), at different blood glucose concentrations in 12 normal subjects. Absorption is slowed significantly ($p < 0.01$) by hyperglycaemia. From Groop *et al.* [180], with permission from Eisevier © 1989

concentrations of orally administered drugs. This may be particularly important when a rapid onset of drug effect is desirable, as with some oral hypoglycaemic drugs (Figure 4.10). There is relatively little information about drug absorption in patients with diabetic gastroparesis [179] and additional studies are required. However, changes in gastric emptying would not be expected to have a major effect on steady-state blood concentrations of drugs that have longer half-lives, including prokinetic drugs.

Impact of gastric emptying on glycaemic control

Although Kassander observed in 1958 that 'the retention of stomach contents in a diabetic may cause confusion as far as food intake and utilisation are concerned' [6], the potential impact of upper gastrointestinal motor function on postprandial glycaemia has, until recently, received little attention. This is despite the recognition that there is a close association between both the development and progression of diabetic micro- (and possibly macro-)vascular complications and average glycaemic control, as assessed by glycated haemoglobin [53,54]. Glycated haemoglobin is influenced by both fasting and postprandial glucose levels; while their relative contributions have not been defined precisely [181], it is clear that improved overall glycaemic control, as assessed by glycated haemoglobin, can be achieved by lowering postprandial blood glucose concentrations, even at the expense of higher fasting glucose levels [182]. Accordingly, the control of postprandial blood glucose levels, as opposed to glycated haemoglobin, now represents a specific target for treatment; this forms the primary rationale for the development and current use of short-acting forms of insulin, such as lispro and aspart, to replace soluble insulin, and short-acting insulin secretagogues, such as repaglinide. It remains to be established whether postprandial glycaemia *per se*, including the magnitude of postprandial hyperglycaemic spikes, has a distinct role in the pathogenesis of diabetic complications, but there is increasing data to support this concept [181,183,184]. It is also possible that the extent of blood glucose fluctuations is an independent determinant of the risk for long-term diabetic complications [184].

As discussed in Chapter 8, postprandial blood glucose levels are potentially determined by a number of factors, including preprandial glucose concentrations, the glucose content of a meal, small intestinal delivery and absorption of nutrients, insulin secretion, hepatic glucose metabolism and peripheral insulin sensitivity. Although the relative contribution of these factors remains controversial, and is likely to vary with time after a meal, it is now recognised that gastric emptying accounts for at least 35% of the variance in peak glucose levels after oral glucose (75 g) in both healthy individuals and patients with type 2 diabetes [46,73,79,185] (Figure 4.11). It is also clear that even modest perturbations in gastric emptying of carbohydrate have a major effect on postprandial glycaemia [76,79]. Although the number of studies is limited, it appears that much of the observed variation in the glycaemic response to different food

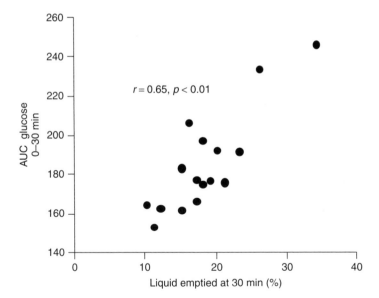

Figure 4.11   Relationship between the glycaemic response (AUC of blood glucose concentrations between 0 and 30 min) and gastric emptying (amount emptied at 30 min) of 75 g glucose dissolved in 350 ml water in 16 healthy subjects. Gastric emptying accounts for 36% of the variance in the AUC of blood glucose. From Horowitz *et al.* [73], with permission from Springer-Verlag © 1993

types ('glycaemic indices') in both normal subjects and patients with diabetes is attributable to differences in rates of gastric emptying [103]. It is also likely that a lack of standardisation of the volume of water ingested in the oral glucose tolerance test (usually an oral glucose load of 75 g) accounts for some of its documented variability—an increase in volume is associated with higher peak blood glucose, presumably as a result of more rapid gastric emptying [186].

In type 1 patients with gastroparesis, as would be predicted, less insulin is initially required to maintain euglycaemia after a meal when compared to those with normal gastric emptying [187]. Slowing of gastric emptying [79] may potentially account for the documented improvement in glycaemic control induced by caloric restriction in type 2 patients [188]. Conversely, acceleration of gastric emptying of high fat/carbohydrate meals induced by the lipase inhibitor, Orlistat (which is used frequently for the treatment of obesity in type 2 patients) has the potential to increase postprandial blood glucose concentrations [189]. There are numerous uncontrolled reports supporting the concept, initially suggested by Kassander [6], that in type 1 patients gastroparesis is a risk factor for poor glycaemic control.

Diagnosis

The decision of when to evaluate diabetic patients for disordered gastric motility is not always easy. As discussed, upper gastrointestinal symptoms occur frequently in patients with diabetes but are not strongly predictive of disordered gastric emptying or motility. Furthermore, it is not known whether asymptomatic type 1 patients with suboptimal and erratic glycaemic control (in particular, unexplained hyperglycaemia or hypoglycaemia) should be screened for disordered gastric emptying, although such an approach would be reasonable. In any diabetic patient who presents with upper gastrointestinal symptoms, a comprehensive history and examination should be performed, focusing on symptoms, including postprandial hypoglycaemia, and evidence of peripheral and autonomic impairment, such as orthostatic hypotension and bladder and erectile dysfunction. Occasionally the vomitus contains food that has been eaten many hours earlier, which is suggestive of gastroparesis. This should be followed by appropriate investigation to identify other causes of upper gastrointestinal symptoms. Physical examination is, however, usually unremarkable, except in severe cases where a succession splash and/or gastric distension may be evident. Upper gastrointestinal endoscopy is usually required to exclude gastric outlet or duodenal obstruction, as well as mucosal disorders [190]. It is important to recognise that there are many causes of gastroparesis apart from diabetes (a comprehensive list is provided in Table 4.1) and that the latter may be acute as well as chronic (defined arbitrarily as a disorder persisting for more than 3 months)—while diabetes may be the most common cause of chronic gastroparesis, gastric emptying is delayed in 20–50% of patients with functional

Table 4.1   Causes of gastroparesis and rapid gastric emptying

---

Transient delayed gastric emptying

   Drugs: e.g. opioids, anticholinergics, nicotine, dopaminergics, cytotoxics,
   β-adrenergic antagonists
   Postoperative ileus
   Viral gastroenteritis
   Electrolyte abnormalities—hyperglycaemia, hypokalaemia,
   hypomagnesaemia
   Hypothyroidism, hyperthyroidism, hypopituitarism, Addison's disease
   Herpes zoster
   Critical illness
   Pregnancy

Chronic gastric stasis

   Diabetes mellitus
   Idiopathic/functional dyspepsia
   Post-surgical, e.g. vagotomy
   Gastro-oesophageal reflux
   Atrophic gastritis
   Progressive systemic sclerosis
   Chronic idiopathic intestinal pseudo-obstruction
   Myotonia dystrophica
   Dermatomyositis/polymyositis
   Systemic lupus erythematosus
   Duchenne's muscular dystrophy
   Amyloidosis
   Autonomic degeneration
   Spinal cord disease
   Tumour-associated
   Anorexia nervosa and bulimia nervosa
   Central nervous system disease, brain stem lesions, Parkinson's disease
   Post-irradiation
   HIV infection
   Porphyria
   Liver disease
   Heart and lung transplantation

Rapid gastric emptying

   Post-surgical
   Pancreatic insufficiency (fat)
   ? 'Early' type 2 diabetes
   Zollinger–Ellison syndrome
   Duodenal ulcer disease (modest increase)

---

dyspepsia [127]. Chronic gastroparesis is a common accompaniment of diseases which cause motor dysfunction throughout the gastrointestinal tract, such as progressive systemic sclerosis [70]. In acute gastroparesis, correction of the underlying aetiology is usually associated with restoration of gastric motor function. It is particularly important to recognise that gastroparesis may be drug-induced; while in some patients it may prove difficult to withdraw medication that could slow gastric emptying, this should be attempted. Other reversible causes of gastroparesis, such as an electrolyte abnormality, adrenal insufficiency or hypothyroidism, must be identified and treated. Paradoxically, in patients with diabetes resulting from exocrine pancreatic insufficiency, gastric emptying of high-fat meals is abnormally rapid because of diminished small intestinal feedback [191].

Several techniques may be used to assess gastroduodenal motor function in humans, and these can be broadly divided into three categories: (a) measurement of gastric emptying; (b) measurement of gastric intraluminal pressures or contractions; and (c) measurement of gastric myoelectrical activity (Table 4.2). In research studies, a number of techniques are frequently used concurrently. Scintigraphic measurement of gastric emptying is the most accurate and, arguably, the only clinically useful assessment of gastric motility at present [70] (Figure 4.2), although other techniques, particularly ultrasound and carbon breath tests, show considerable promise [70,192]. While it has been suggested that the use of radio-opaque markers is a sensitive technique for the evaluation of gastric emptying in diabetes [193], this probably primarily assesses the integrity of late

Table 4.2 Methods to assess gastric motor function

Gastric emptying

   Scintigraphy
   Ultrasound (Doppler)
   Carbon breath tests
   Radiology
      Liquid barium sulphate
      Radio-opaque markers
   Applied potential tomography/epigastric impedance
   Pharmacokinetics of oral drug absorption
   Intubation and aspiration of gastric contents
   CT scanning
   Magnetic resonance imaging (MRI)

Contractile activity

   Manometry (lumen-occlusive contractions)
   Ultrasound (2D and 3D)
   Barostat (fundic tone)
   Scintigraphy
   Magnetic resonance imaging (MRI)
   Single photon-emission computed tomography (SPECT)

Myoelectrical activity

   Cutaneous electrodes (electrogastrography)
   Mucosal/serosal electrodes

---

phase 2 and phase 3 activity (the latter, as discussed, is suppressed by hypergly-caemia [150], and does not assess small intestinal feedback mechanisms). There is known to be a poor correlation between gastric emptying of digestible and non-digestible solids in diabetes [11]. Scintigraphy is relatively easy to perform and non-invasive. Radiopharmaceuticals have been developed to measure gastric emptying of solids, liquids and fat. The radiation dose approximates that received from a single abdominal radiograph. Measurement of gastric emptying should ideally be performed during euglycaemia, but at a minimum with regular blood glucose monitoring. Unfortunately, there is a lack of standardisation of scintigraphic techniques, with substantial variation between different centres, particularly in relation to the volume and composition of the test meal, the posture of the subject during the gastric emptying measurement, the duration of data acquisition and the calculation of gastric emptying rates [70,194]. This renders comparisons between studies performed in different centres difficult and usually dictates the need for each laboratory to have access to an appropriate control range. The test meal should be palatable and perhaps 300–500 ml in volume, with a total caloric content > 300 kcal. While there is some evidence that the use of test meals designed to provoke symptoms (e.g. high-fat meals) may be more sensitive, this has not clearly been established. Studies are usually performed with the subject upright, either sitting or standing. While a dual isotope technique, using different isotope markers to measure both solid and nutrient liquid emptying simultaneously, may be preferable because of greater sensitivity, this adds significantly to the complexity of the test. If it is only feasible for a single isotope to be used, gastric emptying of solids (or semi-solids) is usually measured; in this situation, more prolonged observations may increase the precision of the test [195], particularly as in many patients with gastroparesis the 50% gastric emptying time is not reached for many hours. In such cases attempts to derive a 50% emptying time by extrapolation may be associated with substantial errors [195]. It should be recognised that, while considerable attention has been given to gastric emptying of solids, including approaches to simplify the measurements, e.g. by minimising the duration of use of the gamma camera [195], there is little evidence that this approach offers any advantage over the use of a nutrient liquid or semi-solid meal (water should not be used, as it does not stimulate small intestinal mechanisms which retard gastric emptying). Moreover, as discussed, gastric emptying of liquids is dependent on different mechanisms from that of solids [70], and if the liquid contains carbohydrate it may be the major determinant of the postprandial glycaemic response [29,31,32,47]. Gastric emptying in diabetes appears to be relatively reproducible in the short term [196], perhaps because blood glucose control tends to be similar during repeat tests [28,52].

Scintigraphy also allows the assessment of intragastric meal distribution [31,34] as well as the frequency and amplitude of antral contractions (by quantifying changes in radioactivity in small regions of the antrum) [18,33,197,198], but the clinical utility of these methods has not been established.

Carbon breath tests have recently been used to quantify solid and/or liquid gastric emptying [12,19,192]; these are cheaper and simpler than external scintigraphy and, with the use of stable isotopes, avoid the use of irradiation. There is some ongoing debate as to the appropriate method of data analysis, and studies in patients with diabetes are limited [12,19,192,199]. Additional validation of these methods in patients with gastroparesis, particularly those in whom gastric emptying is markedly delayed, is required before their use can be advocated. However, it seems likely that carbon breath tests will prove to be useful as a screening test for gastroparesis, and in large epidemiological studies [19].

Ultrasonography (two- or three-dimensional) allows the non-invasive measurement of gastric emptying, gastric contractile activity, gastric volume and (with the use of Doppler) the velocity and direction of episodes of transpyloric flow [60,61,200,201]. Ultrasound is only suited to measurement of gastric emptying of liquids where both low- and high-nutrient liquids have been used, and may be technically difficult in obese subjects.

Magnetic resonance imaging (MRI) allows non-invasive assessment of gastric emptying as well as gastric volume and gastric contractile activity [67,202]. While it is a promising research technique, the costs are substantial and the required equipment has limited availability; subjects are usually also required to lie supine. Although it has been used widely in the past, indirect measurement of gastric emptying by quantification of the absorption kinetics of orally administered solutes (most frequently paracetamol) cannot be recommended for either clinical or research purposes [70].

Manometry is a complex technique which can be used to record pressures resulting from phasic contractions in the antrum, pylorus and duodenum that cause occlusion of the lumen. While both solid-state and water-perfused manometric catheters are potentially applicable, in most studies, a multi-lumen catheter incorporating an array of close-spaced water-perfused side-holes is used. The system is connected to a perfusion pump with a water reservoir. It is impossible to position a recording sidehole in the pylorus accurately because it is a narrow and mobile structure, and a 'sleeve' sensor (as used for measurement of lower oesophageal sphincter pressures) or multiple, closely spaced sideholes are required to record pyloric pressures [203]. Proximal gastric tone, including gastric accommodation, as well as perception of distension can be measured using the barostat—a thin-walled polyethylene bag is placed in the proximal stomach and linked to the barostat device, which consists of a pressure transducer linked by an electronic relay to an air injection system [63]. When the pressure in the bag is made constant (often 2 mmHg above basal intragastric pressure), changes in intrabag volume reflect proximal gastric tone, i.e. if the stomach relaxes, air is injected into the gastric bag to maintain the pressure, while air is withdrawn when the stomach contracts. The application of antropyloroduodenal manometry, as well as the barostat, has yielded important insights into the gastric motor and sensory dysfunctions associated with diabetes—both techniques have been used extensively in research studies carried out by specialised centres. However, their place in the clinical investigation of gastric function in patients with diabetes has not been defined. The barostat method is particularly invasive and may affect gastric emptying [204], as well as intragastric meal distribution and antral area [201]. For these reasons, it is likely that non-invasive techniques, including ultrasonography [200], MRI [202] and single-photon-emission computed tomography (SPECT) imaging [205], will be increasingly used in research studies to measure gastric volumes. The clinical utility of these techniques remains to be established.

As discussed, the activity of the gastric pacemaker (slow-wave) can be recorded using electrodes attached to the abdominal skin—so-called cutaneous electrogastrography (EGG) [206]. The EGG does not allow assessment of gastric contractile activity or the rate of gastric emptying [206], despite claims to the contrary. It remains an interesting research tool.

Modulation of gastric emptying to improve glycaemic control

The potential for the modulation of gastric emptying, by dietary or pharmacological means, to minimise postprandial glucose excursions and optimise glycaemic control, represents a novel approach to the optimisation of glycaemic control in diabetes, which is now being explored actively. It is important to appreciate that the underlying strategies are likely to differ fundamentally between type 1 and type 2 diabetes. In type 1 diabetes, interventions that improve the coordination between nutrient absorption and the action of exogenous insulin are likely to be beneficial, even in those patients who have delayed gastric emptying, i.e. by accelerating or even slowing gastric emptying, so that the rate of nutrient delivery (and hence absorption) is more predictable. In contrast, in type 2 diabetes, it may be anticipated that slowing of the absorption of nutrients would be desirable, as insulin release is both diminished and delayed. Such permutations need to take into account the differential emptying rates of various meal components, discussed previously, e.g. acceleration of gastric emptying of high-carbohydrate liquid components of a meal may, potentially, have a greater impact on postprandial blood glucose than that of solids.

Non-pharmacological approaches

In the treatment of type 2 diabetes mellitus, dietary modifications potentially represent a more attractive and cost-effective approach than drugs and warrant increased attention. A number of dietary strategies may slow carbohydrate absorption. For example, in patients with type 2 diabetes, an increase in dietary fibre benefits glycaemic control; the magnitude of this improvement, which is likely to be primarily attributable to soluble, rather than insoluble, fibre, is comparable to that achieved by oral hypoglycaemic agents [207]. Slowing of gastric emptying is likely to be important in mediating this effect [208]. The reduced glycaemic response to ingestion of bread containing sodium propionate appears to be related to slowing of gastric emptying [209]. Fat is a potent inhibitor of gastric emptying and, as discussed, these effects may be dependent on posture [77]; there is the potential for relatively small quantities of fat given immediately before consumption of, or with, a meal to slow gastric emptying of other meal components, so that the postprandial rise in blood glucose is minimised [210] (this is analogous to the slowing of alcohol absorption and liquid gastric emptying when alcohol is ingested after a solid meal, rather than in the fasted state [75]). As discussed, the presence of nutrients in the small intestine slows gastric emptying; it is therefore not surprising that small intestinal infusion of fat blunts the glycaemic response to a carbohydrate-containing meal in healthy subjects [211]. Rather then favouring weight gain, there is evidence that the suppression of subsequent food intake by the addition of fat to a meal may exceed the caloric value of the fat load [212].

In the broadest sense, the glycaemic response to a meal is also likely to be critically dependent on whether food from the previous meal is still present in the stomach and/or small intestine at the time of its ingestion, so that glucose tolerance may be expected to be worse in the fasted state (e.g. during an oral glucose tolerance test) than after a meal. The observation that the non-absorbable polysaccharide, guar gum, improves second-meal tolerance to glucose in healthy subjects by decreasing glucose absorption is consistent with this concept [213]; the effects of guar are likely to relate to increases in both the viscosity of gastric contents and small intestinal feedback [156]. Hence, an understanding of the interaction between concomitantly ingested solid and liquid meal components has substantial implications for the management of postprandial glycaemia [76].

Pharmacological interventions

A number of pharmacological agents which modify gastric emptying have been shown to affect glycaemic control acutely in patients with type 1 or type 2 diabetes; these include prokinetic drugs (e.g. erythromycin, cisapride, metoclopramide) [32,214,215] and agents which slow gastric emptying [e.g. cholecystokinin, the amylin agonist pramlintide, and glucagon-like peptide-1 (GLP-1)] [185,216,217].

Prokinetics Large-scale studies, based on adequate power calculations, are required to determine the potential for prokinetic drugs to improve chronic glycaemic control in diabetes. At present it is not known whether normalisation of gastric emptying in either type 1 or type 2 patients with gastroparesis improves glycaemic control. While treatment with levosulpiride, a D_2 dopamine receptor antagonist, for 6 months has been reported to improve both gastric emptying and glycated haemoglobin in type 1 patients with delayed gastric emptying [218], in studies of type 1 patients with unstable glycaemic control, cisapride had no effect on glycaemic variability after 4–8 weeks of treatment [32,219], possibly because the magnitude of the observed acceleration of gastric emptying was relatively modest. In a recent study administration of cisapride for 12 months had no effect on glycaemic control in nine type 1 patients with gastroparesis, despite sustained improvements in both gastric emptying and symptoms. However, in interpreting these observations it should be recognised that the group was relatively small and had reasonable glycaemic control at baseline (glycated haemoglobin of 7.6–8.2%) [199]. Hence, it would have been difficult to demonstrate a significant change. Intuitively, prokinetic drugs would not be expected to have a beneficial effect on glycaemic control in type 2 patients who are not using insulin. Erythromycin may, however, as a result of its interaction with motilin receptors, also stimulate insulin secretion (and potentially improve glycaemic control by this mechanism) in type 2 diabetes [220]; further studies are indicated to explore this issue—in particular it remains to be determined whether the effects of erythromycin, or other motilin agonists, on insulin secretion are sustained in the long term.

Agents that slow gastric emptying   The amylin analogue pramlintide, which is administered by subcutaneous injection, slows gastric emptying in healthy subjects [221,222] and patients with both type 1 and type 2 diabetes, possibly by a centrally mediated mechanism [222]; its use in the longer term is associated with a modest improvement in glycaemic control, as assessed by glycated haemoglobin [223–226]. Animal studies suggest that pramlintide does not impair the acceleration of gastric emptying induced by hypoglycaemia [227], but this remains to be established in humans. The use of pramlintide is intuitively attractive as type 1 (and some type 2) patients are amylin- as well as insulin-deficient. Pramlintide also suppresses postprandial glucagon secretion and may cause weight loss; both mechanisms may contribute to a reduction in postprandial blood glucose concentrations [223,226]. Pramlintide is not yet available for clinical use.

The use of glucagon-like peptide-1 (GLP-1) represents another potential strategy, particularly in type 2 patients [228]. As an incretin hormone, GLP-1 augments the postprandial insulin response, as well as suppressing both glucagon secretion and, probably, food intake [229]. GLP-1 may also stimulate pancreatic β-cell proliferation. The predominant effect of GLP-1 on postprandial glycaemia is, however, probably mediated through slowing of gastric emptying [217]. In a recent study, subcutaneous administration of GLP-1 for 6 weeks improved glycaemic control in a small cohort of type 2 patients [230]. The short half-life of GLP-1 limits its potential therapeutic use and longer-acting analogues have been developed [231]. Dipeptidyl peptidase IV (DPP-IV) degrades the active form of GLP-1 (GLP-1 7–36) to the inactive form (GLP-1 9–36); DPP-IV inhibitors are also being evaluated [232,233]. Exendin-4, which is produced by the salivary glands of the Gila monster lizard, is structurally similar to GLP-1 and shares several biological properties, but may be a more potent insulinotropic agent than GLP-1. In type 2 patients exendin reduces postprandial glycaemia after subcutaneous administration [226,234] and, at least in the short term, improves glycated haemoglobin in type 2 patients with suboptimal glycaemic control treated with diet and/or oral agents [234]. Interestingly, it has recently been demonstrated that α-galactosidase inhibitors, such as acarbose and miglitol, stimulate GLP-1 secretion, presumably because of the presence of unabsorbed carbohydrate in the distal small intestine [235–237] and slow gastric emptying [236,238]; both properties may be relevant to their efficacy. It has been suggested that the beneficial effects of α-galactosidase inhibitors on postprandial glycaemia in type 2 patients may also be greater when gastric emptying is initially relatively more rapid [239]. Metformin also increases postprandial GLP-1 levels, possibly by acting as a DPP-IV inhibitor [240]—the significance of this effect is uncertain. While all of these agents present exciting possibilities for the management of diabetes, with the possible exception of pramlintide, prospective studies are required to demonstrate sustained effects on glycaemic control before considering their therapeutic application. It should also be recognised that any drug that slows gastric emptying has the potential to induce or exacerbate upper gastrointestinal symptoms, delay oral drug absorbtion and impair the counter-regulation of glycaemia. Hence it may be important to determine the magnitude of effects on normal, as well as delayed, gastric emptying.

Management of gastroparesis associated with gastrointestinal symptoms

Management of symptomatic diabetic gastroparesis/disordered gastric motility is often challenging. Paradoxically, as discussed, delayed gastric emptying *per se* does not appear to be associated with a poor prognosis [52,241] and there are anecdotal observations that even severe symptoms not infrequently remit. It is, however, likely that patients in whom gastric emptying is grossly delayed have a worse prognosis. Interventions may potentially be most effective if targeted to those with fluctuating, rather than chronic, symptoms; this hypothesis requires evaluation.

In considering management options it should be recognised that diabetes is associated with an increased prevalence of oesophageal (as well as gastric) candidiasis, oesophageal reflux (Chapter 3) and gastric bezoars [190]. The latter are usually responsive to mechanical or chemical dissolution performed endoscopically—most recently, nasogastric lavage with Coca-Cola has been reported to be effective [190]! Hence (as discussed on p. 140) in most patients upper gastrointestinal endoscopy is required and, not infrequently, abdominal ultrasound as well. When the above investigations are unremarkable, gastric emptying should ideally be measured by scintigraphy (and possibly in the future by a carbon breath test), as this enables therapy to be targeted. Because of the poor predictive value of symptoms, objective measurement is required for the diagnosis of gastroparesis; non-specific terminology, such as 'gastropathy' and 'gastroparesis symptoms' [242], while appealing, is probably best avoided. Despite these considerations, it may be argued that provided that endoscopy is unremarkable, it is reasonable to give an empirical trial of prokinetic therapy for perhaps 4 weeks, while recognising that there is a substantial placebo response, that at present there are no objective data to support the cost-effectiveness of such an approach, and that probably the majority of patients will require prolonged therapy. Gastric emptying must be measured if symptoms fail to improve, or recur following the cessation of therapy (and in all patients who have had previous gastric surgery, as it is not feasible to discriminate between abnormally slow and more rapid emptying on the basis of symptoms). Vigorous attempts should be made to optimise glycaemic control [103], while recognising that there are no persuasive data to support this approach; it may prove necessary to maintain blood glucose levels close to the euglycaemic range to facilitate symptomatic improvement. If this proves to be the case, symptomatic gastroparesis would represent an indication for insulin pump therapy, rather than multiple injections of insulin each day. While the use of an insulin pump should result in the achievement of good blood glucose control, despite a variable oral intake, it is essential that patients are motivated and possess the technical ability to operate a pump. It is not known whether the remission/relapse of symptoms is related to fluctuations in blood glucose concentrations.

The identification and correction of malnutrition also represent an important component of therapy. While it is appropriate, and logical, to suggest a dietary intake of small, low-fibre and low-fat meals, with homogenised solid foods and increased nutrient liquids, no controlled study has been performed to establish that such an approach is useful. Patients may need to modify their insulin/oral hypoglycaemic therapy to adjust for increased meal frequency. It is not known whether an increase in dietary fibre intake, which has been shown to improve glycaemic control in type 2 diabetes [207], has the potential to exacerbate either symptoms or the delay in gastric emptying. Elemental diets can be used to accelerate an adequate oral intake in both the short and long term; however, unpalatability limits their use. There is limited evidence that walking after a meal may facilitate gastric emptying in some patients [243] but this has not been shown to improve symptoms. Patients with very severe symptoms may require hospitalisation and intravenous fluids. The acute gastric dilatation of ketoacidosis characteristically responds to nasogastric intubation and correction of hyperglycaemia and electrolyte abnormalities [51]. Anecdotal evidence suggest that dietary modification alone is successful in only a minority of patients and that most will require drug treatment. In patients with severe nausea, antiemetics such as ondansetron appear to be of limited efficacy but may warrant a trial.

Use of prokinetic drugs

At present, the use of prokinetic drugs (mainly cisapride, domperidone, meto-clopramide and erythromycin) forms the mainstay of therapy [167,244–259], and most patients will require drug treatment. In general, these drugs all result in dose-related improvements in gastric emptying after acute admin-istration, although their mechanisms of action differ (Table 4.3); involving simulation of 5-HT$_4$ receptors (cisapride and metoclopramide) [244,245,249], dopamine (dopamine 2) receptor blockade (domperidone and metoclopramide) [70,246,248] and stimulation of motilin receptors (erythromycin) [246,247,257]. The response to prokinetic therapy (magnitude of acceleration in gastric emp-tying) tends to be greater when gastric emptying is more delayed. It should be recognised that relatively few controlled studies have evaluated the effects of 'prolonged' (> 8 weeks) prokinetic therapy, that in many studies the sample sizes have been small, and that the assessments of gastrointestinal symptoms have, not infrequently, been suboptimal; furthermore, the results of some of these studies have been negative [32]. There have hitherto been relatively few randomised controlled trials of high quality, and those that are available differ substantially in design. Not infrequently, it is unclear whether a study has been designed primarily to evaluate the effects of a drug on symptoms or gastric emptying—in view of the poor concordance [9,12,28,46,56] between the two, such a distinction is important. Prokinetic drugs may also affect gastric electrical activity and potentially improve symptoms by this mechanism [248].

With the possible exception of erythromycin, all of these drugs have been shown to improve symptoms in short-term studies [167,251–253]. A beneficial effect on quality of life has also been evident in some studies, although this issue has not been evaluated widely [168,252,253]. In general, there is a poor cor-relation between effects on symptoms and gastric emptying—prokinetic drugs may improve symptoms by effects unrelated to acceleration of gastric emptying or central anti-emetic properties [254]. There is little information as to whether the symptomatic response may differ between patients with and without delayed emptying or between type 1 and type 2 diabetes; it appears that some patients who have normal gastric emptying, but significant upper gastrointestinal symp-toms, also respond to prokinetic therapy [253]. While there is some evidence

Table 4.3 Prokinetic drugs used in the treatment of diabetic gastroparesis

Drug	Mechanism of action	Route of administration	Oral dose
Cisapride	5-HT$_4$ receptor agonist	p.o.	10–20 mg t.i.d
Domperidone	Dopamine D$_2$ receptor antagonist	p.o.	10–20 mg b.i.d.-q.i.d.
Metoclopramide	5-HT$_4$ receptor agonist, D$_2$ antagonist	p.o., s.c., i.m., i.v.	10 mg t.i.d.
Erythromycin	Motilin receptor agonist	p.o. or i.v.	250–500 mg t.i.d.

that tolerance/tachyphylaxis may develop to the gastrokinetic effects of metoclopramide [255], domperidone [251] and erythromycin [256] (the latter may potentially reflect 'downregulation' of motilin receptors), blood glucose levels were not controlled in any of these studies. The mechanical effects of prokinetic drugs that are responsible for faster gastric emptying are poorly defined; the dominant effect is likely to relate to a change in the organisation of antroduodenal contractions to an expulsive pattern, although proximal stomach motility is also affected [45,141,257]. As discussed in Chapter 5, some prokinetic drugs also affect proximal small intestinal transit and motility.

Erythromycin is the most potent gastrokinetic drug when given intravenously (in doses of < 3 mg/kg) [247] and for this reason may be particularly useful in the initial phase of management [258]. When used orally, erythromycin may have greater efficacy as a suspension, rather than as a tablet [259], but is probably less effective than when given intravenously [256]. A beneficial effect of erythromycin, when administered chronically, on symptoms has not been clearly established [256]. The gastric motor response to erythromycin is also critically dependent on the dosage [139,257]. Erythromycin may retard small intestinal transit, which may be undesirable [260]. It has also recently been demonstrated, in both healthy subjects [106,261,262] and patients with diabetes [263,264], that the effects of erythromycin on gastric emptying and gastric motility are attenuated markedly during acute hyperglycaemia; this may also be the case with other prokinetic drugs, including cisapride [265]. Variations in the blood glucose concentration may, accordingly, account for the negative outcome of some studies relating to the effect of prokinetic therapies on gastric emptying in diabetes, particularly longer-term studies [32,256,266–268,273]. It is not known whether the action of drugs that slow gastric emptying is potentiated by hyperglycaemia.

The drug of first choice for oral administration, at least until recently, was cisapride, which has been subjected to the most comprehensive studies, and appears to have the most diffuse gastrointestinal effects, as well as sustained efficacy [14,199,249,250,268,269]. While cisapride has been well tolerated in clinical trials (mild diarrhoea is a well-recognised side effect), there have been recent reports of cardiac arrhythmias, including deaths [270,271]. It has now been established that cisapride has the potential to induce cardiac adverse effects, usually as a result of prolongation of the cardiac action potential (leading to lengthening of the electrocardiographic Q–T interval and torsades de pointes), which are probably related to Class III anti-arrhythmic properties, rather than 5-HT$_4$ receptor activation [270] (other substituted benzamides, including metoclopramide, apparently do not have Class III anti-arrhythmic effects). The clinical relevance of the cardiac effects of cisapride is still uncertain, particularly as the majority of patients who have died while taking cisapride had other risk factors for cardiac disease and were taking the drug in high dosage (~ 80 mg/day), although concerns about this issue have led to substantial restrictions in its use in many countries. There is no doubt that the potential for cardiotoxicity dictates that the use of cisapride should be more circumspect than previously recommended. Children with diabetes and people with idiopathic, congenital or acquired long Q–T syndrome, may be at particular risk for cardiac toxicity. Drugs that inhibit cisapride metabolism, such as ketoconazole, erythromycin and clarithromycin, or may prolong the Q–T interval, should ideally not be used concurrently [270,271], and before initiating therapy with cisapride it is appropriate to perform an electrocardiogram (a Q–T interval > 450 ms represents a relative contraindication to its use) and electrolyte screen (including measurement of plasma potassium and magnesium). An attempt should also be made to use relatively low doses of cisapride; if high doses are required, the electrocardiogram should be repeated at regular intervals during therapy. The risk:benefit ratio is particularly difficult to calculate in patients with diabetes mellitus, particularly those with severe symptoms associated with impaired quality of life and frequent hospitalisations, given the high prevalence of symptomatic and asymptomatic cardiac disease, and there is little information to guide the clinician.

Metoclopramide appears to be less effective in accelerating gastric emptying than cisapride and data relating to its long-term efficacy are limited [272,273], although it has the advantage of being available for parenteral use and having central anti-emetic properties. Some 20% of patients taking metoclopramide experience central nervous system side effects [273]. It would not be surprising if the use of domperidone, which has been shown to improve quality of life in diabetic patients with upper gastrointestinal symptoms [168,253] and is better tolerated than metoclopramide because of the reduced risk of central nervous system side effects, will increase. There is limited evidence that domperidone may be more effective than cisapride [274].

Refractory cases

Treatment of symptomatic gastroparesis is certainly not uniformly satisfactory, particularly in the subgroup of patients who have intractable bouts of nausea and vomiting lasting a number of days. It has been suggested that the efficacy of currently available prokinetic drugs is marginal [246]. If symptoms are refractory to prokinetic therapy (including intravenous erythromycin and intravenous or subcutaneous metoclopramide), placement of a feeding jejunostomy positioned by an endoscopic or laparoscopic approach (and sometimes parenteral nutrition) may be required to maintain nutrition [275]. These measures may be accompanied with a continuous subcutaneous insulin infusion. Because of the high prevalence of small intestinal dysmotility in diabetes (Chapter 5), the placement of a jejunal feeding tube should probably be deferred until after a successful trial of naso-enteric feeding. In most cases surgery is to be avoided vigorously; this may be associated with deterioration, as well as a high risk of nosocomial infections [276]. The anecdotal evidence of an unpredictable clinical course in cases of gastroparesis associated with severe symptoms also argues against the use of aggressive therapy. If surgery is performed (most frequently a $\sim 70\%$ gastric resection, including antrum and pylorus, with a Roux-en-Y jejunal loop), this should be done in specialised centres, and there is anecdotal evidence that this may be associated with sustained symptomatic improvement [277]. There may be a place for small intestinal manometry (Chapter 5) in the evaluation of such patients, although it has not been clearly established that the presence of severe small intestinal motor abnormalities represents contraindication to subtotal gastrectomy. There are uncontrolled data to suggest that pancreatic transplantation, which is known to have beneficial effects on autonomic function, may improve both gastric emptying and symptoms [82,117].

Future therapeutic options

There is a need for novel therapeutic options, particularly for long-term therapy. Dopamine (D_2) antagonists, such as levosulpiride [218], and 5-HT_4 agonists that do not effect cardiac function, such as tegaserod [277], are currently in development. Tegaserod has been shown to accelerate gastric emptying in normal subjects [278]; studies in patients with diabetes are awaited. There may be therapeutic advantages in combining drugs that have different mechanisms of action, the most logical probably being cisapride with domperidone (the combination of cisapride with erythromycin is contraindicated [271]). The recognition of the importance of sensory nerves in signalling information to the central nervous system suggests that drugs designed to modulate sensory feedback from the gastrointestinal tract, such as 5-HT_3 antagonists and κ opiate agonists, may have a therapeutic role. However, the outcome of a recent study which evaluated the effects of the κ opiate agonist, fedotozine, in patients with diabetic gastroparesis, was disappointing [279]. Therapies designed to relax the proximal (and possibly distal) stomach (and thereby reduce gastric wall tension), such as sumatriptan [280], could potentially be beneficial if symptoms reflect an increase in the sensitivity of gastric mechanoreceptors, as appears to be the case in some patients with functional dyspepsia. It has been suggested that clonidine, an α-adrenergic agonist with central and peripheral actions, which may be effective in the treatment of diabetic diarrhoea (Chapter 5), also has efficacy in the treatment of upper gastrointestinal symptoms in diabetes [281], but further studies are required. A beneficial effect of clonidine may potentially relate to a reduction in gastric wall tension [282] or central anti-emetic properties—while the available data are limited and inconsistent, clonidine (0.3 mg p.o.) appears to slow, rather than accelerate, gastric emptying [283]. As discussed, the phosphodiesterase-5 inhibitor, sildenafil (trade name Viagra) accelerates gastric emptying in diabetic mice [99], but its use in humans is recognised to be associated with upper gastrointestinal side effects and, as is the case with sumatriptan (and probably other phosphodiesterase inhibitors), it is likely to slow gastric emptying. Since administration of erythromycin is associated with the risks of long-term antibiotic use and, possibly, diminished efficacy, potent motilides that lack antibiotic activity and may not exhibit tachyphylaxis have been developed; a recent study using one of these drugs for the treatment of upper gastrointestinal symptoms in a large cohort of type 1 patients was, however, negative [284]; it has been suggested that this may relate to an adverse effect of motilin agonists on fundic relaxation [246]. The effect of cholecystokinin antagonists remains to be evaluated.

There are recent uncontrolled observations to suggest that intrasphincteric injection of botulinum toxin into the pylorus may improve both symptoms and gastric emptying in patients with diabetic gastroparesis [285]. Further evaluation is required before clinical use can be contemplated.

There is renewed interest in the potential role of gastric electrical stimulation as a therapy—using either neural electrical stimulation at a high frequency (which probably stimulates vagal sensory nerves and may suppress the vomiting centre [286]) or gastric electrical pacing, in which electrical stimulation of cholinergic motor neurones approximates the physiological frequency (~ 3 cycles/min) [287,288]. The latter approach is based primarily on the rationale that diabetic gastroparesis is associated with impaired gastric myoelectrical activity, although, as discussed, the available evidence suggests that this is only the case during hyperglycaemia [146,172]. While there are observations to suggest that both approaches may be beneficial, controlled trials are required [288].

A number of other agents (e.g. aldose reductase inhibitors, antioxidants such as α-lipoic acid, aminoguanidine, angiotensin-converting enzyme inhibitors, neurotrophins and PKCβII inhibitors) are being evaluated for the prevention and treatment of peripheral and autonomic neuropathy associated with diabetes; such therapies may potentially have application for the treatment of gastroparesis [92]. It also remains to be established whether other potential methods of insulin delivery (e.g. inhaled, intraperitoneal, transdermal and oral) will facilitate the achievement of good glycaemic control in type 1 or type 2 patients with gastroparesis.

Gastric secretion in diabetes

The human stomach has the capacity to secrete a variety of substances, including hydrochloric acid, pepsinogen, mucus, bicarbonate, intrinsic factor, prostaglandins and regulatory peptides. The gastric mucosa, which is responsible for this, consists of rugae (vascular folds) invaginated by gastric pits; each pit serves four or five gastric glands, which contain a variety of cells with specialised functions. The parietal cells, which are abundant in the gastric mucosa, are responsible for the secretion of hydrochloric acid.

Physiology of gastric acid secretion

Neural, humoral and chemical factors contribute to the regulation of gastric acid secretion. Neuronal control is exerted by long reflexes, which are vagally mediated, as well as local intragastric reflexes. Humoral substances act either in an endocrine fashion (e.g. gastrin) or in a paracrine way (e.g. histamine). In addition to these two mechanisms, gastric acid secretion is also modulated by chemical factors, e.g. acid secretion is stimulated by amino acids and amines are suppressed by acid.

Basal, or interprandial, acid secretion follows a circadian rhythm with the maximal secretion at night and the least early in the morning [289]. This rhythm is interrupted by food intake. Food-induced gastric acid stimulation can be considered in three phases; 'cephalic', 'gastric' and 'intestinal'. The vagal nerves appear to be the sole gastrocephalic link in postprandial acid secretion [290] and act directly on the parietal cells, since vagal denervation of the antrum which abolishes the gastrin response does not reduce acid secretion [291]. However, gastrin does form the second pathway in the cephalic phase; thought, smell and sight of food increase serum gastrin levels [292]. When food enters the stomach the second, or gastric, phase of acid secretion is initiated, induced by gastric distension as well as chemical factors. Mechanoreceptors and vagovagal reflexes modulate acid secretion in response to distension [293]. The third, or intestinal, phase, in postprandial acid secretion is initiated by food entering the proximal small intestine—the major stimulatory factors are distension, proteins and their products [294,295].

Gastric acid secretion in diabetes

Since gastric acid secretion is dependent on the integrity of the vagal nerves, chemo- and mechanoreceptors, neuropeptides and hormones, an effect of diabetes is to be expected. Although there is a lack of comprehensive studies, there is evidence that this is the case. In so-called 'early' diabetes, peak acid output was reported to be normal after histamine and pentagastrin administration, but the response to sham feeding or insulin-induced hypoglycaemia was reduced [296,297]. These observations suggest that vagal impairment may be responsible for a decreased peak acid output. In patients with long-standing type 1 diabetes mellitus complicated by autonomic neuropathy, the acid response to direct stimulation of the parietal cells appears to be attenuated [87,297–300]. These studies suggest that 'irreversible' autonomic neuropathy may be associated with decreased acid secretion in both the cephalic and gastric phases. However, it should be recognised that impairment of the gastric acid secretory responses to sham feeding [88] and other stimuli may potentially be due to hyperglycaemia [88] rather than irreversible vagal neuropathy.

The pathophysiology of altered acid secretion in diabetes mellitus has been investigated extensively in rodent models. While the applicability of these observations to human diabetes should be viewed circumspectly (as discussed in Chapter 2), these studies have established that in streptozotocin-induced diabetes, acid secretion induced by electrical stimulation of the vagus nerves or insulin-induced hypoglycaemia is attenuated [301,302]. The gastric acid secretory response to hypoglycaemia is mediated by the ventral medial hypothalamus, lateral hypothalamus and nucleus tractus solitarius [303]. Hence, these observations suggest that both autonomic neuropathy and impaired central regulation may be responsible for the reduction in gastric acid secretion. The outcome of rodent studies that have evaluated the response to direct stimulation of parietal cells have been conflicting. In some studies the acid secretory response to histamine was suppressed, while others reported the opposite [301,304], possibly due to differences in the duration of diabetes. In the study by Tashima *et al.* [301], both pentagastrin administration and intragastric installation of peptone enhanced gastric acid secretion in diabetic rats.

Hence, current evidence suggests that the decreased acid secretion in diabetes *per se* reflects a reduction in the cephalic phase and may not be clinically significant, while intragastric and intestinal phases remain intact or are only affected in long-standing disease.

Gastritis

Helicobacter pylori infection is currently regarded as the main causative factor for gastritis and is responsible for the vast majority of the peptic ulcers. Theoretically, it may be expected that the immunosuppression of diabetes mellitus would predispose to *H. pylori.* infection. However, studies investigating the association of *H. pylori* infection with diabetes have yielded inconsistent results, with a substantial variation in the reported prevalence from 30% to 80% [176,177,305–309]. Accordingly, *H. pylori* infection has been reported to be more prevalent in patients with diabetes in some studies [306,307,309] but not others [176,305]. When methodological limitations and differences in these studies are taken into account, a reasonable conclusion is that the prevalence of *H. pylori* infection is comparable to the general population, or only slightly higher.

As discussed, observations relating to the relation between *H. pylori* infection and dyspeptic symptoms are also inconsistent. Gasbarrini *et al.* reported a higher prevalence of dyspeptic upper gastrointestinal symptoms, particularly bloating, pyrosis and epigastric pain, in *H. pylori*-positive, compared to *H. pylori*-negative, patients with diabetes [308], but these observations were not confirmed by Xia *et al.*, who reported no difference in upper gastrointestinal symptoms between *H. pylori*-positive- and *H. pylori*-negative patients [176].

The prevalence of peptic ulcers in diabetes mellitus has not been assessed in the post-*H. pylori* era. However, *H. pylori* is responsible for up to 90% of peptic ulcers and, as there is no clear increase in the prevalence of *H. pylori* in diabetes, it is probable that the frequency of *H. pylori*-related peptic ulceration in patients with diabetes is comparable to that in the general population [311,312]. However, it should be recognised that the use of non-steroidal anti-inflammatory drugs (NSAIDs) may be increased in diabetes as a result of non-gastrointestinal complications, and there may be an increased incidence of NSAID-related gastric complications, including gastroduodenal bleeding [313,314]. It may be argued that strategies to prevent NSAID-induced upper gastrointestinal toxicity, using misoprostol or proton pump inhibitors, should be used with a low threshold in diabetic patients [315].

As in patients with functional dyspepsia, the presence of *H. pylori* in patients with diabetes probably favours eradication therapy. There is evidence that effective treatment of *H. pylori* infection in patients with diabetes mellitus may prove to be more cumbersome than in non-diabetic subjects. Gasbarrini *et al.* reported an eradication rate of 65% in diabetic patients compared to 92% in non-diabetic patients, using triple therapy of amoxycillin (1 g b.i.d.), clarithromycin (250 mg t.i.d.) and pantoprazole (40 mg b.i.d.) [310]. There are several potential mechanisms that may underlie the apparent reduction in eradication rate, including disordered gastric emptying, impaired antibiotic absorption and the development of resistant strains due to frequent use of antibiotics. The apparently lower success of *H. pylori* eradication therapy in diabetes also dictates that follow-up should be rigorous.

Association of pernicious anaemia and atrophic gastritis with diabetes mellitus

Autoimmune factors are well recognised to play a role in the aetiology of type 1 diabetes [316,317]. In such patients there is an increased prevalence of autoimmune aggression against non-endocrine tissues, including the gastric mucosa. The reported prevalence of parietal cell antibodies in patients with type 1 diabetes is in the range 5–28%, compared to 1.4–12% in non-diabetic controls [318–323]; the prevalence of parietal cell antibodies is not apparently related to either the duration of disease, age of onset or gender [323]. The autoimmune response to parietal cell antibodies may lead to atrophic gastritis, pernicious anaemia and iron deficiency anaemia [320,321,324,325]. The antibodies affect the gastric proton pump, the H^+/K^+-adenosine triphosphatase, which results in decreased gastric acid secretion and increased gastrin levels [326].

Iron deficiency anaemia can be treated successfully by iron supplementation [327]. Parietal cell antibodies can inhibit the secretion of intrinsic factor, which is necessary for the absorption of vitamin B_{12}, potentially resulting in pernicious anaemia. The prevalence of latent and overt pernicious anaemia in type 1 diabetes has been reported to be 1.6–4% and 0.4%, respectively [321,327–329]. The presence of atrophic gastritis in patients with parietal cell antibodies is not known. However, it is conceivable that this will be higher than in the general population, since in a study by De Block *et al.* subgroup analysis suggested that, in type 1 diabetic patients with dyspeptic symptoms and parietal cell antibodies, the prevalence of atrophic gastritis is about 60% [323].

Taking the aforementioned studies into account, screening for parietal cell antibodies in patients with type 1 diabetes currently appears inappropriate. However, there should be a low threshold for further investigation in those patients presenting with anaemia, since both iron deficiency and pernicious anaemia may affect many systems, including cellular immunity, intestinal function, growth, cardiopulmonary status and the central and peripheral nervous systems [330–332]. Finally, atrophic gastritis *per se* is associated with adenocarcinoma of the stomach [333].

Gastric blood supply in diabetes

The arterial blood supply of the stomach is derived from the coeliac axis through six major arteries. The left and right gastric arteries supply the lower third of the oesophagus and the lesser curvature of the stomach, and extend over the anterior and posterior stomach wall. The blood supply to the greater curvature is derived from the left and right gastroepiploic arteries. Short gastric arteries that originate from the splenic artery supply the upper part of the stomach, while the gastro-duodenal artery supplies the gastroduodenal region. The right and left gastric veins, draining the lesser curvature of the stomach, enter directly into the portal vein. The short gastric veins, which drain the gastric fundus and the upper portion of the greater curvature, join in the splenic vein. Blood from the lower end of the greater curvature is drained by the right gastric epiploic vein and enters the superior mesenteric vein. Mucosal blood flow accounts for more than 70% of total gastric blood flow in the fasting and postprandial states. The increase in blood flow after a meal is at least in part secondary to the increase in gastric acid [334]. Apart from the effect of gastric acid, the microcirculation of the stomach is innervated by sympathetic nerve fibres that decrease mucosal blood flow [335].

Since the arterial blood supply of the stomach originates from multiple arteries, gastric ischaemia is relatively uncommon—the latter has been reported in critically ill patients and patients with clinical relevant stenoses of the coeliac or mesenteric arteries. There is no apparent association between microvascular abnormalities and gastric ischaemia; therefore, patients with diabetes do not appear to have an increased incidence of gastric abnormalities related to insufficient arterial blood supply.

Acknowledgements

Our work in this area has been supported by the National Health and Medical Research Council of Australia. We wish to thank Mrs S. Suter for typing the manuscript.

References

1. Rundles RW, Diabetic neuropathy. *Medicine* 1945; **24**: 111–60.
2. Boas I. *Diseases of the Stomach*, 9th edn. Georg Thieme: Leipzig, 1925; 200.
3. Ferroir J. The Diabetic Stomach. Thesis in Medicine, Paris, France, 1937.
4. Saltzman MB, McCallum RW. Diabetes and the stomach. *Yale J Biol Med* 1983; **56**: 179–87.
5. Hodges FJ, Rundles RW, Hanelin J. Roentgenologic study of small intestine II. Dysfunction associated with neurologic diseases. *Radiology* 1947; **49**: 659–73.
6. Kassander P. Asymptomatic gastric retention in diabetics: gastroparesis diabeticorum. *Ann Int Med* 1958; **48**: 797–812.
7. Domstad PA, Kim E, Coupal JJ, Beihn R *et al.* Biologic gastric emptying time in diabetic patients using ^{99m}Tc-labeled resin oatmeal with and without metoclopramide. *J Nucl Med* 1980; **21**: 1098–100.
8. Horowitz M, Harding PE, Maddox A, Maddern GJ *et al.* Gastric and oesophageal emptying in insulin-dependent diabetes mellitus. *J Gastroenterol Hepatol* 1986; **1**: 97–113.
9. Keshavarzian A, Iber FL, Vaeth J. Gastric emptying in patients with insulin-requiring diabetes mellitus. *Am J Gastroenterol* 1987; **82**: 29–35.
10. Gilbey SG, Watkins PJ. Measurement by epigastric impedance of gastric emptying in diabetic autonomic neuropathy. *Diabet Med* 1987; **4**: 122–6.
11. Caballero-Plasencia AM, Muros-Navarro MC, Martin-Ruiz JC, Valenzuela-Barranco M *et al.* Gil-Extremera B. Gastroparesis of digestible and indigestible solids in patients with insulin-dependent diabetes mellitus or functional dyspepsia. *Dig Dis Sci* 1994; **39**: 1409–15.
12. Ziegler D, Schadewaldt P, Pour Mirza A *et al.* (^{13}C)Octanoic acid breath test for non-invasive assessment of gastric emptying in diabetic patients; validation and relationship to gastric symptoms and cardiovascular autonomic function. *Diabetologia* 1996; **39**: 823–30.
13. Lipp RW, Schnedl WJ, Hammer HF, Kotanko P *et al.* Evidence of accelerated gastric emptying in longstanding diabetic patients after ingestion of a semi-solid meal. *J Nucl Med* 1997; **38**: 814–18.
14. Dutta U, Padhy AK, Ahuja V, Sharma MP. Double-blind controlled trial of cisapride on gastric emptying in diabetics. *Trop Gastroenterol* 1999; **20**: 116–19.
15. Loo FD, Palmer DW, Soergel K, Kalbfleisch JH, Wood CM. Gastric emptying in patients with diabetes mellitus. *Gastroenterology* 1984; **86**: 485–94.
16. Merio R, Festa A, Bergmann H, Eder T *et al.* Slow gastric emptying in type 1 diabetes: relation to autonomic and peripheral neuropathy, blood glucose, and glycemic control. *Diabetes Care* 1997; **20**: 419–23.
17. De Block CE, De Leeuw IH, Pelckmuns PA, Callens D *et al.* Delayed gastric emptying and gastric autoimmunity in type 1 diabetes. *Diabetes Care* 2002; **25**: 912–17.
18. Meier M, Linke R, Tatsch K, Standl E, Schnell O. An advanced approach for the assessment of gastric motor function in long-term type 1 diabetes mellitus with and without autonomic neuropathy. *Clin Auton Res* 2002; **12**: 197–202.
19. Samsom M, Vermeijden R, Smout AJPM, Van Doorn E *et al.* Prevalence of delayed gastric emptying in diabetic patients and relationship to dyspeptic symptoms: a prospective study in unselected diabetic patients. *Diabetes Care* 2003; **26**: 3116–22.
20. Iber FL, Parveen S, Vandrunen M, Sood KB *et al.* Relation of symptoms to impaired stomach, small bowel, and colon motility in long-standing diabetes. *Dig Dis Sci* 1993; **38**: 45–50.

21. Horowitz M, Harding PE, Maddox AF, Akkermans LM *et al.* Gastric and oesophageal emptying in patients with type 2 (non-insulin-dependent) diabetes mellitus. *Diabetologia* 1989; **32**: 151–9.

22. Wegener M, Borsch G, Schaffstein J, Luerweg C, Leverkus F. Gastrointestinal transit disorders in patients with insulin-treated diabetes mellitus. *Dig Dis Sci* 1990; **8**: 23–36.

23. Cotroneo P, Grattagliano A, Rapaccini GL, Manto A *et al.* Gastric emptying rate and hormonal response in type II diabetics. *Diabetes Res* 1991; **17**: 99–104.

24. Annese V, Bassotti G, Caruso N, De Cosmo S *et al.* Gastrointestinal motor dysfunction, symptoms, and neuropathy in non-insulin-dependent (type 2) diabetes mellitus. *J Clin Gastroenterol* 1999; **29**: 171–7.

25. Chang C-S, Kao C-H, Wang Y0S, Cheng G-H, Wang S-J. Discreant pattern of solid and liquid gastric emptying in Chinese patients with type II diabetes mellitus. *Nucl Med Commun* 1996; **17**: 60–65.

26. Qi HB, Luo JY, Zhu YL, Wang XQ. Gastric myoelectrical activity and gastric emptying in diabetic patients with dyspeptic symptoms. *World J Gastroenterol* 2002; **8**: 180–82.

27. Zotimer BR, Gramm HF, Kozak GR. Gastric neuropathy in diabetes mellitus: clinical and radiological observations. *Metabolism* 1968; **17**: 199–213.

28. Horowitz M, Maddox AF, Wishart JM, Harding PE *et al.* Relationships between oesophageal transit and solid and liquid gastric emptying in diabetes mellitus. *Eur J Nucl Med* 1991; **18**: 229–34.

29. Weytjens C, Keymeulen B, van Haleweyn C, Somers G, Bossuyt A. Rapid gastric emptying of a liquid meal in long-term type 2 diabetes mellitus. *Diabet Med* 1998; **15**: 1022–7.

30. Wright RA, Clemente R, Wathen R. Diabetic gastroparesis: an abnormality of gastric emptying of solids. *Am J Med Sci* 1985; **289**: 240–42.

31. Jones KL, Horowitz M, Wishart JM, Maddox AF *et al.* Relationships between gastric emptying, intragastric meal distribution and blood glucose concentrations in diabetes mellitus. *J Nucl Med* 1995; **35**: 2220–28.

32. Stacher G, Shernthaner G, Francesconi M, Kopp H-P *et al.* Cisapride versus placebo for 8 weeks on glycemic control and gastric emptying in insulin-dependent diabetes: a double-blind cross-over trial. *J Clin Endocrinol Metab* 1999; **84**: 2357–62.

33. Urbain JL, Vekemans M, Bouillon R, van Cauteren J *et al.* Characterisation of gastric antral motility disturbances in diabetes using scintigraphic technique. *J Nucl Med* 1993; **34**: 576–81.

34. Stacher G, Lenglinger J, Bergmann H, Schneider C *et al.* Gastric emptying: a contributory factor in gastro-oesophageal reflux activity. *Gut* 2000; **47**: 661–6.

35. Lluch I, Ascaso JF, Mora F, Minguez M *et al.* Gastroesophageal reflux in diabetes mellitus. *Am J Gastroenterol* 1999; **94**: 919–24.

36. Lyrenas EB, Olsoon E, Arvidsson U, Orn TJ, Spjutii JH. Prevalence and determinants of solid and liquid gastric emptying in unstable type 1 diabetes. Relationship to postprandial blood glucose concentrations. *Diabetes Care* 1997; **20**: 413–18.

37. Reid B, DiLorenzo C, Travis L, Flores AF *et al.* Diabetic gastroparesis due to postprandial antral motility in childhood. *Pediatrics* 1992; **90**: 43–6.

38. Vaisman N, Weintrob N, Blumenthal A, Yosefsbeog Z, Vardi P. Gastric emptying in type 1 diabetes mellitus. *Ann NY Acad Sci* 1999; **873**: 506–11.

39. Cucchiara S, Franzese A, Salvia G, Alfonsi L *et al.* Gastric emptying delay and gastric electrical derangement in IDDM. *Diabetes Care* 1998; **21**: 438–43.

40. Young AA, Gedulin B, Vine W, Percy A, Rink TJ. Gastric emptying is accelerated in diabetic BB rats and is slowed by subcutaneous injections of amylin. *Diabetologia* 1995; **38**: 642–8.

41. Green GM, Guan D, Schwartz JG, Phillips WT. Accelerated gastric emptying of glucose in Zucker type 2 diabetic rats: role in postprandial hyperglycaemia. *Diabetologia* 1997; **40**: 136–42.

42. Abell TL, Cardoso S, Schwartzbaum J, Familoni B *et al.* Diabetic gastroparesis is associated with an abnormality in sympathetic innervation. *Eur J Gastroenterol Hepatol* 1994; **6**: 241–7.

43. Nowak TV, Johnson CP, Kalbfleisch JH, Weisbrack JP *et al.* Highly variable gastric emptying in patients with insulin-dependent diabetes mellitus. *Gut* 1995; **37**: 23–9.

44. Oliveira RB, Troncon LE, Meneghelli VG, Dantas RO, Goody RA. Gastric accommodation to distension and early gastric emptying in diabetics with neuropathy. *Braz J Med Biol Res* 1984; **17**: 49–53.

45. Werth B, Meyer-Wyss B, Spinas GA, Drewe J, Beglinger C. Non-invasive assessment of gastrointestinal motility disorders in patients with and without cardiovascular signs of autonomic neuropathy. *Gut* 1992; **33**: 1199–203.

46. Jones KL, Horowitz M, Carney BI, Wishart JM *et al.* Gastric emptying in early non insulin-dependent diabetes mellitus. *J Nucl Med* 1996; **37**: 1643–48.

47. Phillips WT, Schwartz JG, McMahan CA. Rapid gastric emptying of an oral glucose solution in type 2 diabetic patients. *J Nucl Med* 1992; **33**: 1496–1500.

48. Schwartz JG, Green GM, Guan D, McMahan CA, Phillips WT. Rapid gastric emptying of a solid pancake meal in type II diabetic patients. *Diabetes Care* 1996; **19**: 468–71.

49. Frank JW, Saslow SB, Camilleri M, Thomforde GM *et al.* Mechanism of accelerated gastric emptying of liquids and hyperglycaemia in patients with type II diabetes mellitus. *Gastroenterology* 1995; **109**: 755–65.

50. Bertin E, Schneider N, Abdelli N, Wampach H *et al.* Gastric emptying is accelerated in type 2 diabetic patients without autonomic neuropathy. *Diabetes Metab* 2001; **27**: 357–64.

51. Scott J, Lloyd-Mostyn RH. Acute autonomic dysfunction in diabetic ketoacidosis. *Lancet* 1976; **1**: 590.

52. Jones KL, Russo A, Berry MK, Stevens JE *et al.* A longitudinal study of gastric emptying and upper gastrointestinal symptoms in patients with diabetes mellitus. *Am J Med* 2002; **113**: 448–55.

53. The Diabetes Control and Complications Trial Research Group. The effect of intensive treatment of diabetes on the development and progression of long-term complications in insulin-dependent diabetes mellitus. *N Engl J Med* 1993; **329**: 977–86.

54. UKPDS, Group UPDS. Intensive blood-glucose control with sulphonylureas or insulin compared with conventional treatment and risk of complications in patients with type 2 diabetes. *Lancet* 1998; **352**: 837–53.

55. Kim CH, Kennedy FP, Camilleri M, Zinsmeister A, Ballard DJ. The relationship between clinical factors and gastrointestinal dysmotility in diabetes mellitus. *J Gastroint Motil* 1991; **3**: 268–72.

56. Samsom M, Jebbink RJA, Akkermans LMA, van Berge-Henegouwen GP, Smout AJPM. Abnormalities of antroduodenal motility in type 1 diabetes. *Diabetes Care* 1996; **19**: 21–27.

57. Hebbard GS. Physiology and pathophysiology of gastric emptying. *Gastroenterol Int* 1998; **11**: 150–60.

58. Horowitz M, Dent J, Fraser R, Sun WM, Hebbard G. Role and integration of mechanisms controlling gastric emptying. *Dig Dis Sci* 1994; **39**: S7–13.

59. Malbert C-H, Mathis C. Antropyloric modulation of transpyloric flow of liquids in pigs. *Gastroenterology* 1994; **107**: 37–46.

60. Hausken T, Odegaard S, Matre K, Berstad A. Antroduodenal motility and movements of luminal contents studied by duplex sonography. *Gastroenterology* 1992; **102**: 1583–90.

61. Kawagishi T, Nishizawa Y, Okuno Y, Shimada H *et al.* Antroduodenal motility and transpyloric fluid movement in patients with diabetes studied using duplex sonography. *Gastroenterology* 1994; **107**: 403–9.

62. Wood JD, Alpers DH, Andrews PLR. Fundamentals of neurogastroenterology. *Gut* 1999; **45**(suppl 11): II6–16.

63. Azpiroz F, Malagelada J-R. Gastric tone measured by an electronic barostat in health and postsurgical gastroparesis. *Gastroenterology* 1987; **92**: 934–43.

64. Der-Silaphet T, Malysz J, Hagel SL, Arsenault A, Huizinga JD. Interstitial cells of Cajal direct normal propulsive activity in the mouse small intestine. *Gastroenterology* 1998; **114**: 724–36.

65. Code CF, Marlett JA. The interdigestive myoelectric complex of the stomach and small bowel of dogs. *J Physiol* 1975; **246**: 289–309.

66. Sun WM, Hebbard GS, Malbert CH, Jones KL *et al.* Spatial patterns of fasting and fed antropyloric pressure waves in humans. *J Physiol (Lond)* 1997; **503**: 455–62.

67. Indireschkumar K, Brasseur JG, Faas H, Hebbard GS *et al.* Relative contributions of 'pressure pump' and 'peristaltic pump' to gastric emptying. *Am J Physiol* 2000; **278**: G604–16.

68. Hausken T, Mundt M, Samsom M. Low antroduodenal pressure gradients are responsible for gastric emptying of a low-caloric meal in humans. *Neurogastroenterol Motil* 2002; **14**: 97–105.

69. Andrews JM, Doran S, Hebbard GS, Malbert CH *et al.* Nutrient-induced patterning of human duodenal motor function. *Am J Physiol* 2001; **280**: G501–9.

70. Horowitz M, Dent J. Disordered gastric emptying: mechanical basis, assessment and treatment. *Baillière's Clin Gastroenterol* 1991; **5**: 371–407.

71. Collins PJ, Houghton LA, Read NW, Horowitz M *et al.* Role of the proximal and distal stomach in mixed solid and liquid meal emptying. *Gut* 1991; **32**: 615–19.

72. Lin HC, Doty JE, Reedy TJ, Meyer JH. Inhibition of gastric emptying by glucose depends on length of intestine exposed to nutrient. *Am J Physiol* 1989; **256**: G404–11.

73. Horowitz M, Edelbroek M, Wishart JM, Straathof JW. Relationship between oral glucose tolerance and gastric emptying in normal healthy subjects. *Diabetologia* 1993; **36**: 857–62.

74. Cuche G, Malbert CH. Ileal short-chain fatty acids inhibit transpyloric flow in pigs. *Scand J Gastroenterol* 1999; **34**: 149–55.

75. Horowitz M, Maddox A, Bochner M, Wishart J *et al.* Relationships between gastric emptying of solid and caloric liquid meals and alcohol absorption. *Am J Physiol* 1989; **257**: G291–8.

76. Berry M, Russo A, Wishart J, Tonkin A *et al.* Effect of a solid meal on gastric emptying of, and the glycemic and cardiovascular responses to, liquid glucose in older subjects. *Am J Physiol* 2003; **284**: G655–62.

77. Horowitz M, Jones K, Edelbroek MA, Smout AJ, Read NW. The effect of posture on gastric emptying and intragastric distribution of oil and aqueous meal components and appetite. *Gastroenterology* 1993; **105**: 382–90.

78. Horowitz M, Cunningham KM, Wishart J, Jones KL, Read NW. The effect of short-term dietary supplementation with glucose on gastric emptying of glucose and fructose and oral glucose tolerance in normal subjects. *Diabetologia* 1996; **39**: 481–6.

79. Beckoff K, MacIntosh CG, Chapman IM, Wishart JM *et al.* Effects of glucose supplementation on gastric emptying, blood glucose homeostasis, and appetite in the elderly. *Am J Physiol* 2001; **280**: R570–6.

80. Corvilain B, Abramowicz M, Fery F, Schoutens A. Effect of short-term starvation on gastric emptying in humans: relationship to oral glucose tolerance. *Am J Physiol* 1995; **269**: G512–17.

81. Yeap B, Russo A, Fraser RJ, Wittert GA, Horowitz M. Hyperglycemia affects cardiovascular autonomic nerve function in normal subjects. *Diabetes Care* 1996; **19**: 880–82.

82. Gaber AO, Oxley D, Karas J, Cardoso S *et al.* Changes in gastric emptying in recipients of combined pancreas–kidney transplants. *Dig Dis* 1991; **9**: 437–43.

83. Sampsom MJ, Wilson S, Karagiannis P, Edmonds M, Watkins PJ. Progression of diabetic autonomic neuropathy over a decade in insulin-dependent diabetics. *Qu J Med* 1990; **75**: 635–46.

84. Kawagishi T, Nishizawa Y, Emoto M, Maekawa K *et al.* Gastric myoelectrical activity in patients with diabetes: role of glucose control and autonomic nerve function. *Diabetes Care* 1997; **20**: 848–54.

85. Buysschaert M, Moulart M, Urbain JL, Pauwels S *et al.* Impaired gastric emptying in diabetic patients with cardiac autonomic neuropathy. *Diabetes Care* 1987; **10**: 448–52.

86. Migdalis L, Thomaides T, Chairopoulos C, Kalogeropulou C *et al.* Changes of gastric emptying rate and gastrin levels are early indicators of autonomic neuropathy in type II diabetic patients. *Clin Auton Res* 2001; **11**: 259–63.

87. Hosking DJ, Mood F, Stewart IM, Atkinson M. Vagal impairment of gastric secretion in diabetic autonomic neuropathy. *Br Med J* 1975; **2**: 588–90.

88. Lam WF, Masclee AA, de Boer SY, Lamers CB. Hyperglycemia reduces gastric secretory and plasma pancreatic polypeptide responses to modified sham feeding in humans. *Digestion* 1993; **54**: 48–53.

89. Belai A, Calcutt NA, Carrington AL, Diemel LT *et al.* Enteric neuropeptides in streptozocin-diabetic rats; effects of insulin and aldose reductase inhibition. *J Auton Nerv Syst* 1996; **58**: 163–9.

90. Ordog T, Takayama I, Cheung WK, Ward SM, Sanders KM. Remodelling of networks of interstitial cells of Cajal in a marine model of diabetic gastroparesis. *Diabetes* 2000; **49**: 1731–9.

91. Lincoln J, Bokor JT Crowe R, Griffith SG *et al.* Myenteric plexus in streptozotocin-treated rats: neurochemical and histochemical evidence for diabetic neuropathy of the gut. *Gastroenterology* 1984; **86**: 654–61.

92. Soediono P, Belai A, Burnstock G. Prevention of neuropathy in the pyloric sphincter of streptozotocin-diabetic rats by gangliosides. *Gastroenterology* 1993; **104**: 1072–82.

93. Guy RJC, Dawson JL, Garrett JR, Laws JW *et al.* Diabetic gastroparesis from autonomic neuropathy: surgical considerations and changes in vagus nerve morphology. *J Neurol Neurosurg Psychol* 1984; **47**: 686–91.

94. Britland ST, Young RJ, Sharma AK, Lee D. Vagus nerve morphology in diabetic gastropathy. *Diabet Med* 1990; **7**: 780–87.

95. Yoshida, MM, Schuffler MD, Sumi SM. There are no morphological abnormalities of the gastric wall or abdominal vagus in patients with diabetic gastroparesis. *Gastroenterology* 1988; **94**: 907–14.

96. He C-L, Soffer E, Ferris C, Walsh RM *et al.* Loss of interstitial cells of Cajal and inhibitory innervation in insulin-dependent diabetes. *Gastroenterology* 2001; **121**: 427–34.

97. Russo A, Fraser R, Adachi K, Horowitz M, Boeckxstaens G. Evidence that nitric oxide mechanisms regulate small intestinal motility in humans. *Gut* 1999; **44**: 72–6.

98. Takahashi T, Nakamura K, Itoh H, Sima AA, Owyang C. Impaired expression of nitric oxide synthase in the gastric myenteric plexus of spontaneously diabetic rats. *Gastroenterology* 1997; **113**: 1535–44.

99. Watkins CC, Sawa A, Jaffrey S, Blackshaw S *et al.* Insulin restores neuronal nitric oxide synthase expression and function that is lost in diabetic gastropathy. *J Clin Invest* 2000; **106**: 373–84.

100. Sun WM, Doran S, Jones K, Ooi E *et al.* Effects of nitroglycerin on liquid gastric emptying and antropyloroduodenal motility. *Am J Physiol* 1998; **275**: G1173–8.

101. Konturek JW, Fischer H, Gromotka PM, Konturek SJ, Domschke W. Endogenous nitric oxide in the regulation of gastric secretory and motor activity in humans. *Aliment Pharmacol Ther* 1999; **13**: 1683–91.

102. Soler NG. Diabetic gastroparesis without autonomic neuropathy. *Diabetes Care* 1980; **3**: 200–201.

103. Rayner CK, Samsom M, Jones KL, Horowitz M. Relationships between upper gastrointestinal motor and sensory function with glycemic control (review). *Diabetes Care* 2001; **24**: 371–81.

104. Schvarcz E, Palmer M, Aman J, Horowitz M *et al.* Physiological hyperglycaemia slows gastric emptying in normal subjects and patients with insulin-dependent diabetes mellitus. *Gastroenterology* 1997; **113**: 60–66.

105. Andrews JM, Rayner CK, Doran S, Hebbard GS, Horowitz M. Physiological changes in blood glucose affect appetite and pyloric motility during antroduodenal lipid infusion. *Am J Physiol* 1998; **275**: G797–804.

106. Jones KL, Kong MF, Berry MK, Rayner CK *et al.* The effect of erythromycin on gastric emptying is modified by physiological changes in the blood glucose concentration. *Am J Gastroenterol* 1999; **94**: 2074–9.

107. MacGregor IL, Gueller R, Watts HD, Meyer JH. The effect of acute hyperglycemia on gastric emptying in man. *Gastroenterology* 1976; **70**: 190–96.

108. Oster-Jorgensen E, Pedersen SA, Larsen ML. The influence of induced hyperglycemia on gastric emptying in healthy humans. *Scand J Lab Clin Invest* 1990; **50**: 831–6.

109. Fraser R, Horowitz M, Maddox A, Chatterton B *et al.* Hyperglycaemia slows gastric emptying in type 1 diabetes mellitus. *Diabetologia* 1990; **30**: 675–80.

110. Samsom M, Akkermans LM, Jebbink RJ, van Isselt H *et al.* Gastrointestinal motor mechanisms in hyperglycaemia-induced delayed gastric emptying in type 1 diabetes mellitus. *Gut* 1997; **40**: 641–6.

111. Morgan LM, Tredger JA, Hamptom SM, French AP *et al.* The effect of dietary modification and hyperglycaemia on gastric emptying and gastric inhibitory polypeptide (GIP) secretion. *Br J Nutr* 1988; **60**: 29–37.

112. El-Salhy M, Sitohy B. Abnormal gastrointestinal endocrine cells in patients with diabetes type 1: relationship to gastric emptying and myoelectrical activity. *Scand J Gastroenterol* 2001; **36**: 1162–9.

113. Ishiguchi T, Tada H, Nakagawa K, Yamamura T, Takahashi T. Hyperglycemia impairs antro-pyloric coordination and delays gastric emptying in conscious rats. *Auton Neurosci* 2002; **95**: 112–20.

114. Schvarcz E, Palmer M, Aman J, Berne C. Hypoglycemia increases the gastric emptying rate in healthy subjects. *Diabetes Care* 1995; **18**: 674–6.

115. Schvarcz E, Palmer M, Aman J, Lindkvist B, Beckman KW. Hypoglycaemia increases the gastric emptying in patients with type 1 diabetes mellitus. *Diabet Med* 1993; **10**: 660–63.

116. Holzapfel A, Festa A, Stacher-Janotta G, Bergmann H *et al.* Gastric emptying in type II (non-insulin dependent) diabetes mellitus before and after therapy readjustment: no influence of actual blood glucose concentration. *Diabetologia* 1999; **42**: 1410–12.

117. Hathaway DK, Abell TL, Cardoso S, Hartwig MS *et al.* Improvement in autonomic and gastric function following pancreas–kidney vs. kidney-alone transplantation and the correlations with quality of life. *Transplantation* 1994; **57**: 816–22.

118. Mizuno Y, Oomura Y. Glucose responding neurons in the nucleus tractus solitarius of the rat: *in vitro* study. *Brain Res* 1984; **307**: 109–116.

119. Song Z, Levin BG, McArdle JJ, Bakhos N, Routh VH. Convergence of pre- and post-synaptic influences on glucosensing neurons in the ventromedial hypothalamic nucleus. *Diabetes* 2001; **50**: 2673–81.

120. Routh VH. Glucose-sensing neurons. Are they physiologically relevant? *Physiol Behav* 2002; **76**: 403–13.

121. de Boer SY, Masclee AA, Lam WF, Lamers CB. Effects of acute hyperglycemia on esophageal motility and lower esophageal sphincter pressure in humans. *Gastroenterology* 1992; **103**: 775–80.

122. de Boer SY, Masclee AA, Lam WF, Lemkes HH *et al.* Effect of hyperglycaemia on gallbladder motility in type 1 (insulin-dependent) diabetes mellitus. *Diabetologia* 1994; **37**: 75–81.

123. Liu M, Seino S, Kirchgessner AL. Identification and characterization of glucoresponsive neurons in the enteric nervous system. *J Neurosci* 1999; **19**: 10305–17.

124. Hasler WL, Soudah HC, Dulai G, Owyang C. Mediation of hyperglycaemia-evoked gastric slow-wave dysrhythmias by endogenous prostaglandins. *Gastroenterology* 1995; **108**: 727–36.

125. Kong M, King P, Macdonald I, Blackshaw P *et al.* Euglycaemic hyperinsulinaemia does not affect gastric emptying in type I and type II diabetes mellitus. *Diabetologia* 1999; **42**: 365–72.

126. Jones KL, Russo A, Stevens JE, Wishart JM *et al.* Predictors of delayed gastric emptying in diabetes mellitus. *Diabetes Care* 2001; **24**: 1264–9.

127. Stanghellini V, Tosetti C, Paternico A, Barbara G *et al.* Risk indicators of delayed gastric emptying of solids in 343 patients with functional dyspepsia. *Gastroenterology* 1996; **110**: 1036–42.

128. Achem-Karam SR, Funakoshi A, Vinik AI, Owyang C. Plasma motilin concentrations and interdigestive migrating motor complex in diabetic gastroparesis: effect of metoclopramide. *Gastroenterology* 1985; **88**: 492–9.

129. Kawagishi T, Nishizawa Y, Okuno Y, Sekiya K, Morii H. Effect of cisapride on gastric emptying of indigestible solids and plasma motilin concentration in diabetic autonomic neuropathy. *Am J Gastroenterol* 1993; **88**: 933–8.

130. Funakoshi A, Glowniak J, Owyang C, Vinik AI. Evidence for cholinergic and vagal noncholinergic mechanisms mediating plasma motilin-like immunoreactivity. *J Clin Endocrinol Metab* 1982; **54**: 1129–34.

131. Jones KL, Wishart JM, Berry M, Russo A *et al. Helicobacter pylori* infection is not associated with delayed gastric emptying or upper gastrointestinal symptoms in diabetes mellitus. *Dig Dis Sci* 2002; **47**: 704–9.

132. de Luis DA, Cordero JM, Caballero C, Boixeda D *et al.* Effect of treatment of *Helicobacter pylori* infection on gastric emptying and its influence on the glycaemic control in type 1 diabetes mellitus. *Diabetes Res Clin Pract* 2001; **52**: 1–9.

133. Ejskjaer NT, Bradley JL, Buxton-Thomas MS, Edmonds ME *et al.* Novel surgical treatment and gastric pathology in diabetic gastroparesis. *Diabet Med* 1999; **16**: 488–95.

134. Abell TL, Camilleri M, Hench V, Malagelada J-R. Gastric electromechanical function and gastric emptying in diabetic gastroparesis. *Eur J Gastroenterol Hepatol* 1991; **3**: 163–7.

135. Camilleri M, Malagelada JR. Abnormal intestinal motility in diabetics with the gastroparesis syndrome. *Eur J Clin Invest* **14**: 420–27.

136. Mearin F, Camilleri M, Malagelada J-R. Pyloric dysfunction in diabetics with recurrent nausea and vomiting. *Gastroenterology* 1986; **90**: 1919–25.

137. Fox S, Behar J. Pathogenesis of diabetic gastroparesis: a pharmacologic study. *Gastroenterology* 1980; **88**: 933–38.

138. Tack J, Janssens J, Vantrappen G, Peeters T *et al*. Effect of erythromycin on gastric motility in controls and in diabetic gastroparesis. *Gastroenterology* 1992; **103**: 72–9.

139. Samsom M, Salet GAM, Roelofs, JMM, Akkermans LMA *et al*. Compliance of the proximal stomach and dyspeptic symptoms in patients with type I diabetes mellitus. *Dig Dis Sci* 1995; **40**: 2037–42.

140. Samsom M, Roelofs JMM, Akkermans LMA, van Berge-Henegouwen GP, Smout AJPM. Proximal gastric motor activity in response to a liquid meal in type 1 diabetes mellitus with autonomic neuropathy. *Dig Dis Sci* 1998; **43**: 491–6.

141. Fraser R, Horowitz M, Maddox A, Dent J. Postprandial antropyloroduodenal motility and gastric emptying in gastroparesis—effects of cisapride. *Gut* 1994; **35**: 172–8.

142. Undeland KA, Hausken T, Svebakk S, Aanerud S, Berstad A. Wide antral area and low vagal tone in patients with diabetes mellitus compared to patients with functional dyspepsia and healthy individuals. *Dig Dis Sci* 1996; **41**: 9–16.

143. Undeland KA, Hausken T, Aanerud S, Berstad A. Lower postprandial gastric volume response in diabetic patients with vagal neuropathy. *Neurogastroenterol Motil* 1997; **9**: 19–24.

144. Nguyen HN, Silny J, Wuller S, Marschall H-V *et al*. Abnormal postprandial duodenal chyme transport in patients with longstanding insulin dependent diabetes mellitus. *Gut* 1997; **41**: 624–31.

145. Samsom M, Jebbink HJA, Akkermans LMA, van Berge-Henegouwen GP, Smout AJPM. Oral erythromycin improves antroduodenal motility and reduces dyspeptic symptoms in type I diabetics with autonomic neuropathy. *Diabetes Care* 1997; **20**: 129–34.

146. Jebbink RJ, Samsom M, Bruijs PP, Bravenboer B *et al*. Hyperglycaemia induces abnormalities of gastric myoelectric activity in patients with type I diabetes mellitus. *Gastroenterology* 1994; **107**: 1390–97.

147. Pfaffenbach B, Wegener M, Adamek RJ, Schaffstein J *et al*. Antral myoelectric activity, gastric emptying and dyspeptic symptoms in diabetes. *Scand J Gastroenterol* 1995; **30**: 1166–71.

148. Hebbard GS, Samson M, Sun WM, Dent J, Horowitz M. Hyperglycaemia affects proximal gastric motor and sensory function during small intestinal triglyceride infusion. *Am J Physiol* **271**; G814–19.

149. Rayner CK, Verhagen MA, Hebbard GS, DiMatteo AC *et al*. Proximal gastric compliance and perception of distension in type 1 diabetes mellitus: effects of hyperglycaemia. *Am J Gastroenterol* 2000; **95**: 1175–83.

150. Barnett JL, Owyang C. Serum glucose concentration as a modulator of interdigestive gastric motility. *Gastroenterology* 1988; **94**: 739–44.

151. Fraser R, Horowitz M, Dent J. Hyperglycaemia stimulates pyloric motility in normal subjects. *Gut* 1991; **32**: 475–8.

152. Verhagen MAMT, Rayner CK, Andrews JM, Hebbard GS *et al*. Physiological changes in blood glucose do not affect gastric compliance and perception in normal subjects. *Am J Physiol* 1999; **276**: G761–6.

153. Brady PG, Richardson R. Gastric bezoar formation secondary to gastroparesis diabeticorum. *Arch Int Med* 1977; **137**: 1729.

154. Jansen RW, Lipsitz LA. Postprandial hypotension: epidemiology, pathophysiology and clinical management. *Ann Int Med* 1995; **122**: 286–95.

155. Jones KL, Tonkin A, Horowitz M, Carney BI *et al*. The rate of gastric emptying is a determinant of postprandial hypotension in non-insulin-dependent diabetes mellitus. *Clin Sci* 1998; **94**: 65–70.

156. Russo A, Stevens J, Wilson T, *et al*. Guar attenuates fall in postprandial blood pressure and slows gastric emptying of oral glucose in type 2 diabetes. *Dig Dis Sci* 2003; **48**: 1221–9.

157. Talley NJ, Weaver AL, Zinsmeister AR, Melton LJ. Onset and disappearance of gastrointestinal symptoms and functional gastrointestinal disorders. *Am J Epidemiol* 1992; **136**: 1–13.

158. Bytzer PM, Talley NJ, Hammer J, Young LJ, Jones MP, Horowitz M. Diabetes mellitus is associated with an increased prevalence of gastrointestinal symptoms: a population-based study of 15 000 adults. *Arch Intera Med* 2001; **161**: 1989–96.

159. Bytzer P, Talley NJ, Jones MP, Horowitz M. Oral hypoglycaemic drugs and gastrointestinal symptoms in diabetes mellitus. *Aliment Pharmacol Ther* 2001; **15**: 137–42.

160. Talley NJ, Howell S, Jones MP, Horowitz M. Predictors of turnover of lower gastrointestinal symptoms in diabetes mellitus. *Am J Gastroenterol* 2002; **97**: 3087–94.

161. Schvarcz E, Palmer M, Ingberg CM, Aman J, Berne C. Increased prevalence of upper intestinal symptoms in long-term type 1 diabetes mellitus. *Diabet Med* 1996; **13**: 478–81.

162. Spangeus A, El-Salhy M, Suhr O, Eriksson J, Lithner F. Prevalence of gastrointestinal symptoms in young and middle-aged diabetic patients. Scand J Gastroenterol 1994; **34**: 1196–2002.

163. Maleki D, Locke GR, Camilleri M, Zinsmeister AR *et al*. Gastrointestinal tract symptoms among persons with diabetes mellitus in the community. *Arch Intera Med* 2000; **160**: 2808–16.

164. Kao GT, Chan WB, Chan JC, Tsang LW, Cockram CS. Gastrointestinal symptoms in Chinese patients with type 2 diabetes mellitus. *Diabet Med* 1999; **16**: 670–74.

165. Ricci JA, Siddique R, Stewart WF, Sandler RS *et al*. Upper gastrointestinal symptoms in a US national sample of adults with diabetes. *Scand J Gastroenterol* 2000; **35**: 152–9.

166. Talley NJ, Bytzer P, Hammer J, Young L *et al*. Psychologic distress is linked to gastrointestinal symptoms in diabetes mellitus. *Am J Gastroenterol* 2001; **96**: 1033–8.

167. Stacher G. Diabetes mellitus and the stomach. *Diabetologia* 2001; **44**: 1081–93.

168. Farup CE, Leidy NY, Murray M, Williams GR *et al*. Effect of domperidone on the health-related quality of life of patients with symptoms of diabetic gastroparesis. *Diabetes Care* 1998; **21**: 1699–706.

169. Siddique R, Ricci J, Stewart WF, Sloan S, Farup C. Quality of life in a US national sample of adults with diabetes and motility-related upper gastrointestinal symptoms. *Dig Dis Sci* 2002; **47**: 683–9.

170. Lustman PJ, Frank BL, McGill JB. Relationship of personality characteristics to glucose regulation in adults with diabetes. *Psychosom Med* 1991; **53**: 305–12.

171. Jones KL, Horowitz M, Berry M, Wishart JM, Guha S. The blood glucose concentration influences postprandial fullness in insulin-dependent diabetes mellitus. *Diabetes Care* 1997; **20**: 1141–6.

172. Jebbink RJA, Bruijs PPM, Bravenboer B, Akkermans LMA *et al*. Gastric myoelectrical activity in patients with type 1 diabetes mellitus and autonomic neuropathy. *Dig Dis Sci* 1994; **39**: 2376–83.

173. Clouse RE, Lustman PJ. Gastrointestinal symptoms in diabetic patients: lack of association with neuropathy. *Am J Gastroenterol* 1989; **84**: 868–72.

174. Lingenfelser T, Sun WM, Hebbard GS, Dent J, Horowitz M. Effects of duodenal distension on antropyloroduodenal pressures and perception are modified by hyperglycemia. *Am J Physiol* 1999; **276**: G711–18.

175. Rayner CK, Smout AJ, Sun WM, Russo A *et al*. Effects of hyperglycemia on cortical response to esophageal distension in normal subjects. *Dig Dis Sci* 1999; **44**: 279–85.

176. Xia HH, Talley NJ, Kamm EPY, Young LJ *et al. Helicobacter pylori* infection is not increased or linked to upper gastrointestinal symptoms in diabetes mellitus. *Am J Gastroenterol* 2001; **96**: 1039–42.

177. Dore MP, Bilotta M, Molaty HM, Pacifico A *et al.* Diabetes mellitus and *Helicobacter pylori* infection. *Nutrition* 2000; **16**: 407–10.

178. Van der Does FE, De Neeling JN, Snoek FJ, Kostense PJ *et al.* Symptoms and well-being in relation to glycemic control in type II diabetes. *Diabetes Care* 1996; **19**: 204–10.

179. Hebbard GS, Sun WM, Bochner F, Horowitz M. Pharmacokinetic considerations in gastrointestinal motor disorders. *Clin Pharmacokinet* 1995; **28**: 41–66.

180. Groop LC, Luzi L, DeFronzo RA, Melander A. Hyperglycaemia and absorption of sulphonylurea drugs. *Lancet* 1989; **2**: 129–30.

181. American Diabetes Association. Postprandial blood glucose. *Diabetes Care* 2001; **4**: 775–8.

182. Bastyr EJ, Stuart CA, Brodows RG, Schwartz S *et al.* Therapy focused on lowering postprandial glucose, not fasting glucose, may be superior for lowering HbAlc. *Diabetes Care* 2000; **23**: 1236–41.

183. Saydah SH, Miret M, Sung J, Varas C. Postchallenge hyperglycemia and mortality in a national sample of US adults. *Diabetes Care* 2001; **24**: 1397–402.

184. Del Prato S. In search of normoglycaemia in diabetes: controlling postprandial glucose. *Int J Obesity* 2002; **26**(suppl 3): S9–17.

185. Schwartz JG, Guan D, Green GM, Phillips WT. Treatment with an oral proteinase inhibitor slows gastric emptying and acutely reduces glucose and insulin levels after a liquid meal in type II diabetic patients. *Diabetes Care* 1994; **17**: 255–62.

186. Sievenpiper JL, Jenkins DJ, Josse RG, Vuksan V. Dilution of the 75 g oral glucose tolerance test increases postprandial glycemia: implications for diagnostic criteria. *Can Med Assoc J* 2000; **162**: 993–6.

187. Ishii M, Nakamura T, Kasai F, Onuma T *et al.* Altered postprandial insulin requirement in IDDM patients with gastroparesis. *Diabetes Care* 1994; **17**: 901–3.

188. Wing RR, Blair EH, Bononi P, Marcus MD *et al.* Caloric restriction *per se* is a significant factor in improvements in glycemic control and insulin sensitivity during weight loss in obese NIDDM patients. *Diabetes Care* 1994; **17**: 30–36.

189. Pilichiewicz A, O'Donovan D, Feinle C, Lei Y *et al.* Effect of lipase inhibition on gastric emptying of, and the glycemic and incretin responses to, an oil/aqueous drink in type 2 diabetes mellitus. *J Clin Endocrinol Metab* 2003; **88**: 3829–34.

190. Ladas SD, Triantafyllou K, Tzathas C *et al.* Gastric phytobezoars may be treated by Coca-Cola lavage. *Eur J Gastroenterol Hepatol* 2002; **14**: 801–3.

191. Carney BI, Jones K, Horowitz M, Sun WM *et al.* Gastric emptying of oil and aqueous meal components in pancreatic insufficiency—effect of posture and on appetite. *Am J Physiol* 1995; **268**: G925–32.

192. Lee JS, Camilleri M, Zinsmeister AR, Burton DD *et al.* Towards office-based measurement of gastric emptying in symptomatic diabetics using ^{13}C octanoic acid breath test. *Am J Gastroenterol* 2000; **95**: 2251–61.

193. Feldman M, Smith HJ, Simon TR. Gastric emptying of solid radiopaque markers: studies in healthy subjects and diabetic patients. *Gastroenterology* 1984; **87**: 895–902.

194. Tougas G, Chen Y, Coates G, Paterson W *et al.* Standardisation of a simplified scintigraphic methodology for the assessment of gastric emptying in a multicenter setting. *Am J Gastroenterol* 2000; **95**: 78–86.

195. Camilleri M, Hasler WL, Parkman HP, Quigley EMM, Soffer E. Measurement of gastrointestinal motility in the GI laboratory. *Gastroenterology* 1998; **115**: 747–62.

196. Lartigue S, Bizais Y, Bruley des Varannes S, Murat A *et al.* Inter- and intrasubject variability of solid and liquid gastric emptying parameters—a scintigraphic study in healthy subjects and diabetic patients. *Dig Dis Sci* 1994; **39**: 109–15.

197. Jones K, Edelbroek M, Horowitz M, Sun W-M *et al.* Evaluation of antral motility in humans using manometry and scintigraphy. *Gut* 1995; **37**: 643–8.

198. Bergmann H, Minear G, Kugi A, Stacher G. Evaluation of gastric antral motility in four dimensions. *SPIE* 1994; **2359**: 724–9.

199. Braden B, Enghofer M, Schaub M, Usadel K-H *et al.* Long-term cisapride treatment improves diabetic gastroparesis but not glycaemic control. *Aliment Pharmacol Ther* 2002; **16**: 1341–6.

200. Tefera S, Gilja OH, Olafsdottir E, Hausken T *et al.* Intragastric distribution of a liquid meal in patients with reflux oesophagitis assessed by three-dimensional ultrasonography. *Gut* 2002; **50**: 153–8.

201. Mundt MW, Hausken T, Samsom M. Effect of intragastric barostat bag on proximal and distal gastric accommodation in response to liquid meal. *Am J Physiol* 2002; **283**: G681–6.

202. Marciani L, Gowland P, Spiller RC, Manoj P *et al.* Effect of meal viscosity and nutrients in satiety, intragastric dilution and emptying assessed by MRI. *Am J Physiol* 2001; **280**: G1222–33.

203. Heddle R, Dent J, Toouli J, Read NW. Topography and measurement of pyloric pressure waves and tone in humans. *Am J Physiol* 1988; **255**: G490–97.

204. Ropert A, des Varannes SB, Bizais Y, Roze C, Galmiche JP. Simultaneous assessment of liquid emptying and proximal gastric tone in humans. *Gastroenterology* 1993; **105**: 667–74.

205. Kuiken SD, Samsom M, Camilleri M, Mullan BP *et al.* Development of a test to measure gastric accommodation in humans. *Am J Physiol* 1999; **277**: G1217–21.

206. Verhagen MA, van Schelven LJ, Samsom M, Smout AM. Pitfalls in the analysis of electrogastrographic recordings. *Gastroenterology* 1999; **117**: 453–60.

207. Chandalia M, Garg A, Lutjohann D, von Bergmann K *et al.* Beneficial effects of high dietary fiber intake in patients with type 2 diabetes mellitus. *N Engl J Med* 2000; **342**: 1392–8.

208. Torsdottir I, Alpsten M, Andersson D, Brummer RJ, Andersson H. Effect of different starchy foods in composite meals on gastric emptying rate and glucose metabolism. I. Comparisons between potatoes, rice and white beans. *Hum Nutr Clin Nutr* 1984; **38**: 329–38.

209. Darwiche G, Ostman EM, Liljeberg HG, Kallinen N *et al.* Measurements of the gastric emptying rate by use of ultrasonography: studies in humans using bread with added sodium propionate. *Am J Clin Nutr* 2001; **74**: 254–8.

210. Cunningham KM, Read N. The effect of incorporating fat into different components of a meal on gastric emptying and postprandial blood glucose and insulin responses. *Br J Nutr* 1989; **61**: 285–90.

211. Welch IM, Bruce C, Hill SE, Read NW. Duodenal and ileal lipid suppresses postprandial blood glucose and insulin responses in man: possible implications for the dietary management of diabetes mellitus. *Clin Sci* 1987; **72**: 209–16.

212. Cox TE, Tyler WT, Randick A, Keln GR *et al.* Suppression of food intake, body weight and body fat by jejunal fatty acid infusions. *Am J Physiol* 2000; **278**: R604–10.

213. Trinick TR, Laker MF, Johnston DG, Keir M *et al.* Effect of guar on second-meal glucose tolerance in normal man. *Clin Sci* 1986; **71**: 49–55.

214. Ishii M, Nakamura T, Kasai F, Baba T, Takebe K. Erythromycin derivate improves gastric emptying and insulin requirement in diabetic patients with gastroparesis. *Diabetes Care* 1997; **20**: 1134–7.

215. Thompson DG, Wingate DL, Thomas M, Harrison D. Gastric emptying as a determinant of the oral glucose tolerance test. *Gastroenterology* 1982; **82**: 51–5.
216. Nyholm B, Orskov L, Hove KJ, Gravholt CH *et al.* The amylin analog pramlintide improves glycemic control and reduces postprandial glucagon concentrations in patients with type 1 diabetes mellitus. *Metabolism* 1999; **48**: 935–41.
217. Willms B, Werner J, Holst J, Orskov C *et al.* Gastric emptying, glucose response and insulin secretion after a liquid test meal: effects of exogenous glucagon-like peptide-1 (GLP-1) amide in type 2 (non-insulin dependent) diabetic patients. *J Clin Endocrinol Metab* 1996; **81**: 327–32.
218. Melga P, Mansi C, Ciuchi E, Giusti R. Chronic administration of levosulpiride and glycemic control in IDDM patients with gastroparesis. *Diabetes Care* 1997; **20**: 55–8.
219. Johansson UB, Wredling RA, Adamson UC, Lins PE. A randomised study evaluating the effects of cisapride on glucose variability and quality of life parameters in insulin-dependent diabetes mellitus patients. *Diabetes Metab* 1999; **25**: 314–19.
220. Ueno N, Inui A, Asakawa A, Takao F *et al.* Erythromycin improves glycaemic control in patients with type II diabetes mellitus. *Diabetologia* 2000; 411–5.
221. Samsom M, Szarka LA, Camilleri M, Vella A *et al.* Pramlintide, an amylin analog, selectively delays gastric emptying: potential role of vagal inhibition. *Am J Physiol* 2000; **278**: G946–51.
222. Vella A, Lee JS, Camilleri M, Szarka LA *et al.* Effects of pramlintide, an amylin analogue, on gastric emptying in type 1 and type 2 diabetes mellitus. *Neurogastroenterol Motil* 2002; **14**: 123–31.
223. Thompson RG, Pearson L, Schoenfeld SL, Kolterman OG. Pramlintide, a synthetic analog of human amylin, improves the metabolic profile of patients with type 2 diabetes using insulin. The Pramlintide in type 2 Diabetes Group. *Diabetes Care* 1998; **21**: 987–93.
224. Thompson RC, Gottlieb A, Organ K, Koda J *et al.* Pramlintide: a human amylin analogue reduced postprandial plasma glucose, insulin, and C-peptide concentrations in patients with type 2 diabetes. *Diabet Med* 1997; **14**: 547–55.
225. Ratner RE, Want LL, Fineman MS, Velte MJ *et al.* Adjunctive therapy with the amylin analogue pramlintide leads to a combined improvement in glycemic and weight control in insulin-treated subjects with type 2 diabetes. *Diabetes Technol Ther* 2002; **4**: 51–61.
226. Baron A, Kim D, Weyer C. Novel peptides under development for the treatment of type 1 and type 2 diabetes mellitus. *Curr. Drug Targets Immune Endocr Metab Disord* 2002; **2**: 63–82.
227. Gedulin BR, Young AA. Hypoglycaemia overrides amylin-mediated regulation of gastric emptying in rats. *Diabetes* 1998; **47**: 93–7.
228. Drucker DJ. Biological actions and the therapeutic potential of the glucagon-like peptides. *Gastroenterology* 2002; **122**: 531–44.
229. Nauck MA, Holst JJ, Willms B, Schmiegel W. Glucagon-like peptide 1 (GLP-1) as a new therapeutic approach for type 2 diabetes. *Exp Clin Endocrinol Diabetes* 1997; **105**: 187–95.
230. Zander M, Madsbad S, Madsen JL, Holst JJ. Effect of a 6-week course of glucagon-like peptide 1 on glycaemic control, insulin sensitivity, and β-cell function in type 2 diabetes: a parallel-group study. *Lancet* 2002; **359**: 824–30.
231. Knudsen LB, Nielsen PF, Huusfeldt PO, Johansen NL *et al.* Potent derivatives of glucagon-like peptide-1 with pharmacokinetic properties suitable for once daily administration. *J Med Chem* 2000; **43**: 1664–9.
232. Deacon CF, Knudsen LB, Madsen K, Wiberg FC *et al.* Dipeptidyl peptidase IV resistant analogues of glucagon-like peptide-1 which have extended metabolic stability and improved biological activity. *Diabetologia* 1998; **41**: 271–8.

233. Ahren B, Simonsson E, Larsson H, Landin-Olsson M *et al.* Inhibition of dipeptidyl peptidase IV improves metabolic control over a 4-week study period in type 2 diabetes. *Diabetes Care* 2002; **25**: 869–75.

234. Fineman MS, Bicsak TA, Shen LZ *et al.* Effect on glycemic control of exenatide (synthetic extendin-4) additive to existing metformin and/or sulphonylurea treatment in patients with type 2 diabetes. *Diabetes Care* 2003; **26**: 2370–7.

235. Selfarth C, Bergmann J, Holst JJ, Ritzel R *et al.* Prolonged and enhanced secretion of glucagon-like peptide 1 (7–36 amide) after oral sucrose due to α-galactosidase inhibition (acarbose) in type 2 diabetic patients. *Diabet Med* 1998; **15**: 485–91.

236. Enc FY, Imeryuz N, Akin L, Turoglu T *et al.* Inhibition of gastric emptying by acarbose is correlated with GLP-1 response and accompanied by CCK release. *Am J Physiol* 2001; **281**: G752–63.

237. Lee A, Patrick P, Wishart J, Horowitz M, Morley JE. The effects of miglitol on glucagon-like peptide-1 secretion and appetite sensations in obese type 2 diabetics. *Diabetes Obes Metab* 2002; **4**: 329–35.

238. Ranganath L, Norris F, Morgan L, Wright J, Marks V. Delayed gastric emptying occurs following acarbose administration and is a further mechanism for its antihyperglycaemic effect. *Diabet Med* 1998; **15**: 120–24.

239. Kawagishi T, Nishizawa Y, Taniwaki H, Tanaka S *et al.* Relationship between gastric emptying and α-galactosidase inhibitor effect on postprandial hyperglycemia in NIDDM patients. *Diabetes Care* 1997; **20**: 1529–32.

240. Mannucci E, Ognibene A, Cremasco F, Bardini G *et al.* Effect of metformin on glucagon-like peptide 1 (GLP-1) and leptin levels in obese non-diabetic subjects. *Diabetes Care* 2001; **24**: 489–94.

241. Kong M-F, Horowitz M, Jones KL, Wishart JM, Harding PE. Natural history of diabetic gastroparesis. *Diabetes Care* 1999; **22**: 503–7.

242. Koch KL. Diabetic gastropathy: gastric neuromuscular dysfunction in diabetes mellitus: a review of symptoms, pathophysiology and treatment. *Dig Dis Sci* 1999; **44**: 1061–75.

243. Lipp RW, Schnedl WJ, Hammer HF, Kotanko P *et al.* Effects of postprandial walking on delayed gastric emptying and intragastric meal distribuiton in longstanding diabetes. *Am J Gastroenterol* 2000; **95**: 419–24.

244. Drenth JPH, Engels LGJB. Diabetic gastroparesis—a critical appraisal of new treatment strategies. *Drugs* 1992; **44**: 537–53.

245. Snape WJ, Battle WM, Schwartz SS, Braunstein SM *et al.* Metoclopramide to treat gastroparesis due to diabetes mellitus: a double-blind controlled trial. *Ann Int Med* 1982; **96**: 444–6.

246. Talley NJ. Diabetic gastropathy and prokinetics. *Am J Gastroenterol* 2003; **98**: 264–71.

247. Janssens J, Peeters TL, Vantrappen G, Tack J *et al.* Erythromycin improves delayed gastric emptying in diabetic gastroparesis. *N Engl J Med* 1990; **322**: 1028–31.

248. Koch KL, Stern RM, Stewart WR, Vasey MW. Gastric emptying and myoelectric activity in patients with diabetic gastroparesis: effect of long-term domperidone treatment. *Am J Gastroenterol* 1988; **84**: 1069–75.

249. Briejer MR, Akkermans LMA, Schuurkes JAJ. Gastrointestinal prokinetic benzamides: the pharmacology underlying stimulations of motility. *Pharmacol Rev* 1995; **47**: 631–51.

250. Horowitz M, Maddox A, Harding PE, Maddern GJ *et al.* Effect of cisapride on gastric and esophageal emptying in insulin-dependent diabetes mellitus. *Gastroenterology* 1987; **92**: 1899–907.

251. Horowitz M, Harding PE, Chatterton BE, Collins PJ, Shearman DJC. Acute and chronic effect of domperidone on gastric emptying in diabetic autonomic neuropathy. *Dig Dis Sci* 1985; **30**: 1–9.

252. Soykan I, Sarosiek I, MacCallum RW. The effect of chronic oral domperidone therapy on gastrointestinal symptoms, gastric emptying, and quality of life in patients with gastroparesis. *Am J Gastroenterol* 1997; **92**: 979–80.

253. Silvers D, Kipnes M, Broadstone V, Patterson D *et al*. Domperidone in the management of diabetic gastroparesis: efficacy, tolerability and quality of life outcomes in a multicenter controlled trial. *Clin Therap* 1998; **20**: 438–53.

254. Jones KL, Horowitz M, Carney BI, Sun WM, Chatterton BE. Effects of cisapride on gastric emptying of oil and aqueous meal components, hunger and fullness. *Gut* 1996; **38**: 310–15.

255. Schade RR, Dugas MC, Lhotsky DM, Gavaler J, van Thiel DH. Effect of metoclopramide on gastric liquid emptying in patients with diabetic gastroparesis. *Dig Dis Sci* 1985; **30**: 10–15.

256. Maganti K, Onyemere K, Jones MP. Oral erythromycin and symptomatic relief of gastroparesis: a systematic review. *Am J Gastroenterol* 2003; **98**: 259–63.

257. Coulie B, Tack J, Peeters T, Janssens J. Involvement of two different pathways in the motor effects of erythromycin on the gastric antrum in humans. *Gut* 1998; **43**: 395–400.

258. Di Baise JK, Quigley EMM. Efficacy of long-term intravenous erythromycin in the management of severe gastroparesis: one center's experience. *J Clin Gastroenterol* 1999; **28**: 131–4.

259. Ehrenpreis ED, Zaitman D, Nellans H. Which form of erythromycin should be used to treat gastroparesis? A pharmacokinetic analysis. *Aliment Pharmacol Ther* 1998; **12**: 373–76.

260. Edelbroek M, Horowitz M, Wishart JM, Akkermans LMA. Effect of erythromycin on gastric emptying, alcohol absorption and small intestinal transit in normal subjects. *J Nucl Med* 1993; **34**: 582–8.

261. Jones KL, Berry M, Kong M-F, Kwiatek MA *et al*. Hyperglycaemia attenuates the gastrokinetic effect of erythromycin and affects the perception of postprandial hunger in normal subjects. *Diabetes Care* 1999; **22**: 339–44.

262. Petrakis IE, Kogerakis N, Prokopakis G, Zacharioudakis G *et al*. Hyperglycaemia attenuates erythromycin-induced acceleration of liquid-phase gastric emptying of hypertonic liquids in healthy subjects. *Dig Dis Sci* 2002; **47**: 67–72.

263. Petrakis IE, Chalkiadakis G, Vrachassotakis N, Sciacca V *et al*. Induced hyperglycemia attentuates erythromcyin-induced acceleration of hypertonic liquid-phase gastric emptying in type 1 diabetic patients. *Dig Dis* 1999; **17**: 241–7.

264. Petrakis IE, Vrachassotakis N, Sciacca V, Vassilakis SI, Chalkiadakis G. Hyperglycaemia attenuates erythromycin-induced acceleration of solid-phase gastric emptying in idiopathic and diabetic gastroparesis. *Scand J Gastroenterol* 1999; **34**: 396–403.

265. Horowitz M, Jones KL, Harding PE, Wishart JM. Relationship between the effects of cisapride on gastric emptying and plasma glucose concentrations in diabetic gastroparesis. *Digestion* 2002; **65**: 41–6.

266. Havelund T, Oster-Jorgensen E, Eshoj O, Larsen ML, Lauritsen K. Effects of cisapride on gastroparesis in patients with insulin-dependent diabetes mellitus. A double-blind controlled trial. *Acta Med Scand* 1987; **222**: 339–43.

267. De Caestecker JS, Ewing DJ, Tothill P, Clarke BF, Heading RC. Evaluation of oral cisapride and metoclopramide in diabetic autonomic neuropathy: an eight-week double-blind cross-over study. *Aliment Pharmacol Ther* 1989; **3**: 69–81.

268. Camilleri M, Malagelada J-R, Abell TL, Brown HL *et al*. Effect of six weeks of treatment with cisapride in gastroparesis and intestinal pseudoobstruction. *Gastroenterology* 1989; **96**: 704–12.

269. Abell TL, Camilleri M, Di Magno EP, Hench VS. Long-term efficacy of oral cisapride in symptomatic upper gut dysmotility. *Dig Dis Sci* 1991; **36**: 621–6.

270. Tonini M, De Ponti F, Di Nucci A, Crema F. Review article: cardiac adverse effects of gastrointestinal prokinetics. *Aliment Pharmacol Ther* 1999; **13**: 1585–91.

271. Evans AJ, Krentz AJ. Should cisapride be avoided in patients with diabetic gastroparesis. *J Diabetes Complications* 1999; **13**: 314–15.

272. McHugh S, Lico S, Diamant NE. Cisapride vs metoclopramide. An acute study in diabetic gastroparesis. *Dig Dis Sci* 1992; **37**: 997–1001.

273. Lata PF, Pigarelli DL. Chronic metoclopramide therapy for diabetic gastroparesis. *Dig Dis Sci* 1992; **37**: 122–6.

274. Franzese A, Borelli O, Corrado G, Rea P *et al*. Domperidone may be more effective than cisapride in children with diabetic gastroparesis. *Aliment Pharmacol Ther* 2002; **16**: 951–7.

275. Gentilcore D, O'Donovan D, Jones KL, Horowitz M. Nutrition therapy for diabetic gastroparesis. *Curr Diabetes Rep* 3: 418–26.

276. Yamashita S, Yamaguchi H, Sakaguchi M, Satsumae T *et al*. Longer-term diabetic patients have a more frequent incidence of nosocomial infections after elective gastrectomy. *Anesthet Analges* 2000; **91**: 1176–81.

277. Watkins PJ, Buxton–Thomas MS, Howard ER. Long-term outcome after gastrectomy for diabetic gastroparesis *Diabet Med* 2003; **20**: 58–63.

278. Degen L, Matzinger D, Merz M, Appel-Dingemanse S *et al*. Tegaserod, a 5-HT$_4$ receptor partial agonist, accelerates gastric emptying and gastrointestinal transit in healthy male subjects. *Aliment Pharmacol Ther* 2001; **15**: 1745–51.

279. Jones KL, Wishart JM, Berry MK, Abitbol J-L, Horowitz M. Effects of fedotozine on gastric emptying and upper gastrointestinal symptoms in diabetic gastroparesis. *Aliment Pharmacol Ther* 2000; **14**: 937–43.

280. Tack J, Piessevaux H, Coulie B, Caenepeel P, Janssens J. Role of impaired gastric accommodation to a meal in functional dyspepsia. *Gastroenterology* 1998; **115**: 1346–52.

281. Rosa-e-Silva L, Troncon LEA, Oliveira RB, Iazigi N *et al*. Treatment of diabetic gastroparesis with oral clonidine. *Aliment Pharmacol Ther* 1995; **9**: 179–83.

282. Thumshirn M, Camilleri M, Choi M-G, Zinsmeister AR. Modulation of gastric sensory and motor functions by nitrergic and α_2-adrenergic agents in humans. *Gastroenterology* 1999; **116**: 573–85.

283. Huilgol V, Evans J, Hellman RS, Soergel KH. Acute effect of clonidine on gastric emptying in patients with diabetic gastropathy and controls. *Aliment Pharmacol Ther* 2002; **16**: 945–50.

284. Talley NJ, Verlinden M, McCallum R *et al*. Efficacy of a motilin receptor agonist (ABT-229) for relief of dyspepsia in type 1 diabetes mellitus: a randomised double-blind placebo controlled trial. *Gut* 2001; **49**: 395–401.

285. Ezzeddine D, Jit R, Katz N, Gopalswamy N, Bhutani MS. Pyloric injection of botulinum toxin for treatment of diabetic gastroparesis. *Gastrointest Endosc* 2002; **55**: 920–23.

286. Tougas G, Huizinga JD. Gastric pacing as a treatment for intractable gastroparesis—shocking news? *Gastroenterology* 1998; **114**: 598–601.

287. McCallum RW, Chen JDZ, Lin Z, Schirmer BD *et al*. Gastric pacing improves emptying and symptoms in patients with gastroparesis. *Gastroenterology* 1998; **114**: 456–61.

288. Abell T, McCallum R, Hocking M, Koch K *et al*. Gastric electrical stimulation for medically refractory gastroparesis. *Gastroenterology* 2003; **125**: 421–8.

289. Moore JG, Wolfe M. The relation of plasma gastrin to the circadian rhythm of gastric acid secretion in man. *Digestion* 1973; **9**: 97–105.

290. Farrell JL. Contribution to the physiology of gastric acid secretion. The vagi as the sole efferent pathway of the cephalic phase of gastric acid secretion. *Am J Physiol* 1928; **85**: 685.

291. Tepperman BL, Walsh JH, Preshaw RM. Effect of antral denervation on gastrin release by sham feeding and insulin hypoglycemia in dogs. *Gastroenterology* 1972; **63**: 973–80.

292. Feldman M, Richardson CT. Role of thought, sight, smell, and taste of food in the cephalic phase of gastric acid secretion in humans. *Gastroenterology* 1986; **90**: 428–33.

293. Cotrim E, Zaterka S, Walsh J. Acid secretion and serum gastrin at graded intragastric pressures in man. *Gastroenterology* 1977; **72**: 676–679.

294. Konturek SJ, Kaess H, Kwiecien N, Radecki T *et al*. Characteristics of intestinal phase of gastric secretion. *Am J Physiol* 1976; **230**: 335–40.

295. Isenberg JI, Ippoliti AF, Maxwell VL. Perfusion of the proximal small intestine with peptone stimulates gastric acid secretion in man. *Gastroenterology* 1977; **73**: 746–752.

296. Langer L. Pentagastrin- and insulin-induced secretion in diabetes mellitus. *Acta Med Scan* 1972; **191**: 471–5.

297. Feldman M, Corbett DB, Ramsey EJ, Walsh JH, Richardson CT. Abnormal gastric function in longstanding, insulin-dependent diabetic patients. *Gastroenterology* 1979; **77**: 12–17.

298. Nakamura T, Takebe K, Imamura K, Miyazawa T *et al*. Decreased gastric secretory functions in diabetic patients with autonomic neuropathy. *Tohoku J Exp Med* 1994; **173**: 199–208.

299. Rabinowitch IM, Fowler AF, Watson BA. Gastric acidity in diabetes mellitus: its clinical significance based on study of one hundred cases. *Arch Int Med* 1931; **47**: 384–90.

300. Dotevall G, Fagerberg SE, Langer L, Walen A. Vagal function in patients with diabetic neuropathy. *Acta Med Scand* 1972; **191**: 21–24.

301. Tashima K, Nishijima M, Fujita A, Kubomi M, Takeuchi K. Acid secretory changes in streptozotocin-diabetic rats: different responses to various secretagogues. *Dig Dis Sci* 2000; **45**: 1352–8.

302. Baydoun R, Dunbar JC. Impaired insulin but normal pentagastrin effect on gastric acid secretion in diabetic rats: a role for nitric oxide. *Diabetes Res Clin Pract* 1997; **38**: 1–8.

303. Hersey SJ, Sachs G. Gastric acid secretion. *Physiol Rev* 1995; **75**: 155–89.

304. Ozcelikay AT, Altan VM, Yildizoglu-Ari N, Altinkurt O *et al*. Basal and histamine-induced gastric acid secretion in alloxan diabetic rats. *Gen Pharmacol* 1993; **24**: 121–6.

305. Quatrini M, Boarino V, Ghidoni A, Baldassarri AR *et al*. *Helicobacter pylori* prevalence in patients with diabetes and its relationship to dyspeptic symptoms. *J Clin Gastroenterol* 2001; **32**: 215–17.

306. Oldenburg B, Diepersloot RJ, Hoekstra JB. High seroprevalence of *Helicobacter pylori* in diabetes mellitus patients. *Dig Dis Sci* 1996; **41**: 458–61.

307. Persico M, Suozzo R, De Seta M, Montella F. Non-ulcer dyspepsia and *Helicobacter pylori* in type 2 diabetic patients: association with autonomic neuropathy. *Diabetes Res Clin Pract* 1996; **31**: 87–92.

308. Gasbarrini A, Ojetti V, Pitocco D, De Luca A *et al*. *Helicobacter pylori* infection in patients affected by insulin-dependent diabetes mellitus. *Eur J Gastroenterol Hepatol* 1998; **10**: 469–72.

309. Guvener N, Akcan Y, Paksoy I, Soylu AR *et al*. *Helicobacter pylori*-associated gastric pathology in patients with type II diabetes mellitus and its relationship with gastric emptying: the Ankara study. *Exp Clin Endocrinol Diabetes* 1999; **107**: 172–6.

310. Gasbarrini A, Ojetti V, Pitocco D, Franceschi F *et al*. Insulin-dependent diabetes mellitus affects eradication rate of *Helicobacter pylori* infection. *Eur J Gastroenterol Hepatol* 1999; **11**: 713–16.

311. Graham DY, Lew GM, Klein PD, Evans DG *et al*. Effect of treatment of *Helicobacter pylori* infection on the long-term recurrence of gastric or duodenal ulcer. A randomised, controlled study. *Ann Intern Med* 1992; **116**: 705–8.

312. Rauws EA, Tytgat GN. Cure of duodenal ulcer associated with eradication of *Helicobacter pylori*. *Lancet* 1990; **335**: 1233–5.

313. Weil J, Langman MJ, Wainwright P, Lawson DH *et al*. Peptic ulcer bleeding: accessory risk factors and interactions with non-steroidal anti-inflammatory drugs. *Gut* 2000; **46**: 27–31.

314. Pietzsch M, Theuer S, Haase G, Plath F *et al*. Results of a systematic screening for serious gastrointestinal bleeding associated with NSAIDS in Rostock hopsitals. *Int J Clin Pharmacol Ther* 2002; **40**: 111–15.

315. Rostom A, Wells G, Tugwell P, Welch V *et al*. The prevention of chronic NSAID-induced upper gastrointestinal toxicity: a Cochrane collaboration meta-analysis of randomised controlled trials. *J Rheumatol* 2000; **27**: 2203–14.

316. Eisenbarth GS. Type 1 diabetes mellitus: a chronic autoimmune disease. *N Engl J Med* 1986; **314**: 1360–68.

317. Drell DW, Notkins AL. Multiple immunological abnormalities in patients with type 1 (insulin-dependent) diabetes mellitus. *Diabetologia* 1987; **30**: 132–43.

318. Neufeld M, Maclaren NK, Riley WJ *et al*. Islet cell and other organ-specific antibodies in US Caucasians and Blacks with insulin-dependent diabetes mellitus. *Diabetes* 1980; **29**: 589–92.

319. Betterle C, Zanette F, Pedini B *et al*. Clinical and subclinical organ-specific autoimmune manifestations in type 1 (insulin-dependent) diabetic patients and their first-degree relatives. *Diabetologia* 1984; **26**: 431–36.

320. Riley WJ, Toskes PP, Maclaren NK, Silverstein J. Predictive value of gastric parietal cell autoantibodies as a marker for gastric and hematologic abnormalities associated with insulin-dependent diabetes. *Diabetes* 1982; **31**: 1051–5.

321. Ungar B, Stocks AE, Whittingham S, Martin FIR, Mackay IR. Intrinsic factor antibody, parietal cell antibody, and latent pernicious anaemia in diabetes mellitus. *Lancet* 1968; **2**: 415–17.

322. Vanderkam SG, De Leeuw IH. Insuline dependente diabetes mellitus in associatie met auto-immuun geïnduceerde thyreoiditis en gastritis. *Tijdschr Geneeskunde* 1992; **48**: 925–8.

323. De Block CE, De Leeuw IH, Van Gaal LF. High prevalence of manifestations of gastric autoimmunity in parietal cell antibody-positive type 1 (insulin-dependent) diabetic patients. The Belgian Diabetes Registry. *J Clin Endocrinol Metab* 1999; **84**: 4062–7.

324. Markson JL, Moore JM. 'Autoimmunity' in pernicious anemia and iron deficiency anemia. *Lancet* 1962; **2**: 1240.

325. Shearman DJC, Delamore JW, Gardner DL. Gastric function and structure in iron deficiency anemia. *Lancet* 1966; **1**: 845–8.

326. Burman P, Mardh S, Norberg L, Karlsson FA. Parietal cell antibodies in pernicious anemia inhibit H^+/K^+-adenosine triphosphatase, the proton pump of the stomach. *Gastroenterology* 1989; **96**: 1434–8.

327. Kokkonen J. Parietal cell antibodies and gastric secretion in children with diabetes mellitus. *Acta Paediatr Scand* 1980; **69**: 485–489.

328. Davis RE, McCann VJ, Stanton KG. Type 1 diabetes and latent pernicious anaemia. *Med J Aust* 1992; **156**: 160–62.

329. Munichoodappa C, Kozak GP. Diabetes mellitus and pernicious anemia. *Diabetes* 1970; **19**: 719–22.

330. Dallman PR. Manifestations of iron deficiency. *Semin Hematol* 1982; **19**: 19–30.

331. Cook JD. Clinical evaluation of iron deficiency. *Semin Hematol* 1982; **19**: 6–18.

332. Toh BH, Van Driel IR, Gleeson PA. Mechanisms of disease: pernicious anemia. *N Engl J Med* 1997; **337**: 1441–8.
333. Brinton LA, Gridley G, Hrubec Z, Hoover R, Fraumeni JF Jr. Cancer risk following pernicious anaemia. *Br J Cancer* 1989; **59**: 810–13.
334. Holm M, Perry MA. Role of blood flow in gastric acid secretion. *Am J Physiol* 1988; **254**: 281–6.
335. Furness JB. The adrenergic innervation of the vessels supplying and draining the gastrointestinal tract. *Z. Zellforsch* 1983; **85**: 529–34.

5

Intestinal Function

Melvin Samsom and Mark A. M. T. Verhagen

Prevalence and epidemiology

The major functions of the small intestine are to digest and absorb nutrients, while those of the large bowel are to extract water and process faeces before expulsion. Diabetes mellitus may be associated with both small intestinal and colonic dysfunction, potentially resulting in a wide range of clinical manifestations, including gastrointestinal symptoms, poor nutritional status and impaired glycaemic control. Evaluation of intestinal dysfunction often necessitates the use of sophisticated techniques, the availability of which is limited to specialised centres. Hence it is not surprising that the majority of studies relating to intestinal function in diabetes have to date involved relatively small numbers of patients. The prevalence of small intestinal and colonic dysfunction in diabetes has not been formally evaluated and remains uncertain. However, small intestinal motor abnormalities are evident in about 80% of patients with diabetic gastroparesis,

Gastrointestinal Function in Diabetes Mellitus.   Edited by Michael Horowitz and Melvin Samsom
© 2004 John Wiley & Sons, Ltd   ISBN: 0-471-89916-X

suggesting that the prevalence of intestinal dysmotility is likely to be comparable to the prevalence of gastroparesis in diabetic patients, i.e. 30–50% of unselected patients [1–6].

This chapter includes an overview of the effects of diabetes on small intestinal and colonic motor, sensory, absorptive and vascular function. The clinical sequelae, including the association of diabetes mellitus with coeliac disease, potential diagnostic techniques and the treatment of disordered intestinal function in diabetes, are discussed.

Gastrointestinal symptoms have been used to evaluate the prevalence of intestinal dysfunction in diabetes. However, it should be recognised that symptoms resulting from intestinal dysfunction are not cause-specific and are heterogeneous, potentially giving rise to diverse complaints, including anorexia, nausea, vomiting, constipation, diarrhoea and abdominal pain or discomfort. Furthermore, the type and severity of gastrointestinal symptoms in patients with diabetes mellitus has been shown to vary over time [7]. Both upper and lower gastrointestinal symptoms may also be related to dysfunction of other parts of the digestive tract, especially the stomach and gallbladder.

While the aforementioned limitations of symptom-based studies must be taken into account, it should be recognised that population-based studies provide persuasive evidence that dyspeptic and bowel symptoms occur more frequently in patients with diabetes mellitus, although the increase in prevalence seems to be modest [8–10]. A comprehensive discussion of these studies can be found in Chapter 1.

At present, population-based studies investigating the underlying mechanisms involved in the aetiology of gastrointestinal symptoms in diabetes mellitus are required. Although there is evidence that gastrointestinal dysmotility, increased visceral perception and psychological disorders play a role in the aetiology of gastrointestinal symptoms in diabetes, no studies have focused on the origin of these symptoms in the diabetic population; this information is likely to be fundamental to an improved understanding of prognosis, quality of life and therapy.

Clinical assessment of small intestinal and colonic function

In the last two decades a number of techniques have been developed that allow a comprehensive assessment of small intestinal and colonic function. Several of these techniques are widely available; others can only be performed in specialised centres. At present, assessment of small intestinal and colonic motility and bacterial overgrowth have clinical indications and consequences. Although several techniques are available to measure absorptive function of the small intestine, this will not be discussed, since they currently lack clinical indications.

The main indications for small intestinal manometry and transit studies in diabetic patients are summarised in Table 5.1. Currently, manometry of the colon

Table 5.1 Indications for small intestinal manometry and colonic transit studies in diabetes mellitus

---

Indications for manometry

    Unexplained nausea and vomiting, associated with normal gastric emptying

    To exclude or confirm a more generalised gastrointestinal motor/transit disorder in diabetic patients with gastroparesis

    To exclude or confirm a more generalised gastrointestinal motor/transit disorder in diabetic patients with intractable constipation or diarrhoea

    To distinguish neuropathic from myopathic motility patterns in diabetic patients with documented small bowel stasis (only by small intestinal manometry)

Indications for colonic transit studies

    To exclude or confirm disordered colonic transit in patients with complaints of constipation or diarrhoea

    To exclude or confirm a more generalised gastrointestinal motor/transit disorder in diabetic patients with gastroparesis

---

is not yet considered to be of clinical use, although it has been shown to be a useful tool in a research setting, especially in investigating the motor dysfunctions underlying disordered colonic transit and the mode of action of potential prokinetic drugs [11–13].

Small and large intestinal manometry

Initially, small intestinal manometry was performed using water-perfused systems in a stationary setting [14]. More recently, solid-state catheters have been developed and water-perfused systems refined allowing high-resolution manometry to be performed in ambulatory settings [15,16]. Typically, stationary manometry is performed for 6 h, including a 3 h fasting period and a 3 h postprandial period [17]. In an ambulatory setting several standardised meals can be ingested and interdigestive motility recorded overnight. The latter is particularly important when stationary manometry does not show a complete MMC cycle [18].

Small intestinal motility is considered to be normal when at least one migrating motor complex (MMC) per 24 h is observed, a conversion to the fed motor pattern is seen for at least 2 h after a 1600 kJ meal [19], small intestinal contractions exceed 20 mmHg, and there is no excess of patterns such as 'short' and 'long' bursts. So-called 'neuropathic' motility features, which are frequently observed in diabetes, consist of early recurrence of phase III after a meal, propagating or non-propagating short and long bursts and abnormal propagation of interdigestive phase III activity fronts, and absence of phase III activity. 'Myopathic' motility features, characterised by low-amplitude contractions (<20 mmHg), are less common in diabetes [20].

Scintigraphic assessment of small intestinal and colonic transit

Scintigraphic studies of the small intestine and colon require a large field-of-view gamma camera with a dedicated computer for analysis, which are now widely available [21]. The most commonly used isotopes are ^{99m}technetium (^{99m}Tc) and ^{111}indium (^{111}In). Since the half-life ($t_{1/2}$) of ^{99m}Tc is 6 h, ^{111}In ($t_{1/2}$ approximately 64 h) is employed most frequently to evaluate colonic transit. The radioactive label may be incorporated in a liquid or solid meal, since small bowel transit times of solids and liquids are similar [22]. Small intestinal transit time is estimated by taking the time that elapses between emptying a radiolabelled meal from the stomach and the arrival of radiolabelled chyme in the right colon, and may vary between approximately 80 and 250 min [23,24].

There are several mathematical models that allow calculation of the total small intestinal transit time without providing information about regional transit. The model that is most frequently applied to estimate small bowel transit time was developed by Malagelada and Camilleri; it estimates small intestinal transit time by taking the time at which 10% of a ^{99m}Tc-labelled meal has entered the colon, minus the lag time [22,25–27]. Ileocolonic transit of chyme is characterised by intermittent bolus transfer. The large variation observed in small intestinal transit times may therefore at least in part be caused by transit in the ileocolonic region [28].

The radioactive label ^{111}In may be bound to 0.7 mm resin microspheres or incorporated in a slow-release capsule which allows accurate determination of colon transit, including information about transit through different regions of the colon [29–31]. Scans taken at 4 and 24 h using this technique provide accurate information about total and regional transit times and make the test relatively easy to use [31]. In contrast to transit through the small intestine, calculation of regional transit times in the colon is feasible, although the clinical relevance of such measurements is still uncertain. Regional colonic transit can be estimated by calculation of the geometric centre, which is the weighted average of counts in the different regions of the colon (ascending, transverse, descending, recto-sigmoid) and stool [26] (Figure 5.1).

Radiographic assessment of small intestinal and colonic transit

The most convenient way to assess colonic transit is by using radio-opaque markers [32,33]. In the 'classical' test developed by Hinton and co-workers, slow transit constipation is diagnosed when an abdominal radiograph shows that more than 80% of the markers are retained the colon after 96 h [32]. Metcalf et al. modified the transit test slightly by using 20 markers given on 3 consecutive days [33]. The abdominal radiograph taken on day 4 is divided into three regions and the location of the pellets provides information about regional transit.

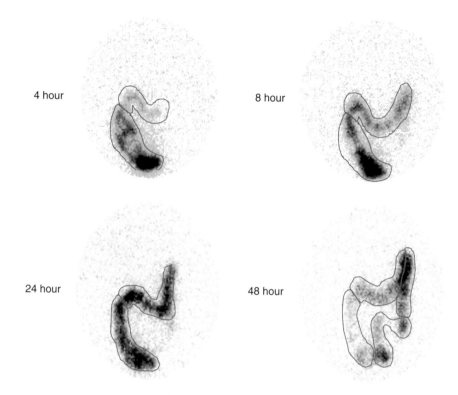

Figure 5.1   Measurement of colonic transit using ^{111}In incorporated in a slow-release capsule. Scintigraphic images were acquired at 4, 8, 24 and 48 h after ingestion of the ^{111}In capsule. The geometric centre is defined as the weighted average of counts in the different regions of the colon [ascending (AC), transverse (TC), descending (DC), rectosigmoid (RS) and stool, 1–5, respectively]. At any time, the proportion of colonic counts in each colonic region is multiplied by its weighting factor using the formula:

$$\text{Geometric Centre} = (\%AC \times 1 + \%TC \times 2 + \%DC \times 3 + \%RS \times 4 + \%\text{Stool} \times 4)/100$$

Although techniques involving radioactive isotopes currently have limited, if any, additional value over pellets when total transit time is taken as the clinical meaningful endpoint, radiographic techniques are likely to be less accurate in calculating regional transit times [29]. The calculation of regional transit times may be of importance when drugs become available that affect colonic transit in one region of the colon more than in another [34–36].

Hydrogen breath test

The use of the hydrogen breath test to evaluate small intestinal transit is based on the fact that some carbohydrates are not absorbed in the small intestine [37–39] and colonic bacteria rapidly ferment these unabsorbed carbohydrates, resulting in the production of gaseous hydrogen. Hydrogen is rapidly absorbed in the intestine and exhaled, so that there is a prompt increase in breath hydrogen once the substrate is fermented.

Measurements of orocaecal transit time usually employ the non-absorbable carbohydrate, lactulose. An increase of hydrogen in breath samples, which are typically obtained every 10–15 min, to a level of ≥ 20 ppm after a lactulose dose of 10 g is indicative of the arrival of the substrate at the right colon. Disadvantages of the hydrogen breath test with respect to scintigraphic methods are: the inability to quantify gastric emptying, which may influence oral–caecal transit; interference by small bowel bacterial overgrowth, which causes a false, 'early' peak in breath hydrogen; and the potential effect of lactulose to accelerate small intestinal transit [38,39].

Glucose is used as a substrate when bacterial overgrowth is suspected [40]. Some patients with bacterial overgrowth have an elevated fasting breath hydrogen. The combination of a high fasting breath hydrogen excretion and an increase of breath hydrogen above 20 ppm after 50 g glucose challenge provides an accurate diagnosis of bacterial overgrowth in about 50% of patients, when compared to the gold standard of jejunal culture [40,41]. One of the pitfalls is that glucose malabsorption may be associated with rapid small bowel transit, resulting in a false-positive outcome of the test [42].

Physiology and pathophysiology of small intestinal and colonic motor function

Small intestinal motor function

After meal ingestion, food is initially stored in the proximal stomach, then triturated in the distal stomach, and finally transported to the small intestine, predominantly as a series of gushes. The major functions of the small intestine are to mix and propel food particles in order to optimise intraluminal digestion and absorption. Those food particles that escape absorption, as well as indigestible solids, are transported to the colon, where water is extracted and faeces processed before expulsion. The motility patterns of the small intestine and colon are designed to efficiently serve these functions of controlled mixing and transport.

When the small intestine is not exposed to nutrients, it exhibits a cyclic pattern of motility (as is the case with the stomach, Chapter 4), termed the migrating motor complex (MMC). The MMC consists of three subsequent phases [43–45]; phase I (about 30 min in duration) is a period of motor quiescence, followed by a period of irregular contractile activity (phase II; about 50 min), culminating in phase III (about 10 min), during which the intestine contracts at its maximum rate (11 or 12 contractions/min in the duodenum and 7 or 8 contractions/min in the ileum). Phase III activity starts in the distal antrum of the proximal intestine and propagates slowly towards the distal ileum. During both phases II and III of the MMC, undigested food particles, enterocytes and bacteria are propelled towards the colon, the so-called 'intestinal housekeeper' function. The length of the MMC cycle shows considerable interindividual and intraindividual variation, but is on average between 80 and 120 min [45–48].

Meal ingestion interrupts the interdigestive motor pattern and induces irregular contractions, resembling phase II. The duration of the postprandial period in the small intestine is dependent on the rate of transport of chyme through the small intestine. The end of the postprandial period is marked by an episode of phase III of the MMC. Small intestinal transit time may vary considerably as a result of the variations in small intestinal motility. Postprandial small intestinal motor activity and transit are influenced by the caloric value and composition of the meal [49].

Studies using ultrasound and Doppler techniques have shown that flow of chyme across the pylorus and the upper part of the duodenum is not unidirectional but to-and-fro, which is likely to optimise the exposure of nutrients to digestive enzymes and the mucosal surface where nutrient-sensing cells that regulate gastric emptying and local motor activity are located [50,51].

Detailed manometric studies have provided insights into the motor correlates of the flow of chyme in the jejunum [45,52,53]—about 50% of all contractions propagate over a distance of less than 1 cm and are responsible for the oral and aboral movement of chyme over short distances. Small intestinal contractions that propagate over longer distances facilitate flow in the aboral direction [52] (Figure 5.2). Flow in the jejunum is typically linear, as a result of the organisation of contractions [54]. This is in contrast to the more pulsatile pattern of flow seen across the ileocaecal valve [28].

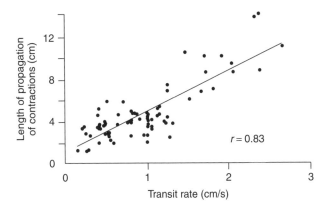

Figure 5.2   Relation between the small intestinal transit and the propagation length of contractions. The rate of transit is highly dependent on the organisation of small intestinal contractions. From Schemann and Ehrlein [52], with permission

Colonic motor function

The major function of the colon is to absorb water and electrolytes in order to concentrate and solidify the intraluminal content. Colonic motility plays an important role in these processes. In contrast to small intestinal motility, colonic motility follows a diurnal rhythm, with relative motor quiescence during sleep [55,56]. The most easily recognisable colonic motor events are high-amplitude peristaltic contractions (HAPCs), which occur infrequently and characteristically after awakening and sometimes in the late postprandial period [55–57]. The HAPCs are propagated aborally over long distances and are responsible for mass movements of faeces in the human colon [55–57].

When HAPCs are not present, colonic motor activity seems disorganised with predominately non-propagating contractions in the colon. These contractions lead to mixing of colonic contents, rather than to propulsion. After meal ingestion, an increase in these segmental contractions occurs as a result of the gastrocolonic reflex [55,56,58,59]. The magnitude of the colonic motor response is dependent on both meal composition and the region of the colon [58,59]. Apart from the effect of a meal on phasic contractile activity, chemical and mechanical stimulation of the upper gut also induces an increase in colonic tone [60,61].

Regulation of intestinal motor function

Transit and absorption of intestinal contents are regulated by the autonomic and enteric nervous systems. The extrinsic nervous system innervates the intestine with sympathetic nerves arising from cell bodies located in the dorsal horn of the spinal cord, which synapse in the coeliac, superior and inferior mesenteric ganglia [62,63]. From these ganglia, postganglionic nerve fibres run with the mesenteric arteries to the colon. The sympathetic input is generally inhibitory to smooth muscle, with the exception of sphincters, to which the input is excitatory. Sympathetic afferent fibres have their cell bodies in the dorsal root ganglia and from these ganglia sensory input reaches the brain via the spinothalamic tract and the reticular formation.

The parasympathetic fibres arising from the dorsal motor nucleus of the vagus supply the small intestine and proximal colon, whereas the distal colon is innervated by parasympathetic efferent nerve fibres from the sacral plexus [62,63]. The parasympathetic nerves innervate the colon muscle with both excitatory enteric, cholinergic nerves and inhibitory non-adrenergic, non-cholinergic (NANC) neurons. Both sympathetic and parasympathetic nerves give input to the enteric nervous system, which consists of two interconnected plexuses, the myenteric and the submucosal plexuses [62,63]. Numerous neuropeptides have been shown to play an important role in controlling the smooth muscle function of the small intestine and colon, e.g. VIP, CCK, CGRP, HT, NO and ENK [63].

Recently, the so-called interstitial cells of Cajal have been identified in the gastrointestinal tract [64–66] and appear to be responsible for the generation of the slow wave activity present in the entire gastrointestinal tract. They are localised to the interface of the circular and longitudinal muscle layer, in close association with the myenteric plexus. The interplay between the enteric nervous system and the interstitial cells of Cajal is essential for normal gut motility.

Although the extrinsic nerves are of importance for fine-tuning postprandial motility [67], the local reflexes within the enteric plexus are indispensable for transport of the intraluminal contents. The local reflexes induce contraction orad to the chyme bolus through excitatory neurotransmitters, such as acetylcholine and substance P, and caudal relaxation through inhibitory neurotransmitters, including vasoactive intestinal peptide and nitric oxide.

The regulation of interdigestive motility involves both extrinsic and enteric neuronal pathways. The extrinsic innervation serves more as a modulator than an initiator of fasting motility [68–70]. Both cholinergic and non-cholinergic pathways are involved in the regulation of the periodicity of the MMC [68,70]. Cholinergic input is essential for the propagation of the MMC, while adrenergic input is involved in the organisation the MMC periodicity [69].

Many gastrointestinal hormones, including somatostatin, secretin, motilin, cholecystokinin and glucose-dependent insulinotropic peptide, are involved in the regulation of both the postprandial and interdigestive motility of the small intestine and colon [71–73]. The endocrine cells responsible for the synthesis of these hormones are scattered among the epithelial cells in the gut and are in close contact with the environment (gut lumen) and the intrinsic and extrinsic nervous systems. Gastrointestinal hormones may also act as neurotransmitters, since they are able to bind to specific receptors located on peptidergic neurons. These neurons are abundantly present in the gut wall and are predominantly of intrinsic origin. Although many of these gastrointestinal hormones or neuropeptides are under investigation, the roles of motilin and cholecystokinin are of particular interest.

Motilin is produced predominantly in the upper part of the small intestine and its release is temporally associated with phase III of antral origin [44,71]. Exogenous motilin has been shown to induce phase III activity, while antibodies to motilin lead to total abolition of phase III; accordingly, it is likely that motilin plays an important role in the periodicity of phase III of the MMC [74]. Cholecystokinin (CCK) seems to be of greater importance in the fed state [75,76]. CCK, which increases more than a five-fold after a meal, interrupts the interdigestive motor pattern and induces an small intestinal contractile activity [77].

Small intestinal and colonic dysmotility in diabetes mellitus

Studies evaluating small intestinal, and especially colonic, motility in diabetes mellitus are limited and the outcomes inconclusive [78–87]. The discrepant observations are at least partially due to the lack of stabilisation of blood glucose concentration during the tests, and the relatively small numbers of patients studied. Furthermore, the variety and insensitivity of techniques that have been applied in cross-sectional studies make comparison and interpretation of the data difficult. True population-based studies and/or longitudinal studies are still lacking; hence the natural history and relation to symptoms and other diabetic complications of small intestinal and colonic dysmotility remain to be determined.

Small intestinal dysmotility

Studies that have investigated small intestinal motility in diabetes mellitus have revealed a wide spectrum of motor patterns, ranging from normal to grossly abnormal motility, as observed in patients with chronic intestinal pseudo-obstruction syndrome secondary to diabetes mellitus.

Camilleri and Malagelada reported that small intestinal motility was abnormal in 80% of patients with long-standing diabetes who had delayed gastric emptying [5]. While these observations suggest that small intestinal dysmotility may be associated with delayed gastric emptying, small intestinal dysmotility is also evident in some patients who have normal gastric emptying [82], indicating that delayed gastric emptying is not a reliable predictor of small intestinal dysmotility.

Postprandial small intestinal motor abnormalities include early recurrence of phase III and burst activity [5,82] (Figure 5.3). The former indicates a premature return of phase III, i.e. before the stomach and small intestine are 'empty'. Bursts are periods of continuous high amplitude and frequency contractions lasting less than 2 min ('short bursts') or at least 2 min ('long bursts'). Although the occurrence of burst activity *per se* is not abnormal, the frequency and duration are indicative of motor disturbances of the small intestine [46]. Both early recurrence of phase III and burst activity are thought to indicate neuropathic changes in either the intrinsic or extrinsic innervation of the gut.

These motility patterns are, however, not specific for diabetes mellitus, since they are also evident in other conditions, including patients with functional bowel diseases and postvagotomy [18,83,84]. Apart from the abnormal motor patterns mentioned above, computerised manometric analyses have also revealed a decrease in the number and amplitude of contractions in the upper part of the small intestine [82]. These qualitative and quantitative motor abnormalities are likely to constitute the mechanical mechanisms involved in abnormal rapid and slow transit through the small intestine, although this has not been formally studied by applying manometric and transit tests concurrently.

The studies that have investigated small intestinal transit in diabetes mellitus have used the breath test or scintigraphic techniques. Using the lactulose breath test in the fasting state, delayed transit was observed in diabetic patients with

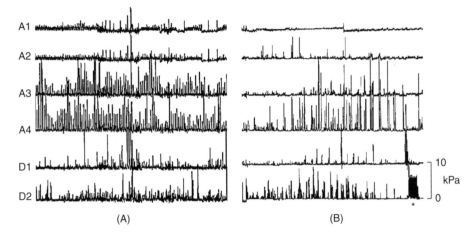

Figure 5.3   A 60 min manometric trace showing four antral and two duodenal recording sites. The tracing in the left panel (A) shows normal postprandial motility with propagated contractions at the level of the antrum and small intestine in a healthy volunteer. The tracing in the right panel (B) shows antral hypomotility and early recurrence of phase III activity in a patient with type 1 diabetes mellitus and gastroparesis. At the time of the duodenal phase III the patient reported nausea (*). From Samsom *et al.* [89] with permission

evidence of autonomic neuropathy, while patients without cardiac autonomic neuropathy showed normal transit times [88]. When the same technique was applied in the postprandial state, both rapid or delayed small intestinal transit was reported in 30–50% of the patients studied [78–80]. Neither the presence of autonomic neuropathy nor gastrointestinal symptoms were found to be related to abnormalities in small intestinal transit times when measured in the postprandial state. The largest study performed to date ($n = 43$) showed delayed small intestinal transit in 23% of the diabetics [3]. However, extrapolation of these data to the diabetic population is difficult, since all patients enrolled in this study were hospitalised for diabetes-related complications, such as poor glycaemic control and hyperosmotic coma. In a study using radiolabelled isotopes, small intestinal transit was accelerated in diabetic patients with autonomic neuropathy, while diabetic patients without autonomic neuropathy showed normal transit times [81].

Fasting small intestinal motility has received even less attention than postprandial motility in diabetes mellitus. At present, only three studies have focused on fasting motility in diabetes and in two of these motor activity was recorded for 24 h [85,89]. Both prolonged manometric studies revealed small intestinal motor abnormalities in the majority of diabetic patients with autonomic neuropathy. The duration of the MMC cycle was abnormally long in most of the patients, reflecting prolongation of phase II without any change in the duration of phases I or III. Phase III activity was more likely to originate in the proximal duodenum than in the gastric antrum when compared to healthy subjects [89]. Total absence of phase III of the MMC was observed in two of the 15 patients studied by Hackelsberger *et al.*, but in none of the patients studies by Samsom *et al.* [89].

The relation between upper gastrointestinal symptoms and abnormal small intestinal transit and motility is largely unknown, apart from anecdotal reports suggesting that early recurrence of phase III after a meal may be associated with nausea [82] (Figure 5.3).

Lower gastrointestinal symptoms, such as diarrhoea, may be related to both rapid and slow small intestinal transit. In the case of rapid intestinal transit, diarrhoea may be the result of a fluid overload of the proximal colon and nutrient malabsorption. Slow intestinal transit may lead to diarrhoea secondary to bacterial overgrowth in the case of slow intestinal transit. As becomes clear from the articles discussed above, studies in well-characterised diabetics are required that focus on the relation between gastrointestinal symptoms and small intestinal motor abnormalities.

Colonic dysmotility

The data relating to colonic function in patients with diabetes mellitus are even more limited than those that exist for the small intestine [79–81,86,87,90]. In the only available study, which was performed more than 20 years ago, colonic myoelectrical and motor activity was recorded in 12 type 1 patients with constipation [87]. A delay in the colonic motor response to a meal was evident in the diabetic patients with mild constipation, while no postprandial increase in colonic motility was observed in patients with severe constipation. Cholinergic stimulation with neostigmine increased colonic motor activity in all diabetics, indicating that the colonic smooth muscle was intact and that the abnormal response to a meal was due to enteric or extrinsic nerve damage [87].

Colonic transit has been assessed in several studies using radio-opaque markers. In studies by Kawagishi *et al.* [86] and Werth *et al.* [80], transit was markedly delayed in patients with evidence of cardiovascular autonomic neuropathy, while normal transit was observed in patients without autonomic neuropathy. The increase in colonic transit time in the patients with autonomic neuropathy was attributable primarily to a delay in transit in the distal colon. Iber *et al.*, also used a radiographic technique to study colonic transit in asymptomatic male type 2 diabetics and those with upper and lower gastrointestinal symptoms [79]. Delayed colonic transit was observed in both groups, particularly in the symptomatic diabetics. The observed absence of lower gastrointestinal symptoms in some of the patients with prolonged colonic transit suggests that symptoms may not be a good indicator of the presence or absence of delayed colonic transit in diabetic patients.

Pathophysiology of small intestinal and colonic dysmotility

The aetiology of intestinal dysmotility in diabetes mellitus is without doubt multifactorial, with two major factors, autonomic neuropathy and prior glycaemic control. Both factors are closely linked and may influence each other and are, therefore, dynamic rather than static entities.

Effect of autonomic neuropathy on intestinal function

Potentially, neuropathy of the autonomic (vagal and sympathetic) and enteric nerves may result in intestinal dysmotility. Autonomic neuropathy at the level of the gut can be assessed using cardiac autonomic nerve (CAN) function tests as a surrogate marker (see Chapter 10). These CAN function tests do not provide direct information about gastrointestinal sympathetic or parasympathetic nerve function, neither do they allow a distinction to be made between autonomic and enteric nerve dysfunction. However, at present CAN function tests are the best tests available in the clinical situation.

Studies using CAN function tests to assess involvement of the autonomic nerve system indicate that in patients with CAN the prevalence and severity of dysmotility of the small intestine and colon is substantially greater when compared to patients with normal CAN function. In a retrospective study by Bharucha *et al.*, a comprehensive assessment of autonomic nerve function was performed in 13 (11 type 1) patients with diabetes mellitus, and a strong association between autonomic neuropathy and small intestinal dysmotility was found [91].

Histological examination of diabetic patients with gastroparesis showed morphological changes of the vagal nerves in some, but not all, patients [92–95]. The observed abnormalities consisted of a reduced number of unmyelinated fibres, degenerated unmyelinated fibres, and capillary basement membrane thickening [93,94]. These findings were, however, not confirmed by Yoshida *et al.* [95], indicating that structural changes of these nerves are not a prerequisite for gastrointestinal motor abnormalities in diabetes.

As discussed in Chapter 2 studies using experimental animal models of diabetes have shown altered activity of many neurotransmitters known to be of importance in preserving the integrity of intestinal motility, such as serotonin, calcitonin-related peptide, substance P, peptide Y and NO [96–98]. The role of NO in diabetes is of particular interest, since non-adrenergic non-cholinergic relaxation of smooth muscle has been shown to be impaired in diabetic rats, which might account for the lack of inhibition of motor activity observed in the human small intestine with diabetes, as evidenced by early recurrence of phase III and postprandial burst activity [98]. A recent study showed that, apart from changes in nerves and neuropeptides, the pacemaker cells of the gut are also affected. The myenteric plexus of the stomach in diabetic mice showed a reduced number of interstitial cells of Cajal [99]. These findings were recently confirmed in human jejunal tissue obtained from a patient with long-standing type 1 diabetes [100]. A full-thickness biopsy showed a reduction of the interstitial cells of Cajal throughout the entire thickness of the jejunum (Figure 5.4). In addition, decreases in neuronal nitric oxide synthase, vasoactive intestinal

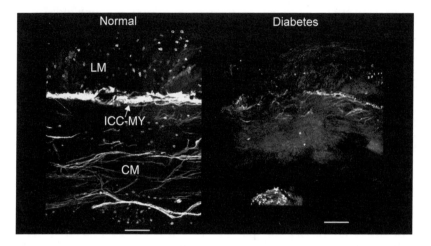

Figure 5.4 Distribution of interstitial cells of Cajal (ICC). Left panel shows distribution of ICC in the normal human jejunum and the right panel shows the distribution in a patient with type 1 diabetes mellitus. C-kit-immunopositive structures, indicating the presence of ICCs, are shown in white. A decrease in C-kit-positive immunoreactivity is seen in all regions of the jejunum in the diabetic patient compared with the control (bar = 100:M). LM, longitudinal muscle; ICC-MY, ICC in the myenteric plexus; CM, circular muscle. From He *et al.* [100] with permission

peptide, PACAP and tyrosine hydroxylase immunopositive nerve fibres were observed in the circular muscle layer, while substance P immunoreactivity was increased. These changes in the interstitial cells of Cajal and the decrease in inhibitory innervation observed in animal models for diabetes and in human tissue may play an important role in the pathophysiology of small intestinal and colonic dysmotility in diabetes mellitus.

Effects of blood glucose concentration on intestinal function

Many studies have shown that the gastrointestinal motor responses to various stimuli are affected by acute hyperglycaemia in both healthy subjects and diabetic patients (discussed in Chapters 3 and 4). The exact mechanism through which glucose influences motor and sensory function of the intestine is still unresolved. Both stimulatory and inhibitory effects occur during hyperglycaemia, indicating that the effects are likely to be mediated by neural or humoral mechanisms, rather than a direct effect on the smooth muscle of the gut.

The profound effect of acute hyperglycaemia on intestinal motor and sensory function has been confirmed in several studies [82,101–107]. These studies showed that blood glucose levels in the range 12–15 mmol reduce the number and propagation of pressure waves in the proximal small intestine [82,103,104], resulting in slower small intestinal transit [104,108]. In the fasting state, hyperglycaemia induces duodenal phase III motor activity [102] and shortens the MMC length [107] (Figure 5.5). Hyperglycaemia blunts the gastrocolonic response evoked by gastric distension and affects reflex pathways within the colon [90]. The effects of hyperglycaemia on colonic transit have not yet been formally assessed, but are likely to increase, rather than decrease, colonic transit times.

Studies in healthy volunteers showed that hyperglycaemia affects not only motor activity, but also perception of the symptoms arising from

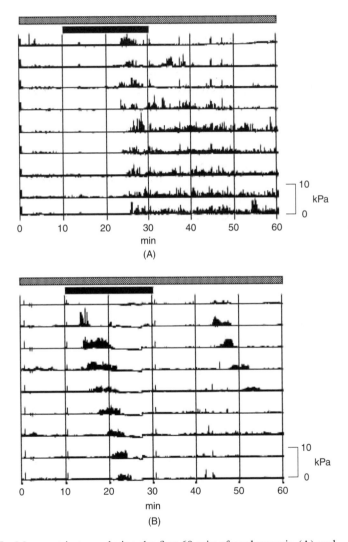

Figure 5.5 Manometric trace during the first 60 min of euglycaemia (A) and hyperglycaemia (B) in a healthy volunteer. Tracings are arranged with the most proximal channel (antrum) at the top and the most distal (jejunal) at the bottom. Time zero marks the start of i.v. infusion and the nutrient liquid meal was infused 10 min later. During hyperglycaemia there is premature onset of phase III and the fed pattern is not evident. From Russo *et al.* [104] with permission

the gut [105,106,109]. Chemical (lipid infusion) and mechanical (balloon distension) stimulation result in more sensations, such as nausea and fullness during hyperglycaemia compared to euglycaemia [105].

Although the effects of hypoglycaemia on small intestinal motility have only been studied in healthy subjects in the fasting state, the effects seem to be less pronounced than those of hyperglycaemia, e.g. insulin-induced hypoglycaemia induces only a transient increase in jejunal motor activity, while no effect on pyloric and duodenal motility or the periodicity of the MMC has been observed [110,111].

The effect of chronic hyperglycaemia on small intestinal and colonic function is much more difficult to assess. The indirect evidence obtained from studies of pancreas–kidney transplantation suggests that, at least in a subset of patients with diabetes mellitus, the autonomic neuropathy is reversible by normoglycaemia, indicating that gut function may improve during long-term stabilisation of blood glucose levels [112,113].

Intraluminal digestion and nutrient absorption

Transport of chyme through the small intestine is closely linked to intraluminal digestion and absorption of nutrients. The efficacy of absorption of nutrients is, therefore, potentially affected by dysmotility of the small intestine observed in diabetes, and by alterations in the transport mechanisms facilitating nutrient uptake across the intestinal membrane. Optimising the conditions for intraluminal digestion and absorption in the small intestine starts once food particles enter the duodenum, where chyme is quickly neutralised. Within a few centimetres the pH rises quickly from low antral values of around pH 2 to high duodenal values (pH 6–7). This increase in pH reflects interplay between motor activity and secretion. Coordinated antroduodenal contractions spread the chyme in the proximal duodenum, while pancreaticobiliary and mucosal bicarbonate secretion buffer the gastric acid [114–118].

Large polymeric molecules (proteins and carbohydrates) that have been partly digested in the stomach are broken down into oligomers in the lumen of the small intestine. Further breakdown takes place at the luminal brush border to enable the absorption of small molecules (amino acids and hexoses). Fatty molecules are dissolved by bile salts and degraded by lipase. The majority of carbohydrate, lipid and protein absorption takes place in the proximal half of the small intestine. Some specific nutrients, such as bile salts and the vitamin B_{12}–intrinsic factor complex, are absorbed only in the ileum.

Digestion and absorption of carbohydrates

Digestion of carbohydrates is initiated in the mouth were food is mixed with salivary secretions that contain amylase; the latter hydrolyses large polymers into smaller fragments [119]. The acidic environment of the stomach facilitates non-enzymatic hydrolysis of some of the disaccharides, such as sucrose. In the small intestine the polysaccharides are broken down by pancreatic amylase, which is secreted by the pancreas in large amounts. Brush border saccharidases present on the apical membrane of enterocytes are responsible for further breakdown of hydrolysis products (i.e. maltose, trimaltose) and disaccharides, with the exception of lactose, which can only be cleaved into glucose and galactose by the enzyme lactase. While passive transport mechanisms might play a role in the absorption of monosaccharides, carrier-mediated and active transport are probably more important [119].

Glucose is the most important monosaccharide and its absorption has been studied extensively [119]. Glucose transport through the enterocyte in the small intestine is mediated by the sodium-glucose co-transporter (SGLT 1) at the luminal membrane, and the glucose transporter (GLUT 2) at the basolateral membrane [120]. Thus, glucose absorption is dependent on the presence of sodium ions in the intestinal lumen [121]. The glucose receptor is physically close to disaccharidases in the brush border. This may account for the more rapid absorption of glucose, which is part of a disaccharide from the intestinal lumen [122]. Monosaccharides are transported into the portal vein and then metabolised in the liver, where they may be taken up and converted to glycogen, or stored via the glucose-6-phosphate pathway, although the majority are available to the systemic circulation.

In contrast to glucose and galactose, most fructose transport is facilitated by GLUT 5, which is located on the brush borders of the enterocytes [123]. Because the glycaemic response to fructose is substantially less than that to glucose, it has been recommended as a substitute for glucose in the diabetic diet [124,125].

Digestion and absorption of proteins

Although digestion of proteins starts in the stomach, where proteins are partially digested by gastric proteinases into smaller polypeptides, most of the breakdown takes place in the small intestine [126,127]. The products of protein digestion by pepsin in the stomach induce a stimulus that initiates the release of cholecystokinin and secretin. These hormones stimulate the production of inactive precursors of proteolytic enzymes (trypsin, chymotrypsin, elastase) in the pancreas, which are activated in the lumen of the proximal small intestine as a result of enzymatic cleavage by trypsin. Activated pancreatic enzymes cleave the polypeptide molecules into small molecules of two to six amino acids or into single amino acids. Amino acids, dipeptides and tripeptides cross the luminal mucosal membrane and are subsequently degraded by intracellular peptidases into single amino acids, which are then transported to the portal vein [126,127]. While the majority of the absorption takes place in the proximal intestine, absorption of amino acids can also take place in the jejunum.

Digestion and absorption of fat

Lipid digestion is a multistep process, starting with emulsification, followed by digestion of long-chain triglycerides, phospholipids and sterol–ester bonds, so-called lipolysis. The lipolytic products are mixed with bile salts and biliary lecithin, resulting in the formation of micelles; the latter require an aqueous milieu, as in the small intestine. Lipid digestion starts in the stomach, where dietary triglycerides are mixed with lecithin, which is the initiation of emulsification. Intragastric lipolysis may account for 20–30% of intraluminal lipid digestion [128–130]. The duodenal pH of 6.0–7.5 is essential for further digestion of lipids; as a result, these fatty acids become ionised and migrate to the surface of the emulsion, where they facilitate the binding of colipase [131]. The colipase–lipase enzyme complex attaches to the triglyceride emulsion for further digestion, resulting in lipolytic products, i.e. monoglycerides and fatty acids. The bile salts enter the duodenum after contraction of the gall bladder. Adequate intraluminal bile salt concentrations are essential for effective solubilisation of lipolytic products. These bile salts have a strong tendency to form negatively charged conglomerates called micelles. Lipids that critically depend on this mechanism include cholesterol, fat-soluble vitamins and plant sterols [132].

The uptake of the triglycerides is to a large extent dependent on their chain length and partially driven by concentration gradients, although specific carriers also play a role in the uptake of long-chain fatty acids. After brush border membrane uptake, long-chain fatty acids and monoglycerides bind to fatty acid-binding proteins (FABPs), which facilitate intracellular transport.

Approximately 75% of absorbed fatty acids are resynthesised into triglyceride and secreted by the enterocytes as lipoprotein, then transported via the lymph vessels or portal vein [133,134]. The remaining 25% serve as substrates for phospholipid and other intracellular lipid resynthesis events, or undergo transport to the liver bound to albumin via the portal vein [135,136].

The products of lipid digestion and absorption released into the intestine are important in the initiation of feedback regulation of gastrointestinal motor function [137,138].

Cholesterol is absorbed by passive diffusion, and its delivery to the brush border lipid bilayer is facilitated by micelle diffusion [139]. The processing of cholesterol by the enterocytes is a major component of the homeostatic control underlying the regulation of cholesterol levels in the human body. The enterocytes receive the bulk of cholesterol from luminal sources (i.e. dietary and biliary), but also have the capacity to synthesise cholesterol. Bile salts are passively absorbed as monomers throughout the upper small intestine, although active transport in the ileum is responsible for approximately 95% of the intraluminal bile salts uptake [140,141]. The absorbed bile salts undergo an efficient process of hepatic uptake after portal vein delivery and re-excretion into bile; they become rapidly available again for intraluminal micelle formation.

Effects of diabetes mellitus on digestion and absorption of nutrients; the role of the small intestine in postprandial glycaemia

The handling of ingested (or intraluminal digested) glucose by the gut is important in the regulation of postprandial glucose concentrations and, hence, glycaemic control. At the level of the liver, processing of glucose is influenced by the glucose gradient between portal venous and hepatic arterial blood [142]; accordingly, high systemic blood glucose levels may favour a decreased availability of absorbed glucose to the systemic circulation. During hepatic glucose uptake, glycogenolysis and gluconeogenesis are concurrently suppressed, limiting the increase in systemic glucose [143,144]. Impairment of this suppression contributes to postprandial hyperglycaemia in diabetes, especially in patients with type 2 diabetes [145,146].

The relative contribution of the stomach and small intestine to postprandial blood glucose concentrations, compared to the liver, is likely to vary over time after a meal. Experimental diabetes in animals has been reported to enhance glucose absorption and increase glucose metabolism [147]. The increase in glucose absorption in the enterocytes [148,149] is accompanied by an increase in the expression of glucose transporters SGLT1 and GLUT2 and their mRNAs in diabetic rats and humans [149,150].

In contrast to these reports, glucose absorption was found to be normal in type 1 patients when studied with a jejunal perfusion technique [151]. These findings were confirmed in a study in which uncomplicated type 1 diabetics received an intraduodenal infusion of the glucose analogue, 3-O-methylglucose (3-OMG); the results showed comparable absorption kinetics of 3-O-methylglucose in type 1 diabetes and healthy subjects [152]. In studies performed in type 2 diabetics glucose absorption was also similar, or at most slightly reduced, when compared to healthy humans [153]. The apparent discrepancies between the observations in animal models and humans may be at least partially explained by differences in actual blood glucose concentrations and prior glycaemic control at the time of the study, since the enhanced uptake of glucose is partially or completely normalised when glycaemic control is improved by treatment with insulin or after islet cell transplantation [152,154,155].

The effect of small intestinal dysmotility in diabetes mellitus on glucose absorption has not been formally studied. However, it has been established that pharmacologically-induced 'dysmotility', as induced by loperamide, slows glucose absorption. These observations suggest that severe small intestinal dysmotility in diabetes may result in less predictable glucose uptake [156].

There is little or no evidence that diabetes *per se* affects protein absorption to a clinically relevant extent. However, when diabetes mellitus is associated with severe pancreatic insufficiency (see Chapter 7), coeliac disease (discussed later in this chapter) or bacterial overgrowth, malabsorption of protein may occur. In diabetic patients with bacterial overgrowth, protein malabsorption is the result of several factors: the abundantly present bacteria compete with the host for proteins; amino acid absorption may be impaired as a result of mucosal damage; and the levels of proteolytic enzymes may be decreased [157–159].

Since lipid absorption is dependent on the interplay of several organs (small intestine, pancreas, liver, gall bladder), diabetes mellitus has the potential to be associated with fat malabsorption, although there is a substantial functional reserve that compensates for minor changes in some of the critical phases of this process. The disorders of the liver, pancreas and gallbladder that may result in fat malabsorption are discussed in Chapter 7. Fat malabsorption may also result from loss of effective absorption surface, as in diabetic patients with co-existent coeliac disease. Although it is not known whether small intestinal dysmotility *per se* can lead to fat malabsorption, it certainly can when the dysmotility is associated with bacterial overgrowth [160,161]. The bacterial deconjugation of bile acids is the primary mechanism for malabsorption of fats and fat-soluble vitamins; anaerobic organisms in particular reduce the level of conjugated bile acids below the critical micelle concentration, leading to steatorrhoea [162–165].

Effects of drugs and fibre on nutrient absorption and glycaemic control

The positive effects of fibre (particularly soluble fibre) on glycaemic control have been well established in both type 1 and type 2 diabetes [166–168]. The beneficial effects of fibre on postprandial hyperglycaemia are likely to reflect an increase in the viscosity of the intraluminal content, inducing a decrease in the rate of gastric emptying and slowing intestinal glucose absorption [169].

The effects of fibre at the level of the small intestine are at least partially due to its effect on small intestinal motility. Fibre treatment has been shown to decrease stationary contractions and to increase the length of propagating contractile activity, resulting in a reduction of the postprandial glycaemic peak [170].

Apart from increasing dietary fibre in order to blunt postprandial hyperglycaemia, manipulation of the intraluminal digestion of carbohydrates has been reported to be an effective therapeutic approach in diabetes mellitus. Inhibition of intestinal α-glucosidase activity by agents such as acarbose is widely used in type 2 diabetes. Acarbose delays the digestion of polysaccharides, resulting in flattening of postprandial glucose curves and a decrease in the gastric emptying rate [171–173].

Recently, drug-induced malabsorption of fat has become a treatment option in diabetes mellitus. The inhibition of pancreatic lipase activity by orlistat prevents the hydrolysis of triglycerides, resulting in fat malabsorption. This approach has been reported to improve glycaemic control in type 2 diabetes, as assessed by glycated haemoglobin, which is likely to be mediated by the loss of body weight as a result of the drug-induced fat malabsorption [174]. As discussed in Chapter 4, orlistat has the potential to exacerbate postprandial glycaemia after ingestion of fatty meals which contain carbohydrate as a meals of more rapid gastric emptying.

Intestinal secretion and permeability

Although the available data are limited, there is evidence that intestinal secretion may be abnormal in diabetes, due to increased secretion of fluids in response to a meal, rather than an increased basal secretory state [176]. In animal models for diabetes there is also increased fluid secretion from small intestinal epithelial cells, and this reflects impaired adrenergic regulation of mucosal ion transport, which is accompanied by net intestinal fluid secretion. This process can be reversed by the α2-adrenergic agonist, clonidine [177]. The impairment of intestinal fluid absorption takes some time to develop and is prevented by insulin treatment [178]. These observations suggest that progressive neuropathy of the enteric and autonomic nervous system is likely to be responsible for the impaired intestinal secretion, rather than hyperglycaemia.

To what extent altered intestinal permeability plays a role in chronic diarrhoea in diabetes is unclear. Small intestinal permeability to cellobiose and mannitol is reported to be slightly higher in patients with uncomplicated type 1 diabetes mellitus [179] and one study reported abnormal permeability in about two/thirds of diabetic patients with chronic diarrhoea [180].

Intestinal blood supply

The splanchnic circulation is essential for oxygenation of the small and large intestine, transport of absorbed nutrients and maintenance of systemic blood pressure, and regulated by neuronal, myogenic and hormonal factors. Blood supply of the gastrointestinal tract is potentially affected in patients with diabetes mellitus, since diabetes may be associated by abnormalities in one or more of these regulatory factors.

Regulation of intestinal blood flow

The superior and inferior mesenteric arteries supply blood to the small and large intestine, while the superior, middle and inferior rectal arteries provide the arterial blood supply of the rectum. About 25% of the cardiac output in the fasting state circulates through the splanchnic arteries [181]. The branches of the superior mesenteric artery supply part of the duodenum, jejunum, ileum and large intestine distal to the splenic flexure [182]. The inferior mesenteric artery supplies the right part of the colon, transverse colon and the upper part of the rectum. The lower part of the rectum is supplied by the middle and inferior rectal arteries, which originate from the internal iliac artery and internal pudendal artery. The mesenteric arteries give rise to numerous branches that supply the layers of the intestine and finally drain via the mesenteric veins into the portal vein.

Sympathetic postganglionic nerve fibres are the most important neuronal input; stimulation results in a reduction in intestinal blood flow [183,184]. Sustained sympathetic stimulation is followed by an autoregulatory escape, during which blood flow increases [184]. The effect of circulating catecholamines is comparable with that of sympathetic stimulation; an autoregulatory response is also evident during prolonged stimulation. In contrast to sympathetic activity, vagal nerve tone has little effect on intestinal blood flow.

Data derived from animal studies indicate that gastrointestinal hormones and neuropeptides, such as insulin, glucagon, somatostatin, cholecystokinin, vasoactive intestinal peptide and neurotensin, increase postprandial blood flow, facilitating nutrient absorption [183,184]. Recently, the role of nitric oxide as a determinant of splanchnic blood flow has been recognised [185]; in pigs the NO synthase inhibitor L-NMMA attenuates the postprandial increase in blood flow [185].

The availability of non-invasive techniques for measuring of intestinal blood flow, such as echo-Doppler, have substantially increased knowledge about the determinants of human splanchnic blood flow under physiological and pathological conditions [186–188]. Using echo-Doppler it has been established that food intake is associated with a doubling of the flow through the mesenteric arteries in humans [186,188]. Both the duration and the magnitude of the increase in blood flow are nutrient-dependent, e.g. after ingestion of a meal rich in carbohydrate, the blood flow returns to baseline after 3 h, whereas after a meal rich in fat, blood flow is still increased at this time [186,188].

An important role for gut hormones in the regulation of splanchnic blood flow remains to be established in human studies. In a study by Sieber *et al.* it was shown that, while a meal increased superior mesenteric blood flow, 'physiological' doses of CCK, secretin and glucagon had no effect on blood flow in healthy volunteers [186].

Effect of diabetes on intestinal blood flow

Animal models of diabetes are associated with abnormalities of neurotransmitters in the mesenteric veins and arteries, including substance P, calcitonin gene-related peptide and vasoactive intestinal peptide and hyperaemia of the small intestine [189]. The latter may reflect an increase in the demand consequent upon hypertrophy of the mucosa, mediated by endogenous prostaglandin and increased sensitivity to NO [190,191].

Human diabetes may be associated with abnormalities in mesenteric blood flow. In diabetic patients with autonomic neuropathy, preprandial superior mesenteric arterial blood flow is greater than that in both control subjects and patients without autonomic neuropathy [192]. After a meal, the peak systolic velocity in the superior mesenteric artery increased in control subjects and in patients without autonomic neuropathy, but not in those with autonomic neuropathy [193]. These observations were in part confirmed by Purewal *et al.*, who reported that flow in the superior mesenteric artery was greater in diabetic patients with autonomic neuropathy under basal conditions, but not after a meal [192]. To what extent, if any, these changes reflect the blood glucose concentrations remains to be investigated. The effects of changes in mesenteric blood flow on gastrointestinal motor and/or sensory function, or on nutrient absorption are also not known.

Mesenteric blood flow may affect systemic blood pressure, particularly when modifications in splanchnic blood flow are not associated with compensatory changes in vascular resistance in the systemic circulation, resulting in postprandial and/or orthostatic hypotension. Those patients with autonomic dysfunction (most frequently due to diabetes) are at particular risk of postprandial hypotension and often exhibit a marked fall in systemic blood pressure after a meal [194]. A recent study, using 24 h ambulatory blood pressure monitoring, showed that diabetes mellitus was an important risk factor for postprandial hypotension in elderly patients with fall or syncope [195]. As discussed in Chapter 4, the magnitude of the postprandial fall in blood pressure is dependent on meal composition (glucose has the greatest effect) and the rate of nutrient entry into the small intestine [196]. When postprandial hypotension becomes symptomatic treatment with the somatostatin analogue octreotide can be considered [197,198]. The beneficial effect of octreotide is likely to be due to a combination of increases in splanchnic and peripheral vascular resistance and cardiac output [199].

Patients with diabetes mellitus also frequently report symptoms attributable to orthostatic hypotension. A large survey of type 1 diabetes mellitus reported that the frequency of feeling faint on standing was 18% [200]. Symptomatic orthostatic hypotension in diabetic patients has been shown to be related to cardiovascular autonomic neuropathy; abnormal blood pressure response to standing (>20 mmHg fall in systolic blood pressure) seems to be the best predictor (see Chapter 9).

Clinical manifestations

Diagnostic work-up and treatment of constipation

Although constipation in diabetic patients is most likely to be due to colonic motor or pelvic floor dysfunction, it is essential to exclude other causes. The latter include intraluminal abnormalities, electrolyte imbalance, hormonal dysfunction (such as hypothyroidism) and side effects of medication. These potential causes of constipation should be excluded by a combination of physical examination (including inspection of the pelvic floor and rectal examination), haematological and biochemical tests. A colonoscopy may be performed at this point, especially if additional risk factors are present or after a treatment trial with laxatives. A lower-cost alternative is a barium enema, but findings such as melanosis coli from excessive use of anthranoids and solitary rectal ulcer may be missed using this technique.

General measures in the treatment of constipation include adequate dietary fibre intake (20–30 g/day) and hydration. Increased consumption of dietary fibre increases stool weight and the frequency of defaecation and decreases colonic transit time [201,202]. Bulk-forming synthetic fibres, such as polycarbophil, psyllium and methylcellulose, should be prescribed in patients who are not able to increase their daily dietary fibre intake. Although high-fibre diets improve bowel habits, they have the potential to increase, rather than decrease, gastrointestinal symptoms, as has been recognised in constipation-predominant irritable bowel syndrome.

When these measures fail to adequately relieve constipation, osmotic laxatives (polyethylene glycol, lactulose, sorbitol) and saline laxatives (magnesium sulphate, magnesium phosphate, magnesium citrate) may improve bowel habits. For diabetic patients with constipation who do not respond to fibre and osmotic laxatives, a transit study and evaluation of the pelvic floor function are indicated. Measurement of colonic transit provides objective information of importance, since the correlation between stool frequency and colon transit is poor [203]. As discussed, colonic transit can be assessed using commercially available radio-opaque markers or by scintigraphy (see above) and will allow diagnosis of slow transit constipation [29,33]. Outlet obstruction, an important cause of constipation in diabetes [204] is discussed separately in Chapter 6.

The use of prokinetic drugs or stimulant laxatives (anthraquinones) in the treatment of diabetic patients with constipation represents the last pharmacological approach, particularly as the efficacy of the available prokinetic drugs in the treatment of constipation in diabetes has not been clearly established. The chronic use of anthraquinones is generally discouraged because of the potential damage to the smooth muscle cells and myenteric plexus [205].

The most widely used prokinetic drugs in diabetic patients with gastrointestinal transit disorders are cisapride, metoclopramide and erythromycin. The benzamide cisapride has been shown to accelerate colonic transit in patients with slow transit constipation, irrespective of its cause [206–208]. Although there are no large studies evaluating the efficacy of cisapride in diabetics with constipation, it is likely to improve bowel habits in these patients. The dosage of cisapride may vary between 5 and 10 mg bid or tid [206–208]. As discussed in Chapter 4, cisapride has the potential to cause cardiac dysrhythmias, which limits its use [209]. The effect of metoclopramide on colonic transit in diabetes has not been investigated, but in a study focusing on gastric emptying, some patients reported an increase in bowel frequency [210]. Reports on the efficacy of the motilin-agonist, erythromycin in patients with constipation are conflicting; some studies have shown an improvement, while others were unable to reproduce these results; studies in constipated diabetics are lacking [211,212].

More promising than the prokinetic drugs mentioned above are the more recently developed full and partial 5-HT$_4$ agonists, Prucalopride and Tegaserod.

Both prokinetics accelerate gastrointestinal and colonic transit in health and in patients with constipation [34–36].

When oral laxatives in combination with prokinetic drugs fail, enemas may be useful. Enemas lower the surface tension of stool, facilitating mixing of aqueous and fatty substances, as well as stimulating intestinal fluid and electrolyte secretion [213].

In the selected and small group in whom slow transit constipation is intractable despite extensive medical treatment, surgery should be considered. In these patients measurement of regional transit times may potentially be helpful in deciding whether subtotal or partial colectomy should be the operation of choice [214,215]. Since the outcome of (sub)total colectomy in slow transit constipation *per se* is often disappointing, with postoperative incontinence in up to 37% and recurrent constipation in up to 32%, this operation should only be performed in centres with extensive expertise in the clinical work-up of these patients [216].

Diagnostic work-up in, and treatment of, diabetic patients with diarrhoea

In contrast to constipation, where the colon is likely to play the central role, the pathogenesis of chronic diarrhoea in diabetes mellitus is multifactorial. As discussed above, colonic transit and colonic motor activities have only been measured in diabetic patients with constipation. It is, therefore, not known to what extent the colon *per se* plays a role in diabetic patients with chronic diarrhoea. A number of factors may lead to diarrhoea in patients with diabetes mellitus; these include food composition, abnormal intestinal motility, small intestinal bacterial overgrowth, excessive loss of bile acids, pancreatic insufficiency, drugs, secretory dysfunction, lactose malabsorption, coeliac disease, hormonal dysfunction (e.g. hyperthyroidism) and anorectal dysfunction.

In diabetic patients, as in healthy subjects, as little as 10 g of sorbitol can induce diarrhoea [217,218]. Many diabetics are unaware of sorbitol in their food and the prevalence of diarrhoea is higher in those patients consuming it [217]. Fructose (as included in corn syrup) may also be malabsorbed and lead to diarrhoea.

As described above, abnormal small intestinal motility occurs frequently in diabetic patients. Both rapid and delayed small intestinal transit may potentially cause diarrhoea; as a result of rapid small intestinal transit, there is an increase in intraluminal contents that reach the caecum, while delayed small intestinal transit potentially causes bacterial overgrowth. The role of bile acids in diabetic diarrhoea is controversial. While Molloy and Tomkin reported that bile acid excretion was increased in type 1 patients with diarrhoea [219], this was not confirmed by others [101]. Other causes of chronic diarrhoea, including pancreatic insufficiency, coeliac disease and anorectal dysfunction, are discussed elsewhere.

A comprehensive history in any diabetic patient with chronic diarrhoea (often defined as more than 200 ml sloppy stool/day) may reveal a high sorbitol intake or the use of other laxative drugs and is, therefore, the first step in diagnosis and treatment. Physical examination should focus on signs of autonomic neuropathy (see Chapter 9) and anorectal function (see Chapter 6). In addition, haematological and biochemical, hormonal screening tests should be performed. The timing and choice of investigations in diabetic patients with diarrhoea is dictated by both the history of the patient and the risk factors involved. In order to exclude other causes of diarrhoea, microbiological investigation of faeces and endoscopic evaluation of the colon should be performed. A jejunal biopsy or serological tests for antigliadin and endomycium antibodies will allow diagnosis of coeliac disease. When no cause is found, dysmotility of the small intestine and colon is likely to play an important role in the aetiology of the diarrhoea.

Bacterial overgrowth has been reported in up to 40% of diabetic patients with chronic diarrhoea [220,221]. Slow small intestinal transit and a decreased frequency of phase III the migrating motor complex are thought to be the underlying mechanisms. Primary treatment of bacterial overgrowth is directed at selectively suppressing the intestinal bacterial flora with antibiotics. Numerous antibiotics have been reported to be effective, including tetracycline, cephalosporines, quinolones and metronidazole. Octreotide is an expensive but effective alternative in the treatment of bacterial overgrowth, most likely due to its stimulatory effect on intestinal motility [160,222]. The beneficial effects of octreotide are dose-dependent; high doses may result in steatorrhoea, slowing of small intestinal transit and bacterial overgrowth [223]. The role of prokinetic drugs in treating bacterial overgrowth remains to be explored. Diabetic patients with rapid intestinal transit frequently respond to loperamide, since it prolongs both small intestinal and large intestinal transit times at doses varying between 2 and 4 mg bid/tid [224]. Furthermore, loperamide increases internal anal sphincter pressure and may, therefore, be of benefit in patients with a combination of diarrhoea and faecal incontinence [225]. Bile salt binders, such as cholestyramine, are the treatment of choice in patients with diarrhoea attributable to an increase in bile acid excretion, which should be distinguished from fatty diarrhoea prior to treatment.

As discussed, loss of adrenergic innervation may lead to increased intestinal secretion in patients with diarrhoea; stimulation of α2-adrenergic receptors by clonidine has been beneficial in some diabetic patients with chronic diarrhoea who failed to respond to other medical therapy, and was found not to cause hypotension [226].

Coeliac disease and diabetes mellitus

Coeliac disease is a chronic condition involving the mucosa of the small intestine, which impairs nutrient absorption. In most patients mucosal damage is reversed by avoidance of wheat gliadins, barley, rye and prolamins in the diet [227]. Coeliac disease may cause severe symptoms of diarrhoea, lassitude and weight loss, but may also be subclinical or even asymptomatic.

The association of coeliac disease and type 1 diabetes mellitus is well established. Both disorders are associated with HLA markers, suggesting a genetic link between the two diseases [228,229]. The recent introduction of serological tests has contributed significantly to knowledge about the prevalence of coeliac disease in children and adults with diabetes mellitus.

The prevalence of coeliac disease in type 1 diabetic children varies from 1.0% to 3.5%, which is at least 15 times higher than the prevalence among children without diabetes [230–235]. Two recent studies have investigated the prevalence of coeliac disease in adults with diabetes mellitus [236,237]. Page et al. screened 1789 diabetic patients (78.2% type 1 and 21.8% type 2) using IgA-antigliadin antibodies; 73 patients had elevated antibody levels and 49 of these patients agreed to undergo a small intestinal biopsy; coeliac disease was diagnosed in 10 type 1 and three type 2 patients. In a study by De Vitis et al. serological screening was performed in 1114 patients with type 1 diabetes [237]; in 121 patients increased IgA antigliadin antibody level, and in 55 patients elevated IgA endomycium antibodies, were found. Villous atrophy was evident in 63 of the 78 patients who agreed to undergo a jejunal biopsy. When the prevalence of coeliac disease in diabetic patients is compared to that present in the healthy adult population, which has been shown to be between 1:950 and 1:1700, it is clear that the prevalence of coeliac disease in type 1 diabetics is about six times higher than in the healthy population [238,239]. The relatively high prevalence of coeliac disease among patients with type 1 diabetes mellitus dictates that the threshold for screening tests for coeliac disease should be low in these patients.

The classical symptoms of coeliac disease are diarrhoea, lassitude and weight loss. However, more recent studies have shown that these symptoms are absent in about 30% of coeliac patients, with and without diabetes [240]. Other symptoms may include abdominal distension, nausea or vomiting, and aphthous stomatitis [241,242] Patients with coeliac disease may also have extra-intestinal symptoms, including muscle cramps, bone pain due to osteoporotic fractures or osteomalacia, and psychiatric disorders including schizophrenia and depression.

The rare condition of intestinal lymphoma may also present with a symptom complex similar to coeliac disease [243,244]. A flat jejunal mucosa found on small intestinal histology is similar to that in coeliac disease. The HLA genotype is identical to that found in coeliac disease, which supports the association between the disorders.

Physical findings in patients with coeliac disease are variable. A body weight of less than 90% of the ideal is evident in 67% of patients showing the classical symptoms and in 31% of patients with subclinical symptoms [245]. Finger clubbing, dryness of the skin, aphthous stomatitis and dermatitis herpetiformis are observed in some patients [246].

Biochemical and haematological abnormalities may consist of low levels of haemoglobin, albumin, calcium, potassium, magnesium and iron. However, such changes may not be evident in patients with subclinical coeliac disease, with the exception of iron deficiency [247]. Anaemia may be due to deficiencies of iron, folic acid and vitamin B [248].

The diagnostic gold standard in coeliac disease is small intestinal biopsy, since the diagnosis is made in morphological terms. The microscopic picture of the mucosa may reveal a spectrum of mucosal abnormalities, varying from total villous atrophy to normal villi and crypts, but with an abnormal high count of lymphocytes [249]. The endoscopic pattern in coeliac disease may show a reduction of duodenal folds, but this finding has a low specificity [250].

The determination of serum IgG and IgA antigliadin and IgA endomycium antibody levels have shown their value as a screening test, with an acceptable sensitivity and specificity for the diagnosis of coeliac disease, especially when used in combination [251–253].

Treatment of coeliac disease does not differ from patients without diabetes. A gluten-free diet is the chosen therapy [254] and in the great majority of patients gluten withdrawal will result in the restoration of the small intestinal mucosa and resolution of symptoms. A recent study reported that the introduction of a gluten-free diet in diabetic patients with coeliac disease has no positive effect on glycaemic control, but is associated with weight gain [240].

In the small group of patients with persistent symptoms and mucosal abnormalities although keeping a strict diet, treatment with prednisolone, azathioprine or cyclosporine may be required [255,256].

References

1. Domstad PA, Kim EE, Coupal JJ, Beihn R *et al.* Biologic gastric emptying time in diabetic patients, using Tc-99 m-labeled resin-oatmeal with and without metoclopramide. *J Nucl Med* 1980; **21**: 1098–100.
2. Horowitz M, Harding PE, Maddox AF, Wishart JM *et al.* Gastric and oesophageal emptying in patients with type 2 (non-insulin-dependent) diabetes mellitus. *Diabetologia* 1989; **32**: 151–9.
3. Wegener M, Borsch G, Schaffstein J, Luerweg C, Leverkus F. Gastrointestinal transit disorders in patients with insulin-treated diabetes mellitus. *Dig Dis* 1990; **8**: 23–36.
4. Horowitz M, Maddox AF, Wishart JM, Harding PE *et al.* Relationships between oesophageal transit and solid and liquid gastric emptying in diabetes mellitus. *Eur J Nucl Med* 1991; **18**: 229–34.
5. Camilleri M, Malagelada JR. Abnormal intestinal motility in diabetics with the gastroparesis syndrome. *Eur J Clin Invest* 1984; **14**: 420–27.
6. Dooley CP, el Newihi HM, Zeidler A, Valenzuela JE. Abnormalities of the migrating motor complex in diabetics with autonomic neuropathy and diarrhea. *Scand J Gastroenterol* 1988; **23**: 217–23.

7. Talley NJ, Howell S, Jones MP, Horowitz M. Predictors of turnover of lower gastrointestinal symptoms in diabetes mellitus. *Am J Gastroenterol* 2002; **97**: 3087–94.
8. Bytzer P, Talley NJ, Leemon M, Young LJ *et al.* Prevalence of gastrointestinal symptoms associated with diabetes mellitus: a population-based survey of 15 000 adults. *Arch Intern Med* 2001; **161**: 1989–96.
9. Janatuinen E, Pikkarainen P, Laakso M, Pyorala K. Gastrointestinal symptoms in middle-aged diabetic patients. *Scand J Gastroenterol* 1993; **28**: 427–32.
10. Schvarcz E, Palmer M, Ingberg CM, Aman J, Berne C. Increased prevalence of upper gastrointestinal symptoms in long-term type 1 diabetes mellitus. *Diabet Med* 1996; **13**: 478–81.
11. Kamm MA, Vander Sijp JR, Lennard-Jones JE. Observations on the characteristics of stimulated defaecation in severe idiopathic constipation. *Int J Colorectal Dis* 1992; **7**: 197–201.
12. der Ohe MR, Camilleri M, Kvols LK, Thomforde GM. Motor dysfunction of the small bowel and colon in patients with the carcinoid syndrome and diarrhea. *N Engl J Med* 1993; **329**: 1073–8.
13. De Schryver AM, Andriesse GI, Samsom M, Smout AJ *et al.* The effects of the specific 5-HT$_4$ receptor agonist, prucalopride, on colonic motility in healthy volunteers. *Aliment Pharmacol Ther* 2002; **16**: 603–12.
14. Arndorfer RC, Stef JJ, Dodds WJ, Linehan JH, Hogan WJ. Improved infusion system for intraluminal esophageal manometry. *Gastroenterology* 1977; **73**: 23–7.
15. Mathias JR, Sninsky CA, Millar HD, Clench MH, Davis RH. Development of an improved multi-pressure-sensor probe for recording muscle contraction in human intestine. *Dig Dis Sci* 1985; **30**: 119–23.
16. Samsom M, Smout AJ, Hebbard G, Fraser R *et al.* A novel portable perfused manometric system for recording of small intestinal motility. *Neurogastroenterol Motil* 1998; **10**: 139–48.
17. Camilleri M, Hasler WL, Parkman HP, Quigley EMM, Soffer E. Measurement of gastrointestinal motility in the GI laboratory. *Gastroenterology* 1998; **115**: 747–62.
18. Verhagen MAMT, Samsom M, Jebbink RJA, Smout AJPM. Clinical relevance of antroduodenal manometry. *Eur J Gastroenterol Hepatol* 1999; **11**: 523–8.
19. Malagelada JR, Camilleri M, Stanghellini V. *Manometric Diagnosis of Gastrointestinal Motility Disorders*. Thieme Medical: New York, 1986.
20. Greydanus MP, Camilleri M. Abnormal postcibal antral and small bowel motility due to neuropathy or myopathy in systemic sclerosis. *Gastroenterology* 1989; **96**: 110–15.
21. Collins PJ, Horowitz M, Cook DJ, Harding PE, Shearman DJ. Gastric emptying in normal subjects—a reproducible technique using a single scintillation camera and computer system. *Gut* 1983; **24**: 1117–25.
22. Malagelada JR, Robertson JS, Brown ML, Remington M. Intestinal transit of solid and liquid components of a meal in health. *Gastroenterology* 1984; **87**: 1255–63.
23. Camilleri M, Zinsmeister AR, Greydanus MP, Brown ML, Proano M. Towards a less costly but accurate test of gastric emptying and small bowel transit. *Dig Dis Sci* 1991; **36**: 609–15.
24. Samsom M, Szarka LA, Camilleri M, Vella A *et al.* Pramlintide, an amylin analog, selectively delays gastric emptying: potential role of vagal inhibition. *Am J Physiol* 2000; **278**: G946–51.
25. Read NW, Miles CA, Fisher D, Holgate AM *et al.* Transit of a meal through the stomach, small intestine, and colon in normal subjects and its role in the pathogenesis of diarrhea. *Gastroenterology* 1980; **79**: 1276–82.

26. Camilleri M, Colemont LJ, Phillips SF, Brown ML *et al.* Human gastric emptying and colonic filling of solids characterized by a new method. *Am J Physiol* 1989; **257**: G284–90.

27. Van der Sijp JR, Kamm MA, Nightingale JM, Britton KE *et al.* Disturbed gastric and small bowel transit in severe idiopathic constipation. *Dig Dis Sci* 1993; **38**: 837–44.

28. Greydanus MP, Camilleri M, Colemont LJ, Phillips SF *et al.* Ileocolonic transfer of solid chyme in small intestinal neuropathies and myopathies. *Gastroenterology* 1990; **99**: 158–64.

29. Van der Sijp JR, Kamm MA, Nightingale JM, Britton KE *et al.* Radioisotope determination of regional colonic transit in severe constipation: comparison with radio-opaque markers. *Gut* 1993; **34**: 402–8.

30. Proano M, Camilleri M, Phillips SF, Brown ML, Thomforde GM. Transit of solids through the human colon: regional quantification in the unprepared bowel. *Am J Physiol* 1990; **258**: G856–62.

31. Camilleri M, Zinsmeister AR. Towards a relatively inexpensive, noninvasive, accurate test for colonic motility disorders. *Gastroenterology* 1992; **103**: 36–42.

32. Hinton JM, Lennard-jones JE, Young AC. A new method for studying gut transit times using radio-opaque markers. *Gut* 1969; **10**: 842–7.

33. Metcalf AM, Phillips SF, Zinsmeister AR, MacCarty RL *et al.* Simplified assessment of segmental colonic transit. *Gastroenterology* 1987; **92**: 40–47.

34. Degen L, Matzinger D, Merz M, Appel-Dingemanse S *et al.* Tegaserod, a 5-HT$_4$ receptor partial agonist, accelerates gastric emptying and gastrointestinal transit in healthy male subjects. *Aliment Pharmacol Ther* 2001; **15**: 1745–51.

35. Prather CM, Camilleri M, Zinsmeister AR, McKinzie S, Thomforde G. Tegaserod accelerates orocecal transit in patients with constipation-predominant irritable bowel syndrome. *Gastroenterology* 2000; **118**: 463–8.

36. Bouras EP, Camilleri M, Burton DD, Thomforde G *et al.* Prucalopride accelerates gastrointestinal and colonic transit in patients with constipation without a rectal evacuation disorder. *Gastroenterology* 2001; **120**: 354–60.

37. Bond JH Jr, Levitt MD, Prentiss R. Investigation of small bowel transit time in man utilizing pulmonary hydrogen (H$_2$) measurements. *J Lab Clin Med* 1975; **85**: 546–55.

38. Rhodes JM, Middleton P, Jewell DP. The lactulose hydrogen breath test as a diagnostic test for small-bowel bacterial overgrowth. *Scand J Gastroenterol* 1979; **14**: 333–6.

39. Miller MA, Parkman HP, Urbain JL, Brown KL *et al.* Comparison of scintigraphy and lactulose breath hydrogen test for assessment of orocecal transit: lactulose accelerates small bowel transit. *Dig Dis Sci* 1997; **42**: 10–18.

40. Kerlin P, Wong L. Breath hydrogen testing in bacterial overgrowth of the small intestine. *Gastroenterology* 1988; **95**: 982–8.

41. Corazza GR, Menozzi MG, Strocchi A, Rasciti L *et al.* The diagnosis of small bowel bacterial overgrowth. Reliability of jejunal culture and inadequacy of breath hydrogen testing. *Gastroenterology* 1990; **98**: 302–9.

42. Sellin JH, Hart R. Glucose malabsorption associated with rapid intestinal transit. *Am J Gastroenterol* 1992; **87**: 584–9.

43. Code CF, Marlett JA. The interdigestive myo-electric complex of the stomach and small bowel of dogs. *J Physiol* 1975; **246**: 289–309.

44. Vantrappen G, Janssens J, Peeters TL, Bloom SR *et al.* Motilin and the interdigestive migrating motor complex in man. *Dig Dis Sci* 1979; **24**: 497–500.

45. Samsom M, Fraser R, Smout AJ, Verhagen MA *et al.* Characterization of small intestinal pressure waves in ambulant subjects recorded with a novel portable manometric system. *Dig Dis Sci* 1999; **44**: 2157–64.

46. Wilmer A, Andrioli A, Coremans G, Tack J, Janssens J. Ambulatory small intestinal manometry. Detailed comparison of duodenal and jejunal motor activity in healthy man. *Dig Dis Sci* 1997; **42**: 1618–27.

47. Husebye E, Skar V, Aalen OO, Osnes M. Digital ambulatory manometry of the small intestine in healthy adults. Estimates of variation within and between individuals and statistical management of incomplete MMC periods. *Dig Dis Sci* 1990; **35**: 1057–65.

48. Kellow JE, Borody TJ, Phillips SF, Tucker RL, Haddad AC. Human interdigestive motility: variations in patterns from esophagus to colon. *Gastroenterology* 1986; **91**: 386–95.

49. Zhao XT, Miller RH, McCamish MA, Wang L, Lin HC. Protein absorption depends on load-dependent inhibition of intestinal transit in dogs. *Am J Clin Nutr* 1996; **64**: 319–23.

50. Hausken T, Odegaard S, Matre K, Berstad A. Antroduodenal motility and movements of luminal contents studied by duplex sonography. *Gastroenterology* 1992; **102**: 1583–90.

51. King PM, Adam RD, Pryde A, McDicken WN, Heading RC. Relationships of human antroduodenal motility and transpyloric fluid movement: non-invasive observations with real-time ultrasound. *Gut* 1984; **25**: 1384–91.

52. Schemann M, Ehrlein HJ. Postprandial patterns of canine jejunal motility and transit of luminal content. *Gastroenterology* 1986; **90**: 991–1000.

53. Hausken T, Mundt M, Samsom M. Low antroduodenal pressure gradients are responsible for gastric emptying of a low-caloric liquid meal in humans. *Neurogastroenterol Motil* 2002; **14**: 97–105.

54. Read NW, Al Janabi MN, Edwards CA, Barber DC. Relationship between postprandial motor activity in the human small intestine and the gastrointestinal transit of food. *Gastroenterology* 1984; **86**: 721–7.

55. Soffer EE, Scalabrini P, Wingate DL. Prolonged ambulant monitoring of human colonic motility. *Am J Physiol* 1989; **257**: G601–6.

56. Narducci F, Bassotti G, Gaburri M, Morelli A. Twenty four hour manometric recording of colonic motor activity in healthy man. *Gut* 1987; **28**: 17–25.

57. Reddy SN, Di Lorenzo C, Yanni G, Bazzocchi G *et al*. A unified technique approach to the study of colonic scintigraphy and intraluminal pressure. *Gastroenterology* 1990; **98**: A383.

58. Kock NG, Hulten L, Leandoer L. A study of the motility in different parts of the human colon. Resting activity, response to feeding and to prostigmine. *Scand J Gastroenterol* 1968; **3**: 163–9.

59. Kerlin P, Zinsmeister A, Phillips S. Motor responses to food of the ileum, proximal colon, and distal colon of healthy humans. *Gastroenterology* 1983; **84**: 762–70.

60. Steadman CJ, Phillips SF, Camilleri M, Talley NJ. Control of muscle tone in the human colon. *Gut* 1992; **33**: 541–6.

61. Ford MJ, Camilleri M, Wiste JA, Hanson RB. Differences in colonic tone and phasic response to a meal in the transverse and sigmoid human colon. *Gut* 1995; **37**: 264–9.

62. Gonella J, Bouvier M, Blanquet F. Extrinsic nervous control of motility of small and large intestines and related sphincters. *Physiol Rev* 1987; **67**: 902–61.

63. Huizinga JD Motor function of the colon. In Phillips S, Pemberton JH, Shorter RG (eds), *Large Intestine—Physiology, Pathophysiology and Disease*, Raven: New York, 1991; 93–114.

64. Langton P, Ward SM, Carl A, Norell MA, Sanders KM. Spontaneous electrical activity of interstitial cells of Cajal isolated from canine proximal colon. *Proc Natl Acad Sci USA* 1989; **86**: 7280–84.

65. Wang XY, Sanders KM, Ward SM. Intimate relationship between interstitial cells of cajal and enteric nerves in the guinea-pig small intestine. *Cell Tissue Res* 1999; **295**: 247–56.

66. Huizinga JD, Thuneberg L, Kluppel M, Malysz J *et al.* W/kit gene required for interstitial cells of Cajal and for intestinal pacemaker activity. *Nature* 1995; **373**: 347–9.

67. Weisbrodt NW, Copeland EM, Moore EP, Kearley RW, Johnson LR. Effect of vagotomy on electrical activity of the small intestine of the dog. *Am J Physiol* 1975; **228**: 650–54.

68. Marik F, Code CF. Control of the interdigestive myoelectric activity in dogs by the vagus nerves and pentagastrin. *Gastroenterology* 1975; **69**: 387–95.

69. Hashmonai M, Go VL, Szurszewski JH. Effect of total sympathectomy and of decentralization on migrating complexes in dogs. *Gastroenterology* 1987; **92**: 978–86.

70. Sarna S, Stoddard C, Belbeck L, McWade D. Intrinsic nervous control of migrating myoelectric complexes. *Am J Physiol* 1981; **241**: G16–23.

71. Itoh Z, Takeuchi S, Aizawa I, Mori K *et al.* Changes in plasma motilin concentration and gastrointestinal contractile activity in conscious dogs. *Am J Dig Dis* 1978; **23**: 929–35.

72. Owyang C, Achem-Karam SR, Vinik AI. Pancreatic polypeptide and intestinal migrating motor complex in humans. Effect of pancreaticobiliary secretion. *Gastroenterology* 1983; **84**: 10–17.

73. Feinle C, D'Amato M, Read NW. Cholecystokinin-A receptors modulate gastric sensory and motor responses to gastric distention and duodenal lipid. *Gastroenterology* 1996; **110**: 1379–85.

74. Lee KY, Chang TM, Chey WY. Effect of rabbit antimotilin serum on myoelectric activity and plasma motilin concentration in fasting dog. *Am J Physiol* 1983; **245**: G547–53.

75. Fargeas MJ, Bassotti G, Fioramonti J, Bueno L. Involvement of different mechanisms in the stimulatory effects of cholecystokinin octapeptide on gastrointestinal and colonic motility in dogs. *Can J Physiol Pharmacol* 1989; **67**: 1205–12.

76. Rodriguez-Membrilla A, Martinez V, Vergara P. Peripheral and central cholecystokinin receptors regulate postprandial intestinal motility in the rat. *J Pharmacol Exp Ther* 1995; **275**: 486–93.

77. Niederau C, Karaus M. Effects of CCK receptor blockade on intestinal motor activity in conscious dogs. *Am J Physiol* 1991; **260**: G315–24.

78. Keshavarzian A, Iber FL. Intestinal transit in insulin-requiring diabetics. *Am J Gastroenterol* 1986; **81**: 257–60.

79. Iber FL, Parveen S, Vandrunen M, Sood KB *et al.* Relation of symptoms to impaired stomach, small bowel, and colon motility in long-standing diabetes. *Dig Dis Sci* 1993; **38**: 45–50.

80. Werth B, Meyer-Wyss B, Spinas GA, Drewe J, Beglinger C. Non-invasive assessment of gastrointestinal motility disorders in diabetic patients with and without cardiovascular signs of autonomic neuropathy. *Gut* 1992; **33**: 1199–203.

81. Rosa-e-Silva L, Troncon LEA, Oliveira RB, Foss MC *et al.* Rapid distal small bowel transit associated with sympathetic denervation in type I diabetes mellitus. *Gut* 1996; **39**: 748–56.

82. Samsom M, Akkermans LM, Jebbink RJ, van Isselt H *et al.* Gastrointestinal motor mechanisms in hyperglycaemia induced delayed gastric emptying in type I diabetes mellitus. *Gut* 1997; **40**: 641–6.

83. Jebbink HJA, Van Berge-Henegouwen GP, Akkermans LMA, Smout AJPM. Small intestinal motor abnormalities in patients with functional dyspepsia demonstrated by ambulatory manometry. *Gut* 1996; **38**: 694–700.

84. Wilmer A, Van Cutsem E, Andrioli A, Tack J *et al.* Ambulatory gastrojejunal manometry in severe motility-like dyspepsia: lack of correlation between dysmotility, symptoms, and gastric emptying. *Gut* 1998; **42**: 235–42.

85. Hackelsberger N, Schmidt T, Renner R, Widmer R *et al.* Ambulatory long-term jejunal manometry in diabetic patients with cardiac autonomic neuropathy. *Neurogastroenterol Motil* 1997; **9**: 77–83.

86. Kawagishi T, Nishizawa Y, Okuno Y, Sekiya K, Morii H. Segmental gut transit in diabetes mellitus: effect of cisapride. *Diabetes Res Clin Pract* 1992; **17**: 137–44.

87. Battle WM, Snape WJ Jr, Alavi A, Cohen S, Braunstein S. Colonic dysfunction in diabetes mellitus. *Gastroenterology* 1980; **79**: 1217–21.

88. Scarpello JH, Greaves M, Sladen GE. Small intestinal transit in diabetics. *Br Med J* 1976; **20**; 2: 1225–6.

89. Samsom M, Jebbink RJ, Akkermans LM, Berge-Henegouwen GP, Smout AJ. Abnormalities of antroduodenal motility in type 1 diabetes. *Diabetes Care* 1996; **19**: 21–7.

90. Sims MA, Hasler WL, Chey WD, Kim MS, Owyang C. Hyperglycemia inhibits mechanoreceptor-mediated gastrocolonic responses and colonic peristaltic reflexes in healthy humans. *Gastroenterology* 1995; **108**: 350–59.

91. Bharucha AE, Camilleri M, Low PA, Zinsmeister AR. Autonomic dysfunction in gastrointestinal motility disorders. *Gut* 1993; **34**: 397–401.

92. Watkins PJ, Thomas PK. Diabetes mellitus and the nervous system. *J Neurol Neurosurg Psychiat* 1998; **65**: 620–32.

93. Guy RJ, Dawson JL, Garrett JR, Laws JW *et al.* Diabetic gastroparesis from autonomic neuropathy: surgical considerations and changes in vagus nerve morphology. *J Neurol Neurosurg Psychiat* 1984; **47**: 686–91.

94. Britland ST, Young RJ, Sharma AK, Lee D *et al.* Vagus nerve morphology in diabetic gastropathy. *Diabet Med* 1990; **7**: 780–78.

95. Yoshida MM, Schuffler MD, Sumi SM. There are no morphologic abnormalities of the gastric wall or abdominal vagus in patients with diabetic gastroparesis. *Gastroenterology* 1988; **94**: 907–14.

96. Belai A, Calcutt NA, Carrington AL, Diemel LT *et al.* Enteric neuropeptides in streptozotocin-diabetic rats; effects of insulin and aldose reductase inhibition. *J Auton Nerv Syst* 1996; **58**: 163–9.

97. Lucas PD, Sardar AM. Effects of diabetes on cholinergic transmission in two rat gut preparations. *Gastroenterology* 1991; **100**: 123–8.

98. Takahashi T, Nakamura K, Itoh H, Sima AA, Owyang C. Impaired expression of nitric oxide synthase in the gastric myenteric plexus of spontaneously diabetic rats. *Gastroenterology* 1997; **113**: 1535–44.

99. Ordog T, Takayama I, Cheung WK, Ward SM, Sanders KM. Remodeling of networks of interstitial cells of Cajal in a murine model of diabetic gastroparesis. *Diabetes* 2000; **49**: 1731–9.

100. He CL, Soffer EE, Ferris CD, Walsh RM *et al.* Loss of interstitial cells of cajal and inhibitory innervation in insulin-dependent diabetes. *Gastroenterology* 2001; **121**: 427–34.

101. Scarpello JH, Hague RV, Cullen DR, Sladen GE. The ^{14}C-glycocholate test in diabetic diarrhoea. *Br Med J* 1976; **2**: 673–5.

102. Fraser R, Horowitz M, Dent J. Hyperglycaemia stimulates pyloric motility in normal subjects. *Gut* 1991; **32**: 475–8.

103. Björnsson ES, Urbanavicius V, Eliasson B, Attvall S *et al.* Effects of hyperglycemia on interdigestive gastrointestinal motility in humans. *Scand J Gastroenterol* 1994; **29**: 1096–104.

104. Russo A, Fraser R, Horowitz M. The effect of acute hyperglycemia on small intestinal motility in normal subjects. *Diabetologia* 1996; **39**: 984–9.
105. Lingenfelser T, Sun WM, Hebbard GS, Dent J, Horowitz M. Effects of duodenal distension on antropyloroduodenal pressures and perception are modified by hyperglycemia. *Am J Physiol* 1999; **276**: G711–18.
106. Hebbard GS, Samsom M, Sun WM, Dent J, Horowitz M. Hyperglycemia affects proximal gastric motor and sensory function during small intestinal triglyceride infusion. *Am J Physiol* 1996; **271**: G814–19.
107. Oster-Jorgensen E, Qvist N, Pedersen SA, Rasmussen L, Hovendal CP. The influence of induced hyperglycemia on the characteristics of intestinal motility and bile kinetics in healthy men. *Scand J Gastroenterol* 1992; **27**: 285–8.
108. De Boer SY, Masclee AAM, Lamers CBHW Effect of hyperglycemia on gastrointestinal and gallbladder motility. *Scand J Gastroenterol* 1992; **27** (suppl 194): 13–18.
109. Hebbard GS, Samsom M, Andrews JM, Carman D *et al*. Hyperglycemia affects gastric electrical rhythm and nausea during intraduodenal triglyceride infusion. *Dig Dis Sci* 1997; **42**: 568–75.
110. Fellows IW, Evans DF, Bennett T, Macdonald IA *et al*. The effect of insulin-induced hypoglycaemia on gastrointestinal motility in man. *Clin Sci (Lond)* 1987; **72**: 743–8.
111. Fraser R, Fuller J, Horowitz M, Dent J. Effect of insulin-induced hypoglycaemia on antral, pyloric and duodenal motility in fasting subjects. *Clin Sci (Lond)* 1991; **81**: 281–5.
112. Nusser J, Scheuer R, Abendroth D, Illner WD *et al*. Effect of pancreatic and/or renal transplantation on diabetic autonomic neuropathy. *Diabetologia* 1991; **34** (suppl 1):S118–20.
113. Hathaway DK, Abell T, Cardoso S, Hartwig MS *et al*. Improvement in autonomic and gastric function following pancreas-kidney vs. kidney-alone transplantation and the correlation with quality of life. *Transplantation* 1994; **57**: 816–22.
114. Knutson L, Flemström G. Duodenal mucosal bicarbonate secretion in man. Stimulation by acid and inhibition by the α2-adrenoreceptor agonist clonidine. *Gut* 1989; **30**: 1708–15.
115. Dalenbäck J, Mellander A, Olbe L, Sjövall H. Motility-related cyclic fluctuations of interdigestive gastric acid and bicarbonate secretion in man. *Scand J Gastroenterol* 1993; **28**: 943–8.
116. Ainsworth MA, Kjelsden J, Olsen O, Chistensen P, Schaffalitzky de Muckadell OB. Duodenal disappearance rate of acid during inhibition of mucosal bicarbonate secretion. *Digestion* 1990; **47**: 121–9.
117. Williams SE, Turnberg LA. Demonstration of a pH gradient across mucus adherent to rabbit gastric mucosa: evidence for a 'mucus-bicarbonate' barrier. *Gut* 1981; **22**: 94–6.
118. Verhagen MAMT, Roelofs JMM, Edelbroek MAL, Smout AJPM, Akkermans LMA. The effect of cisapride on duodenal acid exposure in the proximal duodenum in healthy subjects. *Aliment Pharmacol Ther* 1999; **13**: 621–30.
119. Southgate DA. Digestion and metabolism of sugars. *Am J Clin Nutr* 1995; **62**: 203–10S.
120. Levin RJ. Digestion and absorption of carbohydrates—from molecules and membranes to humans. *Am J Clin Nutr* 1994; **59**: 690–9S.
121. Bieberdorf FA, Morawski S, Fordtran JS. Effect of sodium, mannitol, and magnesium on glucose, galactose, 3-*O*-methylglucose, and fructose absorption in the human ileum. *Gastroenterology* 1975; **68**: 58–66.
122. Kellet GL, Jamal A, Robertson JP, Wollen N. The acute regulation of glucose absorption, transport and metabolism in rat small intestine by insulin *in vivo*. *Biochem J 1984*; **219**: *1027–35*.

123. Sigrist-Nelson K, Hopfer U. A distinct D-fructose transport system in isolated brush border membrane. *Biochim Biophys Acta* 1974; **367**: 247–54.

124. Bantle JP, Laine DC, Thomas JW. Metabolic effects of dietary fructose and sucrose in types I and II diabetic subjects. *J Am Med Assoc* 1986; **19**: 3241–6.

125. Malerbi DA, Paiva ES, Duarte AL, Wajchenberg BL. Metabolic effects of dietary sucrose and fructose in type II diabetic subjects. *Diabetes Care* 1996; **19**: 1249–56.

126. Freeman HJ, Kim YS, Sleisenger MH. Protein digestion and absorption in man. Normal mechanisms and protein-energy malnutrition. *Am J Med* 1979; **67**: 1030–36.

127. Sleisenger MH, Kim YS. Protein digestion and absorption. *N Engl J Med* 1979; **300**: 659–63.

128. Moreau H, Laugier R, Gargouri Y, Ferrato F, Verger R. Human preduodenal lipase is entirely of gastric fundic origin. *Gastroenterology* 1988; **95**: 1221–6.

129. Gooden JM, Lascelles AK. Relative importance of pancreatic lipase and pregastric esterase on lipid absorption in calves 1–2 weeks of age. *Aust J Biol Sci* 1973; **26**: 625–33.

130. Abrams CK, Hamosh M, Lee TC, Ansher AF *et al*. Gastric lipase: localization in the human stomach. *Gastroenterology* 1988; **95**: 1460–64.

131. Carey MC, Small DM, Bliss CM. Lipid digestion and absorption. *Ann Rev Physiol* 1983; **45**: 651–77.

132. Rigler MW, Honkanen RE, Patton JS. Visualization by freeze fracture, *in vitro* and *in vivo*, of the products of fat digestion. *J Lipid Res* 1986; **27**: 836–57.

133. Ikeda I, Tanaka K, Sugano M, Vahouny GV, Gallo LL. Discrimination between cholesterol and sitosterol for absorption in rats. *J Lipid Res* 1988; **29**: 1583–91.

134. Kayden HJ, Senior JR, Mattson FH. The monoglyceride pathway of fat absorption in man. *J Clin Invest* 1967; **46**: 1695–703.

135. Chijiiwa K, Linscheer WG. Mechanism of pH effect on oleic acid and cholesterol absorption in the rat. *Am J Physiol* 1987; **252**: G506–10.

136. Mattson FH, Volpenhein RA. The digestion and absorption of triglycerides. *J Biol Chem* 1964; **239**: 2772–7.

137. Raybould HE, Meyer JH, Tabrizi Y, Liddle RA, Tso P. Inhibition of gastric emptying in response to intestinal lipid is dependent on chylomicron formation. *Am J Physiol* 1998; **274**: R1834–8.

138. Glatzle J, Kalogeris TJ, Zittel TT, Guerrini S *et al*. Chylomicron components mediate intestinal lipid-induced inhibition of gastric motor function. *Am J Physiol* 2002; **282**: G86–91.

139. Liscum L, Dahl NK. Intracellular cholesterol transport. *J Lipid Res* 1992; **33**: 1239–54.

140. Ananthanarayanan M, Bucuvalas JC, Shneider BL, Sippel CJ, Suchy FJ. An ontogenically regulated 48 kDa protein is a component of the $Na^{(+)}$-bile acid cotransporter of rat liver. *Am J Physiol* 1991; **261**: G810–17.

141. von Dippe P, Levy D. Reconstitution of the immunopurified 49 kDa sodium-dependent bile acid transport protein derived from hepatocyte sinusoidal plasma membranes. *J Biol Chem* 1990; **265**: 14812–16.

142. Hsieh PS, Moore MC, Neal DW, Cherrington AD. Importance of the hepatic arterial glucose level in generation of the portal signal in conscious dogs. *Am J Physiol* 2000; **279**: E284–92.

143. Radziuk J, McDonald TJ, Rubenstein D, Dupre J. Initial splanchnic extraction of ingested glucose in normal man. *Metabolism* 1978; **27**: 657–69.

144. Ferrannini E, Bjorkman O, Reichard GA JR, Pilo A *et al*. The disposal of an oral glucose load in healthy subjects. A quantitative study. *Diabetes* 1985; **34**: 580–88.

145. Pehling G, Tessari P, Gerich JE, Haymond MW *et al*. Abnormal meal carbohydrate disposition in insulin-dependent diabetes. Relative contributions of endogenous glucose

production and initial splanchnic uptake and effect of intensive insulin therapy. *J Clin Invest* 1984; **74**: 985–91.

146. Frank JW, Saslow SB, Camilleri M, Thomforde GM *et al.* Mechanism of accelerated gastric emptying of liquids and hyperglycemia in patients with type II diabetes mellitus. *Gastroenterology* 1995; **109**: 755–65.

147. Fujita Y, Kojima H, Hidaka H, Fujimiya M *et al.* Increased intestinal glucose absorption and postprandial hyperglycaemia at the early step of glucose intolerance in Otsuka Long-Evans Tokushima Fatty rats. *Diabetologia* 1998; **41**: 1459–66.

148. Burant CF, Flink S, DePaoli AM, Chen J *et al.* Small intestine hexose transport in experimental diabetes. Increased transporter mRNA and protein expression in enterocytes. *J Clin Invest* 1994; **93**: 578–85.

149. Miyamoto K, Hase K, Taketani Y, Minami H *et al.* Diabetes and glucose transporter gene expression in rat small intestine. *Biochem Biophys Res Commun* 1991; **181**: 1110–17.

150. Dyer J, Wood IS, Palejwala A, Ellis A, Shirazi-Beechey SP. Expression of monosaccharide transporters in intestine of diabetic humans. *Am J Physiol* 2002; **282**: G241–48.

151. Costrini NV, Ganeshappa KP, Wu W, Whalen GE, Soergel KH. Effect of insulin, glucose, and controlled diabetes mellitus on human jejunal function. *Am J Physiol* 1977; **233**: E181–7.

152. Rayner CK, Schwartz MP, van Dam PS, Renooij W, Smet de M, Horowitz M, Wishart JM, Smout AJ, Samsom M. Upper gastrointestinal responses to intraduodenum nutrient in type I diabetes mellitus. *Eur J Gastroenterol Hepatol* 2004; **16**: 1–7.

153. Basu A, Basu R, Shah P, Vella A *et al.* Type 2 diabetes impairs splanchnic uptake of glucose but does not alter intestinal glucose absorption during enteral glucose feeding: additional evidence for a defect in hepatic glucokinase activity. *Diabetes* 2001; **50**: 1351–62.

154. Westergaard H. Insulin modulates rat intestinal glucose transport: effect of hypoinsulinemia and hyperinsulinemia. *Am J Physiol* 1989; **256**: G911–18.

155. Thomson AB, Rajotte RV. Insulin and islet cell transplantation in streptozotocin-diabetic rats: effect on intestinal uptake of hexoses. *Comp Biochem Physiol A* 1985; **82**: 827–31.

156. Samsom M, Benninga M, van Steenderen L, Renooij W *et al.* Inhibition of small intestinal motility decreases glucose absorption in humans. *Gastroenterology* 1999; **116**: A1073.

157. Giannella RA, Rout WR, Toskes PP. Jejunal brush border injury and impaired sugar and amino acid uptake in the blind loop syndrome. *Gastroenterology* 1974; **67**: 965–74.

158. Jonas A, Krishnan C, Forstner G. Pathogenesis of mucosal injury in the blind loop syndrome. *Gastroenterology* 1978; **75**: 791–5.

159. Rutgeerts L, Mainguet P, Tytgat G, Eggermont E. Enterokinase in contaminated small-bowel syndrome. *Digestion* 1974; **10**: 249–54.

160. Soudah HC, Hasler WL, Owyang C. Effect of octreotide on intestinal motility and bacterial overgrowth in scleroderma. *N Engl J Med* 1991; **325**: 1461–7.

161. Husebye E, Skar V, Hoverstad T, Iversen T, Melby K. Abnormal intestinal motor patterns explain enteric colonization with Gram-negative bacilli in late radiation enteropathy. *Gastroenterology* 1995; **109**: 1078–89.

162. King CE, Toskes PP The experimental rat blind loop preparation: a model for small-intestine bacterial overgrowth in man. In Pfeiffer CJ (ed.) *Animal Models for Intestinal Disease.* CRC Press: Boca Raton, FL, 1985; 217.

163. Tabaqchali S, Hatzioannou J, Booth CC. Bile-salt deconjugation and steatorrhoea in patients with the stagnant-loop syndrome. *Lancet* 1968; **2**: 12–16.

164. Simon GL, Gorbach SL. The human intestinal microflora. *Dig Dis Sci* 1986; **31**: 147–62S.

165. Kim YS, Spritz N, Blum M, Terz J, Sherlock P. The role of altered bile acid metabolism in the steatorrhea of experimental blind loop. *J Clin Invest* 1966; **45**: 956–62.

166. Jenkins DJ, Goff DV, Leeds AR, Alberti KG *et al.* Unabsorbable carbohydrates and diabetes: decreased post-prandial hyperglycaemia. *Lancet* 1976; **2**: 172–4.

167. Chandalia M, Garg A, Lutjohann D, von Bergmann K *et al.* Beneficial effects of high dietary fiber intake in patients with type 2 diabetes mellitus. *N Engl J Med* 2000; **342**: 1392–8.

168. Giacco R, Parillo M, Rivellese AA, Lasorella G *et al.* Long-term dietary treatment with increased amounts of fiber-rich low-glycemic index natural foods improves blood glucose control and reduces the number of hypoglycemic events in type 1 diabetic patients. *Diabetes Care* 2000; **23**: 1461–6.

169. Meyer JH, Gu YG, Jehn D, Taylor IL. Intragastric vs. intraintestinal viscous polymers and glucose tolerance after liquid meals of glucose. *Am J Clin Nutr* 1988; **48**: 260–66.

170. Cherbut C, Bruley DV, Schnee M, Rival M *et al.* Involvement of small intestinal motility in blood glucose response to dietary fibre in man. *Br J Nutr* 1994; **71**: 675–85.

171. Bischoff H. Pharmacology of α-glucosidase inhibition. *Eur J Clin Invest* 1994; **24** (suppl 3):3–10 3–10.

172. Uttenthal LO, Ukponmwan OO, Wood SM, Ghiglione M *et al.* Long-term effects of intestinal α-glucosidase inhibition on postprandial glucose, pancreatic and gut hormone responses and fasting serum lipids in diabetics on sulphonylureas. *Diabet Med* 1986; **3**: 155–60.

173. Mertes G. Safety and efficacy of acarbose in the treatment of type 2 diabetes: data from a 5-year surveillance study. *Diabetes Res Clin Pract* 2001; **52**: 193–204.

174. Hollander PA, Elbein SC, Hirsch IB, Kelley D *et al.* Role of orlistat in the treatment of obese patients with type 2 diabetes. A 1-year randomized double-blind study. *Diabetes Care* 1998; **21**: 1288–94.

175. Pilichiewicz A, O'Donovan D, Feinle C, Lei Y, Wishart JM, Bryant L, Meyer JH, Horowitz M, Jones KL. Effect of lipase inhibition on gastric emptying of, and the glycemic and incretin responses to, an oil/aqueous drink in type 2 diabetes mellitus. *J Clin Endocrinol Metab.* 2003; **88**: 3829–34.

176. Whalen GE, Soergel KH, Geenen JE. Diabetic diarrhea. A clinical and pathophysiological study. *Gastroenterology* 1969; **56**: 1021–32.

177. Chang EB, Fedorak RN, Field M. Experimental diabetic diarrhea in rats. Intestinal mucosal denervation hypersensitivity and treatment with clonidine. *Gastroenterology* 1986; **91**: 564–9.

178. Chang EB, Bergenstal RM, Field M. Diarrhea in streptozocin-treated rats. Loss of adrenergic regulation of intestinal fluid and electrolyte transport. *J Clin Invest* 1985; **75**: 1666–70.

179. Carratu R, Secondulfo M, de Magistris L, Iafusco D *et al.* Altered intestinal permeability to mannitol in diabetes mellitus type I. *J Pediatr Gastroenterol Nutr* 1999; **28**: 264–9.

180. Cooper BT, Ukabam SO, O'Brien IA, Hare JP, Corrall RJ. Intestinal permeability in diabetic diarrhoea. *Diabet Med* 1987; **4**: 49–52.

181. Rowell LB, Detry JM, Blackmon JR, Wyss C. Importance of the splanchnic vascular bed in human blood pressure regulation. *J Appl Physiol* 1972; **32**: 213–20.

182. Walls EW The blood and vascular system and lymphatic system. In Cunningham DJ, Romannes GJ (eds), *Cunningham's Textbook of Anatomy.* Oxford University Press: Oxford 1981; 924–31.

183. Norryd C, Dencker H, Lunderquist A, Olin T. Superior mesenteric blood flow in man studied with a dye-dilution technique. *Acta Chir Scand.* 1975; **141**: 109–18.

184. Granger DN, Richardson PD, Kvietys PR, Mortillaro NA. Intestinal blood flow. *Gastroenterology* 1980; **78**: 837–63.

185. Alemany CA, Oh W, Stonestreet BS. Effects of nitric oxide synthesis inhibition on mesenteric perfusion in young pigs. *Am J Physiol* 1997; **272**: G612–16.

186. Sieber C, Beglinger C, Jaeger K, Hildebrand P, Stalder GA. Regulation of postprandial mesenteric blood flow in humans: evidence for a cholinergic nervous reflex. *Gut* 1991; **32**: 361–6.

187. Moneta GL, Taylor DC, Helton WS, Mulholland MW, Strandness DE Jr. Duplex ultrasound measurement of postprandial intestinal blood flow: effect of meal composition. *Gastroenterology* 1988; **95**: 1294–301.

188. Sidery MB, Macdonald IA, Blackshaw PE. Superior mesenteric artery blood flow and gastric emptying in humans and the differential effects of high fat and high carbohydrate meals. *Gut* 1994; **35**: 186–90.

189. Belai A, Milner P, Aberdeen J, Burnstock G. Selective damage to sensorimotor perivascular nerves in the mesenteric vessels of diabetic rats. *Diabetes* 1996; **45**: 139–43.

190. Korthuis RJ, Benoit JN, Kvietys PR, Laughlin MH. Intestinal hyperemia in experimental diabetes mellitus. *Am J Physiol* 1987; **253**: G26–32.

191. Goldin E, Casadevall M, Mourelle M, Cirera I *et al.* Role of prostaglandins and nitric oxide in gastrointestinal hyperemia of diabetic rats. *Am J Physiol* 1996; **270**: G684–90.

192. Purewal TS, Goss DE, Zanone MM, Edmonds ME, Watkins PJ. The splanchnic circulation and postural hypotension in diabetic autonomic neuropathy. *Diabet Med* 1995; **12**: 513–22.

193. Best IM, Pitzele A, Green A, Halperin J *et al.* Mesenteric blood flow in patients with diabetic neuropathy. *J Vasc Surg* 1991; **13**: 84–9.

194. Mathias CJ, da Costa DF, Fosbraey P, Bannister R *et al.* Cardiovascular, biochemical and hormonal changes during food-induced hypotension in chronic autonomic failure. *J Neurol Sci* 1989; **94**: 255–69.

195. Puisieux F, Bulckaen H, Fauchais AL, Drumez S *et al.* Ambulatory blood pressure monitoring and postprandial hypotension in elderly persons with falls or syncopes. *J Gerontol A Biol Sci Med Sci* 2000; **55**: M535–40.

196. Jones KL, Tonkin A, Horowitz M, Wishart JM *et al.* Rate of gastric emptying is a determinant of postprandial hypotension in non-insulin-dependent diabetes mellitus. *Clin Sci (Lond)* 1998; **94**: 65–70.

197. Jansen RW, Peeters TL, Lenders JW, van Lier HJ, v't LA, Hoefnagels WH. Somatostatin analog octreotide (SMS 201–995) prevents the decrease in blood pressure after oral glucose loading in the elderly. *J Clin Endocrinol Metab* 1989; **68**: 752–6.

198. O'Donovan D, Feinle C, Tonkin A, Horowitz M, Jones KL. Postprandial hypotension in response to duodenal glucose delivery in healthy older subjects. *J Physiol* 2002; **540**: 673–9.

199. Hoeldtke RD, Davis KM, Joseph J, Gonzales R *et al.* Hemodynamic effects of octreotide in patients with autonomic neuropathy. *Circulation* 1991; **84**: 168–76.

200. Kempler P, Tesfaye S, Chaturvedi N, Stevens LK, Webb DJ, Eaton S *et al.* Blood pressure response to standing in the diagnosis of autonomic neuropathy: the EURODIAB IDDM Complications Study. *Arch Physiol Biochem* 2001; **109**: 215–22.

201. Burkitt DP, Walker AR, Painter NS. Effect of dietary fibre on stools and the transit times, and its role in the causation of disease. *Lancet* 1972; **2**: 1408–12.

202. Jenkins DJ, Peterson RD, Thorne MJ, Ferguson PW. Wheat fiber and laxation: dose response and equilibration time. *Am J Gastroenterol* 1987; **82**: 1259–63.

203. Ashraf W, Srb F, Lof J. and Quigley EMM. Idiopathic constipation: subjective complaints vs. objective assessment. *Gastroenterology* 1994; **106**: A461.

204. Kuijpers HC. Application of the colorectal laboratory in diagnosis and treatment of functional constipation. *Dis Colon Rectum* 1990; **33**: 35–9.

205. Smith B. Pathologic changes in the colon produced by anthraquinone purgatives. *Dis Colon Rectum* 1973; **16**: 455–8.

206. Krevsky B, Malmud LS, Maurer AH, Somers MB *et al.* The effect of oral cisapride on colonic transit. *Aliment Pharmacol Ther* 1987; **1**: 293–304.

207. Muller-Lissner SA. Treatment of chronic constipation with cisapride and placebo. *Gut* 1987; **28**: 1033–8.

208. Verheyen K, Verkaeke M, Demyttenaere P, Van Mierlo FJ. Double-blind comparison of two weeks cisapride dosage regimens with placebo in the treatment of functional constipation. *Curr Ther Res* 1987; **41**: 978–85.

209. Samsom M, Gooszen HG. Treatment of severely delayed gastric emptying. *Ned Tijdschr Geneeskd* 2000; **144**: 1945–8.

210. Snape WJ Jr, Battle WM, Schwartz SS, Braunstein SN *et al.* Metoclopramide to treat gastroparesis due to diabetes mellitus: a double-blind, controlled trial. *Ann Intern Med* 1982; **96**: 444–6.

211. Yanni G, Snape WJ. Effect of erythromycin on colonic motility in patients with constipation. *Gastroenterology* 1992; **103**: A1384.

212. Jameson JS, Rogers J, Misiewicz JJ, Raimundo AH, Henry MM. Oral or intravenous erythromycin has no effect on human distal colonic motility. *Aliment Pharmacol Ther* 1992; **6**: 589–95.

213. Donowitz M, Binder HJ. Effect of dioctyl sodium sulfosuccinate on colonic fluid and electrolyte movement. *Gastroenterology* 1975; **69**: 941–50.

214. de Graaf EJ, Gilberts EC, Schouten WR. Role of segmental colonic transit time studies to select patients with slow transit constipation for partial left-sided or subtotal colectomy. *Br J Surg* 1996; **83**: 648–51.

215. You YT, Wang JY, Changchien CR, Chen JS *et al.* Segmental colectomy in the management of colonic inertia. *Am Surg* 1998; **64**: 775–7.

216. Lubowski DZ, Chen FC, Kennedy ML, King DW. Results of colectomy for severe slow transit constipation. *Dis Colon Rectum* 1996; **39**: 23–9.

217. Jain NK, Rosenberg DB, Ulahannan MJ, Glasser MJ, Pitchumoni CS. Sorbitol intolerance in adults. *Am J Gastroenterol* 1985; **80**: 678–81.

218. Badiga MS, Jain NK, Casanova C, Pitchumoni CS. Diarrhea in diabetics: the role of sorbitol. *J Am Coll Nutr* 1990; **9**: 578–82.

219. Molloy A, Tomkin G. Altered bile in diabetic diarrhoea. *Br Med J* 1979; **1**:1084.

220. Virally-Monod M, Tielmans D, Kevorkian JP, Bouhnik Y *et al.* Chronic diarrhoea and diabetes mellitus: prevalence of small intestinal bacterial overgrowth. *Diabetes Metab* 1998; **24**: 530–36.

221. Zietz B, Lock G, Straub RH, Braun B *et al.* Small-bowel bacterial overgrowth in diabetic subjects is associated with cardiovascular autonomic neuropathy. *Diabetes Care* 2000; **23**: 1200–120.

222. Tsai ST, Vinik AI, Brunner JF. Diabetic diarrhea and somatostatin. *Ann Intern Med* 1986; **104**: 894.

223. Witt K, Pedersen NT. The long-acting somatostatin analogue SMS 201–995 causes malabsorption. *Scand J Gastroenterol* 1989; **24**: 1248–52.

224. Awouters F, Megens A, Verlinden M, Schuurkes J *et al.* Loperamide. Survey of studies on mechanism of its antidiarrheal activity. *Dig Dis Sci* 1993; **38**: 977–95.

225. Sun WM, Read NW, Verlinden M. Effects of loperamide oxide on gastrointestinal transit time and anorectal function in patients with chronic diarrhoea and faecal incontinence. *Scand J Gastroenterol* 1997; **32**: 34–8.

226. Fedorak RN, Field M, Chang EB. Treatment of diabetic diarrhea with clonidine. *Ann Intern Med* 1985; **102**: 197–9.

227. Trier JS. Celiac sprue. *N Engl J Med* 1991; **325**: 1709–19.

228. Svejgaard A, Platz P, Ryder LP. HLA and disease 1982—a survey. *Immunol Rev* 1983; **70**: 193–218.

229. Caffrey C, Hitman GA, Niven MJ, Cassell PG, Kumar P, Fry L *et al.* HLA-DP and coeliac disease: family and population studies. *Gut* 1990; **31**: 663–7.

230. Thain ME, Hamilton JR, Ehrlich RM. Coexistence of diabetes mellitus and celiac disease. *J Pediatr* 1974; **85**: 527–9.

231. Koletzko S, Burgin-Wolff A, Koletzko B, Knapp M *et al.* Prevalence of coeliac disease in diabetic children and adolescents. A multicentre study. *Eur J Pediat* 1988; **148**: 113–17.

232. Barera G, Bianchi C, Calisti L, Cerutti F *et al.* Screening of diabetic children for coeliac disease with antigliadin antibodies and HLA typing. *Arch Dis Child* 1991; **66**: 491–4.

233. Stenhammar L, Ansved P, Jansson G, Jansson U. The incidence of childhood celiac disease in Sweden. *J Pediat Gastroenterol Nutr* 1987; **6**: 707–9.

234. Pittschieler K, Reissigl H, Mengarda G. Celiac disease in two different population groups of South Tirol. *J Pediatr Gastroenterol Nutr* 1988; **7**: 400–402.

235. Greco L, Tozzi AE, Mayer M, Grimaldi M *et al.* Unchanging clinical picture of coeliac disease presentation in Campania, *Italy Eur J Pediatr* 1989; **148**: 610–3.

236. Page SR, Lloyd CA, Hill PG, Peacock I, Holmes GK. The prevalence of coeliac disease in adult diabetes mellitus. *Qu J Med* 1994; **87**: 631–7.

237. De Vitis I, Ghirlanda G, Gasbarrini G. Prevalence of coeliac disease in type I diabetes: a multicentre study. *Acta Paediatr* 1996; **412**: (suppl) 56–7.

238. Logan RF, Rifkind EA, Busuttil A, Gilmour HM, Ferguson A. Prevalence and 'incidence' of celiac disease in Edinburgh and the Lothian region of Scotland. *Gastroenterology* 1986; **90**: 334–42.

239. Midhagen G, Jarnerot G, Kraaz W. Adult coeliac disease within a defined geographic area in Sweden. A study of prevalence and associated diseases. *Scand J Gastroenterol* 1988; **23**: 1000–1004.

240. Saukkonen T, Vaisanen S, Akerblom HK, Savilahti E. Coeliac disease in children and adolescents with type 1 diabetes: a study of growth, glycaemic control, and experiences of families. *Acta Paediat* 2002; **91**: 297–302.

241. Corazza GR, Frisoni M, Treggiari EA. Clinical features of adult coeliac disease in Italy. In Mearin ML, Mulder CJJ (eds), *Coeliac Disease: 40 Years Gluten Free*. Kluwer Academic: Dordrecht, 1999.

242. Corazza GR, Di Sario A, Sacco G, Zoli G *et al.* Subclinical coeliac disease: an anthropometric assessment. *J Intern Med* 1994; **236**: 183–7.

243. Bayless TM, Kapelowitz RF, Shelley WM, Ballinger WF, Hendrix TR. Intestinal ulceration—a complication of celiac disease. *N Engl J Med* 1967; **276**: 996–1002.

244. Isaacson PG, O'Connor NT, Spencer J, Bevan DH *et al.* Malignant histiocytosis of the intestine: a T-cell lymphoma. *Lancet* 1985; **2**: 688–91.

245. Cooper BT, Holmes GK, Ferguson R, Cooke WT. Celiac disease and malignancy. *Medicine* 1980; **59**: 249–61.

246. Stevens FM. Celiac disease: clinical manifestations. *Pract Gastroenterol* 1980; **4**: 10–15.

247. Corazza GR, Frisoni M, Treggiari EA, Valentini RA *et al.* Subclinical celiac sprue. Increasing occurrence and clues to its diagnosis. *J Clin Gastroenterol* 1993; **16**: 16–21.

248. Hoffbrand AV. Anaemia in adult coeliac disease. *Clin Gastroenterol* 1974; **3**: 71–89.

249. Ferguson A, Arranz E, O'Mahony S. Clinical and pathological spectrum of coeliac disease—active, silent, latent, potential. *Gut* 1993; **34**: 150–51.

250. van Bergeijk JD, Meijer JWR, Mulder CJJ. Endoscopic abnormalities in patients screened for coeliac disease. *J Clin Nutr Gastroenterol* 1993; **8**: 136–9.

251. Cataldo F, Ventura A, Lazzari R, Balli F *et al*. Antiendomysium antibodies and coeliac disease: solved and unsolved questions. An Italian multicentre study. *Acta Paediat* 1995; **84**: 1125–31.

252. Burgin-Wolff A, Gaze H, Hadziselimovic F, Huber H *et al*. Antigliadin and antiendomysium antibody determination for coeliac disease. *Arch Dis Child* 1991; **66**: 941–7.

253. Volta U, Bianchi FB. IgA antibodies to endomysium, gliadin, and reticulin in silent coeliac disease. *Lancet* 1992; **339**: 242.

254. van Berge-Henegouwen GP, Mulder CJ. Pioneer in the gluten free diet: Willem–Karel Dicke 1905–1962, over 50 years of gluten-free diet. *Gut* 1993; **34**: 1473–5.

255. Hamilton JD, Chambers RA, Wynn-Williams A. Role of gluten, prednisone, and azathioprine in non-responsive coeliac disease. *Lancet* 1976; **1**: 1213–16.

256. Longstreth GF. Successful treatment of refractory sprue with cyclosporine. *Ann Intern Med* 1995; **119**: 1014–16.

6

Anorectal Function

Wei Ming Sun and **Nicholas W. Read**

A good set of bowels is worth more to a man than any quantity of brains

Josh Billings (pseudonym of Henry Wheeler Shaw)

Prevalence and epidemiology

Disordered defaecation, characterised by incontinence, constipation and diarrhoea, occurs frequently in patients with diabetes mellitus [1–3] but is often overlooked as a cause of morbidity. For example, in a study of 136 unselected diabetic outpatients referred to a tertiary centre, Feldman and Schiller found that constipation occurred in 60%, diarrhoea in 22% and faecal incontinence in 20% of their patients [1]. Faecal incontinence was twice as common in patients with diarrhoea as in those with constipation. Disordered defaecation appears to be less common among patients with diabetes attending secondary referral centres [4,5], where constipation has been reported in about 20% and faecal incontinence in about 9% [5]. As discussed in Chapter 1, there is relatively little information

Gastrointestinal Function in Diabetes Mellitus. Edited by Michael Horowitz and Melvin Samsom
© 2004 John Wiley & Sons, Ltd ISBN: 0-471-89916-X

about the prevalence of disordered defaecation in diabetic patients managed in the community by primary care physicians. It is likely that, whether in a primary, secondary or tertiary care setting, patients frequently fail to report disturbances in defaecation unless the latter are severe, and that doctors rarely ask.

One study suggested that the prevalence of constipation was higher among patients with type 2 than among those with type 1 diabetes, but the patients with type 2 diabetes were twice as old as those with type 1 diabetes [6]. Defaecation disorders appear to occur more frequently in those patients who have evidence of peripheral and/or autonomic neuropathy. In one study faecal incontinence was reported to occur in 18% of secondary referrals with clinical evidence of peripheral diabetic neuropathy [7]; in another study constipation was more common in patients with autonomic neuropathy than in those without [8]. It would be misleading, however, to imply that such disturbances in colonic function are inevitably caused by diabetes *per se*, as chronic disorders of defaecation occur in up to 20% of the normal population, with an increased prevalence in the elderly [9–11]. In the community the vast majority of such cases have what has become known as irritable bowel syndrome, which has strong associations with emotional upset. Although there are only limited data about the prevalence of irritable bowel syndrome in a diabetic population (Chapter 1), the emotional stress of coping with a serious life-threatening condition may potentially make irritable bowel syndrome more common than in an otherwise healthy population.

Physiology and pathophysiology

In order to understand the pathophysiology of disordered defaecation in a patient with diabetes, it is important to outline the normal physiology of defaecation and faecal continence and to describe how these functions might become disturbed to cause constipation, diarrhoea and faecal incontinence.

Colonic motility

The colon is the dark continent of medicine, a large, stagnant, fermenting vat—a veritable Stygian pool of corruption. As a chemical factory, it has almost limitless potential for microbial salvage of food material that has not been absorbed in the small intestine. The mechanisms by which such salvage takes place are, for the most part, shrouded in mystery, but we can measure what goes in and what comes out. Every day the colon receives about a litre of a rather runny slurry, containing carbohydrates, proteins and fats that have escaped absorption in the small intestine, fibre, mucus and digestive enzymes, bile and salts and water. Most of this material is salvaged in the colon, so that all that remains to be expelled is a solid plug of faeces, composed almost entirely of bacterial cells and indigestible fibre and usually weighing no more than about 100 g. This process normally takes between 1 and 3 days.

The colon may be functionally divided into the proximal portion, where most fermentation takes place, the distal colon, where salt and water is extracted and colonic contents are concentrated and solidified, and the rectum, which is specialised for defaecation. For most of the time, the contractile activity of the colon gently mixes the unabsorbed nutrients with colonic secretions and bacteria and exposes the colonic contents to the mucosal surface. This creates conditions that are sufficiently stagnant for the propagation of bacteria and propels contents distally at a rate consistent with the rates of absorption of fluid, electrolytes and the products of bacterial degradation [12].

Ring-like 'haustral' contractions form and fade and reform a few centimetres away, occasionally propagating a few centimetres in either direction [13]. Their profile seems particularly sharp in the transverse and descending colon, where they appear to dig into the colonic contents and turn them over in much the same way as the gardener might turn over the soil with his spade. The sigmoid colon appears narrower than the rest of the colon. The circular muscle of this region is in a state of tonic contraction for much of the time, and seems to function like a valve, restricting the entry of colonic contents into the rectum [14]. The normal retentive activity of the colon is thought to be under the dominant control of the sympathetic nervous system.

From time to time, but especially first thing in the morning immediately after getting up or after breakfast, the colon assumes a different mode of activity [15–17] that is strongly propulsive. The haustral contractions fade away and broad, powerful contractions develop, often in the transverse or the descending colon, and sweep distally, propelling faeces into the rectum, where their arrival is perceived as a desire to defaecate. These contractions have been termed 'giant migrating contractions' [18] or 'high-amplitude propagated contractions' [17] and the propulsion of colonic contents that they produce is known as a 'mass movement'. Mass movements can be induced by cholinergic agonists, sympathetic antagonists and stimulation of the pelvic parasympathetic nerves. This type of propulsive activity therefore requires a change in autonomic influence favouring dominance of the parasympathetic nervous system.

Defaecation

Defaecation is a complex behavioural sequence, involving integration between the visceral and somatic nervous systems. It is controlled by a collection of neurons in the pons and orchestrated by neural activity in the conus medullaris at the base of the spinal cord. Defaecation is usually triggered by the rapid entry of faeces into the rectum. This event is detected by rapidly adapting mechanoreceptors in the rectum (and possibly the pelvic floor), causing reflex contraction of the rectum and relaxation of the internal anal sphincter (IAS) (the so-called rectoanal inhibitory reflex). These actions propel the stool into the anal canal, where they stimulate the exquisitely sensitive anal receptors and intensify the urge to defaecate [19]. So, if the time and place are appropriate, the subject sits or squats, and contracts the diaphragm, the abdominal muscles and the levatores ani to increase the intra-abdominal pressure. At the same time, the protective contractions of the external anal sphincter (EAS) and puborectalis are suppressed by signals conveyed from the brain via inhibitory spinal pathways. This opens up the anorectal angle and reduces sphincter resistance. Although the force for faecal extrusion may be initially provided by an increase in intra-abdominal pressure, the complete emptying of the rectum and distal colon that often occurs during defaecation can only come about through the agency of a strong propagated colorectal contraction, which, as any veterinary surgeon or neonatal paediatrician can testify, are facilitated by anal stimulation. Thus, defaecation is a complex choreographed sequence that requires exquisite timing and coordination.

Preservation of continence

The entry of faeces into the rectum would inevitably result in defaecation were it not for the fact that human beings are social and territorial. They do not just deposit their faeces anywhere when the urge takes them, like horses and cattle. They share the capability of other territorial species, such as dogs, cats and other primates, to retain their faeces until they find an appropriate time and place to release them. Continence depends on the social awareness of the need to control the contents of the rectum until it is appropriate to evacuate in a controlled manner. It is a conscious function and is conferred by the exquisite sensitivity of the distal rectum and the anal canal and the resistance to the passage of faeces provided by anal sphincter contraction and the acute angulation of anus and rectum caused by contraction of the puborectalis.

Anorectal sensation

Specific sensations are experienced in the rectum with increasing volumes of content (gas, liquid or solid). These are fullness, a desire to defecate, an urgency to defecate, and ultimately pain [19]. It is thought that these sensations are conveyed by simple sensory nerve endings in the rectal wall. These respond to tension, but are sensitised by the chemical milieu of the surrounding tissue. They are, for example, dramatically enhanced by the presence of inflammation [20] or the release of catecholamines [21]. In essence, they act as volume detectors, although receptors situated within the muscle layer also respond to the forces induced by contraction as well as distension. While most of the activity of rectal sensors does not reach consciousness, it may signal local reflexes such as IAS relaxation, rectal contraction and EAS contraction, through enteric and spinal connections [22–23].

Relaxation of the internal anal sphincter causes the anal canal to open in a funnel-like manner, exposing the anal epithelium to faecal contents. Compared with the rectum, the anal canal is exquisitely sensitive. The epithelium is inner-vated with a profusion of sensory nerves, able to appreciate light touch, pain and temperature [24–26]. Recto-anal sensory mechanisms are sensitive enough to discriminate solid faecal material from liquid and gas, so that appropriate action can then take place with confidence.

Anal sphincter contraction

The anal sphincter consists of two concentric sphincters, an inner smooth muscle sphincter and an outer sphincter composed of striated muscle (Figure 6.1). This might be regarded as the 'belt-and-braces' approach to faecal continence, but in this case both mechanisms are essential.

The smooth muscle of the internal anal sphincter (IAS) is tonically active at rest, contributing about to 50–60% of the basal anal pressure and helping to maintain continence during sleep. Its tone is primarily dependent on myo-genic activity and intramural enteric nerves [27–29], but can be enhanced by α-adrenergic influences. Its relaxation during rectal distension is mediated by an enteric nervous reflex and enhanced in conditions that cause enhanced rectal sensitivity.

The striated muscle of the external anal sphincter (EAS) is also tonically active at rest, contributing to 20–30% of the basal anal pressure [30]. It con-tains a high proportion of slow twitch type 1 muscle fibres, which are capable

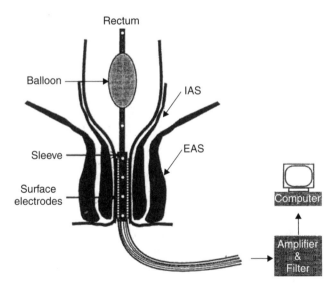

Figure 6.1 Diagram of the anal canal showing the different muscle components and a catheter used to measure pressure in multiple sites in the rectum and anal canal. The balloon is used for rectal distension and the intraluminal surface electrodes are used for recording electrical activity. The sleeve sensor situated in the anal canal records the maximum pressure along its length. IAS, internal anal sphincter; EAS, external anal sphincter

of sustained contraction [31–32], but also some fast twitch type 2 fibres that are able to respond rapidly to events that threaten continence. The protective function of the EAS is supported by corresponding activity in the puborectalis muscle. This is a sling of muscle that forms the innermost aspect of the levator ani complex, which maintains the tone of the pelvic floor. The puborectalis loops around the back of the anorectal junction, pulling it snugly against the bladder neck and uterine cervix and creating an acute angulation between rectum and anus that restricts the passage of rectal contents.

Sphincter muscles would not be able to function unless they had something to close around and 'grip' [33]. This is provided by the bunching and infolding of the anal mucosa and submucosa, and augmented by the presence of three expansile vascular cushions, which provide a hermetic seal at the same time as stretching the muscle so that the circular muscle fibres can contract at a greater mechanical advantage [34–35]. The anal cushions are composed of large blood spaces and are fed by arterioles. Histologically they resemble the erectile tissue of the penis and are therefore well able to confer properties of firmness and solidity. The importance of the anal cushions in preserving continence is emphasised by a high incidence of anal seepage after radical haemorrhoidectomy [36].

Under resting conditions and during sleep, continence is maintained by the conservative and fermentative mode of colonic activity and the tonic contraction of the IAS. Mass movements of faeces are inhibited during sleep by tonic discharge along the sympathetic nerves, although small amounts of faeces may be slowly propelled by sigmoid contractions into the rectum, where they accumulate [37]. The EAS is hypotonic during sleep and does not respond to rectal distension [38]. The IAS is the only barrier maintaining continence during sleep but, provided that the entry of faeces is sufficiently slow, this does not relax. Studies conducted in our laboratory have shown that the rectum can be distended at a slow steady rate of 10 ml/min up to a volume of 200 ml without causing any rectal sensation or relaxation of the internal sphincter [19]. The same volume delivered at a rapid rate, as if by a peristaltic mass movement, would cause instant discomfort and precipitate relaxation of the IAS.

When the subject is awake and active, continence is threatened by rapid rectal distension or rapid increases in intra-abdominal pressure, caused by coughing, laughing, shouting, sitting up or vigorous exercise. Under these conditions, incontinence is prevented by the immediate protective contraction of the EAS and puborectalis, strengthening the sphincter and closing off the anorectal angle. Contraction of these muscles probably also impedes the venous return from the anal cushions, enhancing the turgor of the vascular seal. The responses of the puborectalis and EAS to rectal distension are spinal reflexes, since they can be demonstrated in paraplegic patients. They are, however, so heavily modulated by perception of anorectal sensation that to all intents and purposes they can be regarded as conscious responses [39–40]. Rectal sensitivity and the ability of the striated muscles of the pelvic floor to respond rapidly to the entry of faecal material into the rectum (and to increases in intra-abdominal pressure) are the key elements in the continence response. They gave our ancestors time to seek a quiet bush away from the home base and out of sight of predators. And in this day and age, they allow metropolitan man and woman to undertake journeys on underground railways early in the morning after breakfast without fear of embarrassment.

To summarise, defaecation and the preservation of continence are both complex territorial behaviours in humans. They are generated in the cerebral cortex and are, therefore, markedly influenced by psychosocial factors. The multiple physiological functions required to control the passage of faeces are under the influence of a control centre in the pontine brain stem and orchestrated by the neuronal activity in the terminal expansion of the spinal cord. The instructions are conveyed via pelvic parasympathetic nerves, lumbar sympathetic nerves and sacral somatic nerves, influencing the function of the enteric nervous system and visceral smooth muscle and also the muscles of the pelvic floor. As with many things in life, strength must be combined with sensitivity and timing is crucial. Clearly, the muscles of the colon, abdominal wall and pelvic floor must be able to contract with sufficient power to propel faeces or resist that propulsion. But more important, the arrival of faeces in the rectum or even quite small increases in intra-abdominal pressure need to be detected immediately, so that appropriate responses can be rapidly triggered through spinal and enteric reflexes. These actions can be influenced at many levels by the diabetic process.

Effects of diabetes mellitus on anorectal function

It should be recognised that many previous studies of anorectal function in diabetes have substantial limitations—the techniques used were often suboptimal, only isolated aspects of anorectal function were evaluated and no account was taken of the potential impact of acute or chronic glycaemia.

As discussed, anorectal dysfunction is more common in patients with diabetes who have evidence of neuropathy [7,8]. Diabetic microangiopathy impairs nerve conduction and synaptic transmission [41]; 24–30% of type 1 patients have clinical evidence of peripheral neuropathy and 17% have evidence of autonomic neuropathy [42]. The prevalence of diabetic neuropathy is related to age, duration of diabetes and glycaemic control [43]. As discussed in Chapter 9, autonomic neuropathy is usually diagnosed from measurements of cardiovascular function and, although it seems likely that similar changes must affect gastrointestinal function, there is only a weak correlation between diabetic autonomic neuropathy diagnosed from cardiovascular tests and disturbances in gut motility in other regions, such as gastric emptying [5,44]. There is no such information available for anorectal function.

While disordered gastrointestinal motility in patients with diabetes mellitus has been believed to result from irreversible damage to autonomic nerves, as discussed in Chapters 3 to 6 there is now persuasive evidence that reversible changes in gastrointestinal motility may result from acute alterations in the blood glucose concentration [45,46]. It is likely that some of the abnormalities in anorectal motility observed in diabetic patients reflect hyperglycaemia, rather than diabetes *per se*, particularly in view of observations relating to the effects of hyperglycaemia on anorectal motor and sensory function in healthy subjects [47–50]. We have reported that elevation of the blood glucose to about 12 mmol/l inhibits internal and external anal sphincter function in normal subjects, as evidenced by an increased number of spontaneous anal relaxations and a reduction in squeeze pressure (Figure 6.2), which would predispose to incontinence [47]. In contrast, rectal sensitivity and compliance (ability of the rectum to distend and increase in volume without an increase in pressure) were increased [47]. Chey *et al.* [48] have, however, reported that both the perception of rectal distension and the rectoanal inhibitory reflex were blunted by hyperglycaemia (blood glucose ~ 15 mmol/l) in normal subjects. Another study has established that the central processing of rectal distension (as assessed by measurement of cortical evoked potentials) is affected by hyperglycaemia in

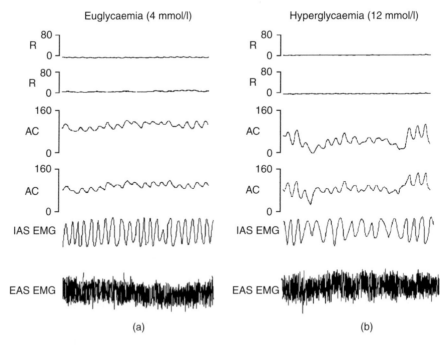

(a)   (b)

Figure 6.2 Recordings of basal pressures in the rectum (R) and anal canal (AC) and electrical activity of the internal (IAS) and external (EAS) anal sphincters in a healthy subject during (a) euglycaemia (blood glucose 4 mmol/l) and (b) hyperglycaemia (blood glucose 12 mmol/l). Hyperglycaemia is associated with a reduction in anal sphincter pressures and instability of the IAS. From Russo *et al.* [50], with permission

healthy subjects [50]. The effects of hyperglycaemia on anorectal function may also be dependent on the methodology used [48]. The gastrocolonic response is blunted by hyperglycaemia in healthy subjects [51]. It seems clear, therefore, that acute elevations of blood glucose have the capacity to cause reversible changes in anorectal function. It is, of course, well documented that the risk of both the development and progression of microangiopathic complications of diabetes, such as retinopathy, nephropathy and neuropathy, is greater in those patients whose disease is poorly controlled and, accordingly, likely that irreversible changes in anorectal motility may occur consequent to chronically poor glycaemic control [52,53]. Studies of the effects of both acute and chronic glycaemia on anorectal function in diabetes are, however, required to address these issues.

Disturbances of defaecation in diabetic patients

Constipation is the thief of time; diarrhoea waits for no man

Since defaecation involves close integration of the peripheral, autonomic and enteric nerves, ischaemic or toxic damage to these nerves caused by the diabetic process must lead to disorders of defaecation that will vary according to the site and type of nerves that are affected. Nevertheless, it is important not to regard the disturbances in defaecation that occur in diabetic patients as necessarily complications of diabetes. As discussed in Chapter 1 Clouse *et al.* have suggested that once the anxiety and depression are taken into account, no specific gastrointestinal symptom is significantly associated with autonomic neuropathy [54].

The pathogenic mechanisms for diabetic diarrhoea have been reviewed in Chapter 5. This chapter will focus on mechanisms of faecal incontinence and retention.

Urgency and faecal incontinence

Faecal incontinence may be provoked by irresistible colonic propulsion and secretion, but it usually also implies a measure of dysfunction in the ano-rectal apparatus for maintaining continence. This might include weakness of the striated musculature of the puborectalis and external anal sphincter, a reduction in internal sphincter tone, a reduction in rectal sensitivity (so that the subject fails to detect the arrival of faecal material) and a failure of recto-anal coordination (so that the patient fails to contract the striated muscles in sufficient time to prevent leakage).

Patients with long-standing diabetes mellitus are more likely to be afflicted by the shame of nocturnal incontinence of faeces than non-diabetics with faecal incontinence. This is best explained by neuropathy involving the sympathetic nerve supply. As discussed, the colon is normally relatively quiescent during sleep, probably as a result of tonic activity in the sympathetic efferent nerves to the colon [37], which reduces propulsion, facilitates fermentation and increases absorption. Accordingly, if the sympathetic nerves supplying the colon are damaged by diabetic microangiopathy, it could unleash mass movements at times when they would not normally occur. Thus, events such as the delivery of ileal contents into the caecum and the build-up of fermentation gases could readily generate colonic mass movements, which would rapidly distend the rectum, causing unrecognised relaxation of the IAS and faecal incontinence. This is particularly important at night, when there is no conscious augmentation of external sphincter contraction in response to rapid entry of faeces into the rectum. Under those conditions, the last barrier protecting continence is the tone of the internal sphincter. Physiological studies have shown that not only is this reduced in diabetes, but that the IAS is also markedly unstable (Figure 6.3) [55]; both abnormalities may be related to neuropathic damage to the sympathetic nerves [56]. Rectal compliance is also impaired, which may be indicative of damage to the enteric nerves. Moreover, as discussed in Chapter 4, ultrastructural degeneration of smooth muscle has been reported in visceral smooth muscle specimens from the stomach of diabetic patients [57].

Impairment of neural function caused by diabetic microangiopathy can affect to a lesser or greater extent all the mechanisms involved in the maintenance of faecal continence. So whether a person develops faecal incontinence or not depends on the interplay between all of these. Physiological studies have demonstrated that cohorts of patients with long-standing diabetes have an abnormally low anal tone, weak squeeze pressures and impaired rectal sensation [58–60]. Anal sensitivity may also be impaired [61–62]. These abnormalities frequently coexist and may be associated with other changes that could threaten continence, in particular the chronic diarrhoea that occurs in some 20% of patients.

Faecal incontinence in diabetic patients is also often associated with urinary incontinence [63]. This association might be explained by damage to the pudendal nerve supplying the muscles of the pelvic floor. Pinna-Pintor and his colleagues have demonstrated that the diabetic process leads to a progressive prolongation of the pudendal nerve terminal motor latency, with consequent weakening of the strength of the EAS [64].

It is important to recognise that the most common factor responsible for pudendal neuropathy in women is, however, damage to the pelvic floor sustained during childbirth. Near the end of the pregnancy, the connective tissue that supports the pelvic floor softens under the influence of the hormone 'relaxin'. Although this facilitates the delivery of the baby's head, the descent of the pelvic floor during delivery can damage the pudendal nerve by stretching it and compressing it where it winds around the iliac spines. Nerve conduction tests have shown that vaginal delivery is inevitably associated with some degree of nerve damage [65]. While this tends to show some recovery, it can

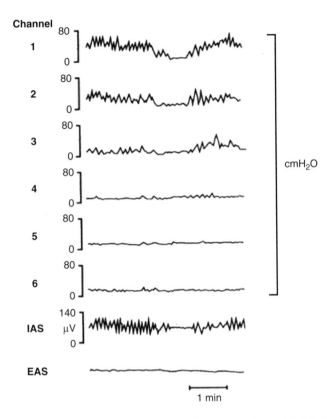

Figure 6.3   Basal recording of anorectal pressure from ports situated 0.5, 1.0, 2.0, 2.5 and 4.5 cm from the anal verge (channels 1–5) and from a rectal balloon (channel 6) 6–11 cm from the anal verge and electrical activity of IAS (raw) and EAS (integrated) in a type 1 patient with faecal incontinence. Note that: (A) anal pressure oscillations and the pressure reduction during spontaneous anal relaxation are associated with changes in electrical activity of the internal, but not external, sphincter; and (B) the anal pressure is lowest during spontaneous anal relaxation. From Sun *et al.* [55], with permission

be exacerbated by subsequent deliveries. The pelvic floor fascia may also be damaged during delivery, leading to permanent descent of the perineum and continued damage to the pudendal nerve. Because the pudendal nerve supplies the external anal sphincter, the external urethral sphincter and part of the puborectalis, pudendal neuropathy induces weakness of both sphincters that increases with age, but especially after the menopause, when loss of oestrogen leads to atrophy of the connective tissue. Severe degrees of perineal descent may also impair continence by opening up the anorectal angle.

   In addition to pudendal neuropathy, the anal sphincter may be torn by the baby's head during an uncontrolled second stage of labour and can also be ruptured during forceps delivery. Endo-anal ultrasonography has shown that 35% of primiparous women tested after delivery had sustained sphincter damage that persisted for at least 6 months [66]. The percentages are higher in those who had undergone forceps delivery and for multiparous women. Such sphincter defects were not found after caesarean section. There was a very strong association between sphincter defects and the development of symptoms of urgency and incontinence [66]. Even moderate degrees of obstetric trauma may be of little consequence in somebody in whom stools are solid and bowel habit is regular, but are nothing short of a disaster in a person with diarrhoea or excessive wind. Diabetic women, especially those with less than optimal diabetic control, are more liable to suffer from obstetric complications, such as traumatic disruption of the anal sphincter or weakness of the pelvic floor, leading to chronic stretching of the pudendal nerve. This is because diabetics tend to give birth to large babies when glycaemic control is poor, and are more likely to experience long and difficult labours and require assisted delivery with forceps or ventouse [67].

In the elderly, faecal incontinence commonly accompanies retention of faeces and is more likely to occur in those who are mentally and physically incapacitated and are institutionalised. The faecal mass distends the rectum and stimulates the secretion of mucus. Although the internal sphincter adapts to maintain its tone even in the presence of quite gross faecal retention [68], quite small increments in distension which might be induced by accumulation of mucus are often sufficient to cause relaxation and incontinence. The association of external sphincter weakness, grossly blunted rectal sensitivity and impaired anal and perianal sensation in these patients suggests the possibility of spinal neuropathy.

Constipation

The three-toed sloth, living upside down high in the dense forest canopy of Amazonas, has to climb down to the ground to defaecate. For the sloth, defaecation is a hazardous procedure, because once on the ground, sloths move ever so slowly and are easy prey. The bowels of the sloth have adapted to this unusual life-style so that it only needs to defaecate once every 9 days. The sloth is probably the most constipated mammal known to man except, perhaps, man himself.

> The world record for constipation was held by a man who resisted the temptation of the toilet for 368 days. He was said to become weak after delivering 36 litres of faeces on June 21st, 1901, but there was much rejoicing in the family (Geib and Jones, 1902 [69]).

Constipation is the opposite of diarrhoea and implies retention of faeces, sluggish movement of intestinal contents, slow colonic transit and an enhanced absorption, leading to hard desiccated stools that are difficult to evacuate. Instead of the gut being programmed for evacuation, it is programmed for retention.

Defaecation can be interrupted by neuromuscular disturbances occurring at any level in this heirarchy of control and operating at any stage in the choreographed sequence of coordinated events. Constipation may therefore be caused by neurological lesions affecting the pontine control centre and the complex integrations within the cauda equina. It may reflect damage to the pelvic parasympathetic nerves that induce colonic propulsion, a myopathy causing weakness of colonic contraction, and an increase in sympathetic nerve activity which impairs colonic propulsion by inducing non-propagated contractions in the sigmoid colon and increases anal tone. Anal mechanisms causing constipation also include blunted rectal sensation, impaired IAS relaxation in response to rectal distension similar to that described in Hirschsprung's disease, and impaired relaxation of the EAS and puborectalis during attempts to defaecate [70]. The latter, which is known as anismus [71], has been described in patients with chronic idiopathic constipation. Finally, defaecation may be obstructed mechanically by expansion of the anal cushions to create haemorrhoids and partial prolapse of the rectum into the anal canal [72]. Thus, constipation may be caused by disease affecting the brain and spinal cord, the somatic, autonomic and enteric nerves, the smooth muscle of the colon and anal sphincter, striated muscle of the pelvic floor and other vascular and connective tissue structures. It is not surprising, therefore, that textbooks of gastroenterology provide long and detailed differential diagnoses.

Little is known about the exact mechanism of diabetic constipation, but much can be inferred from knowledge of the normal physiology. The pelvic parasympathetic nerves that mediate colonic propulsion can be damaged by diabetic neuropathy, but why some patients seem to suffer more from damage to the parasympathetic nerves and constipation while others suffer from sympathetic neuropathy and diarrhoea is unclear. Combined myoelectric and manometric studies have demonstrated blunting of the gastrocolonic response to a meal in some patients with diabetic constipation, although contractile activity could still be elicited by neostigmine, suggesting the presence of autonomic neuropathy [73].

Autonomic neuropathy would be expected to cause reductions in the sensory and motor responses to rectal distension. Sarna and co-workers have suggested that perception and nociception are well preserved in diabetics, even in those with evidence of neuropathy [74], but we found that 81% of diabetic patients with faecal incontinence had impaired rectal sensitivity and 42% of them failed to relax the IAS in response to rectal distension [55]. Such alternations in rectal physiology could lead to the accumulation of faeces.

Constipation is a common symptom, affecting up to 20% of otherwise healthy people. This usually does not have an obvious pathological basis and is regarded as a behavioural or functional disease. Patients with idiopathic constipation show physiological abnormalities of most, if not all, components of the defaecation sequence. Measurements of colonic motility show delayed transit through the colon, infrequent colonic propulsion and increased obstructive contractions in the sigmoid colon. Rectal distension reveals that higher volumes are required to induce an urge to defaecate, a rectal contraction and a relaxation of the IAS. Anal manometry shows an elevated anal tone and paradoxical contraction of the

EAS and puborectalis during attempts to defaecate [75]. This latter phenomenon (anismus) represents failure to activate descending inhibitory spinal pathways that facilitate defaecation. This combination of abnormalities might suggest a lesion in the brain or spinal cord, but investigations are invariably negative. Physiological tests of spinal reflexes have been shown to be abnormal [39], but this may not so much indicate a neurological disease as a failure to activate the programmed sequence of defaecatory behaviour because of a psychological block. It is as if the fear of expression has laid its heavy hand on the pontine switch for defaecation and, as such, resembles the difficulties that some men have when they have to 'pee' in public. This notion of idiopathic constipation as a behavioural disease would explain the remarkable success of biofeedback training and the disappointing results of surgery.

Constipation is particularly common at the extremes of life. Most cases of faecal retention in childhood, however, respond to the sensitive application of behavioural techniques and rarely continue in adulthood. Thus, most paediatricians would assume faecal impaction in infants to be a behavioural abnormality, the way in which the infant resists parental control. Elderly patients with faecal impaction may also suffer from behavioural problems, brought about by the combination of mental and physical infirmity, immobility and the combination of cold weather and outside toilets [76]. Physiological studies, however, suggest the possibility of a neurological lesion. Elderly patients with faecal impaction have considerable blunting of rectal sensitivity. Volumes of half a litre or more may have to be introduced into the rectum before any sensation is induced [77]. Unlike younger women, the defect in rectal sensitivity in the elderly is associated with a corresponding attenuation of peri-anal sensation, an abnormal increase in rectal compliance and a weak external sphincter. This combination of motor and sensory abnormalities, involving both somatic and visceral nerves, suggests the possibility of a neurological defect in the integrating centre in the conus medullaris, the terminal expansion of the spinal cord.

Clinical assessment

The objective of clinical assessment of defaecation disorders is to identify conditions that may respond to specific treatment. Many techniques have been employed as research tools to elucidate the pathophysiology of faecal incontinence or constipation, but few have clinical use.

Faecal incontinence

Patients are more likely to suffer from faecal incontinence and seepage if their faeces are liquid. So patients with severe diarrhoea who pass large amounts of liquid motions require investigation and treatment of their diarrhoea before any specific investigation of anorectal function, since in many cases the incontinence will cease to be a problem if the diarrhoea is treated satisfactorily. The investigation and management of diarrhoea in diabetic patients is described in Chapter 5. This section is concerned with the investigation of faecal incontinence when stool output is relatively low and which does not respond to treatment of diarrhoea. Under these conditions, it is important to identify obstetric trauma, since this can be treated surgically. It is also important to identify specific neurological causes of incontinence, and not to miss faecal impaction with overflow.

Inspection of the perineum and digital examination of the anorectum is essential and should be carried out in all patients with faecal incontinence. With the patient lying in the left lateral position, he/she should be asked to bear down. Normally the perineum descends no more than a centimetre. Any more movement than this indicates an abnormal degree of perineal descent and suggests pudendal neuropathy consequent upon obstetric weakness of the pelvic floor. The degree of perineal descent can be measured more accurately using a St Marks perineometer, which consists of a rod with two adjustable legs which are placed on the patient's ischial tuberosities, and a central graduated cylinder, the tip of which is placed on the anus. When the patient bears down the extent to which the perineum descends can be measured accurately on the graduated cylinder. Bearing down may also reveal the existence of rectal prolapse, which is frequently associated with sphincter weakness and is a frequent cause of seepage. The presence of obvious external haemorrhoids is also a common cause of anal seepage of mucus. Digital examination of the rectum is a useful and simple means of assessing resting anal tone and the strength of conscious contraction. Patients with anal seepage caused by haemorrhoids, anal fistula and anal fissure have an enhanced anal tone [78–79], while anal tone is often very weak in patients with frank incontinence. Pulling back on the sphincter with a finger in the anus or parting the buttocks may elicit gaping of the sphincter, a sign that the external sphincter is particularly weak [80]. Since direct obstetric injury to the anal sphincter characteristically occurs in the anterior position between the anus and vaginal introitus, we have found it useful to examine the thickness of sphincter muscle in this region by means of a bidigital examinal, with the thumb in the anus and the index finger in the vagina. Digital examination of the rectum may also reveal the presence of tumours, solitary rectal ulcer and rectal intussusception, all of which may be associated with leakage of mucus, as well as faecal impaction.

Proctoscopy and/or sigmoidoscopy is also essential part of the investigation of patients with faecal incontinence. These may reveal not only haemorrhoids, fistulae and fissures, but also solitary rectal ulcer, proctitis, tumours and the discrete patches of inflammation and ulceration associated with Crohn's disease. All of these may give rise to rectal seepage. There are no specific findings on clinical examination that indicate anorectal dysfunction caused by diabetes.

Clinical investigation of faecal incontinence might include anorectal manometry, endoanal ultrasonography and X-ray defaecography [81]. Anorectal manometry is usually recorded with either multiple low-compliance perfused catheters, microballoons and/or miniature strain gauge transducers [82]. The measurements obtained depend as much on the method used as the physiological function being measured, and they all have their limitation(s). It is important that investigators using these techniques establish their own normal ranges, since there is little concordance in the results obtained from different laboratories. Our laboratory has substantial experience with a set-up that incorporates an array of perfused catheters with side holes situated 0.5 cm apart in the anorectum, a rectal balloon, so that rectal sensitivity and the recto-anal pressure responses to rectal distension can be measured, and a wire electrode in the EAS to record EAS activity [22]. Using this technique, basal and squeeze pressures are measured on three separate occasions and the sensory and rectal, IAS and EAS pressure responses to graded stepwise rectal distension can be recorded (Figure 6.1). We have found that this combination of measurements provides a comprehensive assessment of anorectal function and can indicate different functional abnormalities in a variety of clinical conditions. For example, we have found that the unstable oscillations of IAS tone and electrical activity occur more frequently in diabetic patients with faecal incontinence than in any other group [55]. Patients with spinal lesions, on the other hand, all show a combination of impaired rectal sensitivity and weak or absent squeeze pressures; in those with high spinal lesions there are exaggerated EAS electrical responses to rectal distension, while in those with low spinal lesions the EAS electrical responses are markedly attenuated [23]. Patients with anal seepage caused by anal fissures, fistulae and haemorrhoids exhibit particularly high resting sphincter pressures, while those with obstetric injury have very low sphincter pressures [58,73]. Neither finding is, however, diagnostic and may in any case be elicited by careful clinical examination.

Endo-anal ultrasound is the only technique that satisfactorily identifies the present of a defect in the sphincter ring caused by obstetric or other trauma (Figure 6.4) [81,82]. A rotating ultrasound probe is inserted into the anus—no bowel preparation is required and it is no more uncomfortable than a digital rectal examination. Endo-anal ultrasound should be conducted in all women with faecal incontinence who have undergone vaginal deliveries and have low sphincter pressures.

Defaecography is a radiographic technique. The rectum is filled with radio-opaque medium, which subjects are asked to evacuate under direct X-ray screening. This is a useful method to assess the dynamics of defaecation [83]. It can assess the degree of perineal descent and reveal the presence of partial rectal prolapse and rectal intussusception, both of which may be associated with seepage.

Other techniques that have been used in some laboratories include the measurement of pudendal nerve terminal motor latency, by the use of a special glove with a stimulating electrode on the tip of the index finger and recording electrodes at the base of the finger [84]. The finger is inserted into the anal canal and the pudendal nerve is located as it enters the pelvis under the ischial spine, so that the recording electrodes are now enclosed by the sphincter and record the

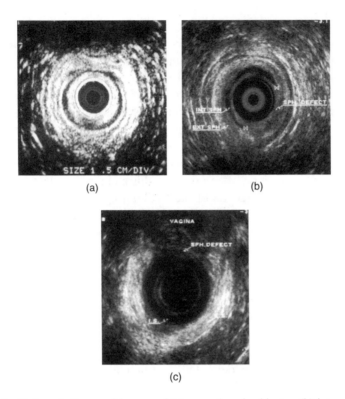

(a)

(b)

(c)

Figure 6.4   Endoanal ultrasound images of (a) normal anal sphincter; (b) internal sphincter defect (region between the crosses); and (c) anterior external anal sphincter defect

myoelectrical response to stimulation. Prolongation of nerve conduction is seen in severe nerve damage and may herald a poor outcome following post-anal, or sphincter, repair.

Investigation of constipation

Visual inspection of the perineum is important to identify degrees of perineal descent, which may be associated with obstructive lesions, such as intussusception and rectovaginal prolapse, and to elicit the presence of external haemorrhoids. Digital examination of the anus may reveal increased tone, found in patients with haemorrhoids, fistulae and fissures. The examination is likely to be painful in all of these conditions, particularly anal fissures. As discussed, increased tone is also a feature of some patients with idiopathic constipation, but others have a very weak sphincter. The latter might also suggest spinal lesions, especially when associated with impaired rectal sensitivity.

Combined anorectal function testing [22] is particularly useful to identify impaired internal sphincter relaxation in the rare patient with short-segment Hirshsprung's disease, to indicate the possibility of undetected spinal lesions (such as a prolapsed lumbar disc affecting the cauda equina, cervical spondylosis, disseminated sclerosis, brain stem tumours or syringomyelia), and to demonstrate the paradoxical sphincter contraction during attempts to defaecate in patients with idiopathic constipation. For the latter, we use a stool-shaped silicone envelope, modified from an Angelchik prosthesis, with a tail-like tape attached to one end of it [85]. We call it the rectal 'mouse'. This pseudo-rodent is generously lubricated and inserted into the rectum. A wire electrode is also inserted into the EAS. The patient then ascends an elevated commode and, with the investigator behind a screen, is instructed to evacuate the simulated stool. Patients with idiopathic constipation often fail to do this and the myoelectrical recording reveals a paradoxical contraction of the EAS during attempts to defaecate.

Defaecography is particularly useful in constipated patients as it demonstrates mechanical lesions that obstruct defaecation, such as partial rectal prolapse, rectocoele and rectal intussusception [83]. A barium enema is essential in patients with constipation, since it may reveal obstructing lesions such as tumours, Crohn's disease or ischaemic strictures and endometriosis, and distinguishes between the grossly dilated megacolon that is suggestive of visceral myopathy or neuropathy and the elongated narrowed multihaustral colon found in many patients with chronic idiopathic constipation.

Colonic transit is usually measured by asking the subject to ingest a known quantity of radio-opaque markers and then taking abdominal X-rays over the next few days to determine the passage of these markers and where they might be accumulating. An alternative is the use of radio-isotopes. There are several ways of conducting a radiographic marker test. The most accurate and reproducible method may be to take 20 markers every day for 5 days and then take a single X-ray at the end of that time; transit is determined by dividing the number of markers in the abdomen by the number ingested daily [86]. This test provides an objective assessment of whether there is impairment of colonic propulsion. Accumulation of the markers in the rectum is suggestive of faecal impaction. Some years ago, constipation was divided into different types according to the distribution of markers [87]. There now seems to be little utility in this assessment, although patients with ulcerative colitis and those with irritable bowel syndrome often have hold-up in the proximal colon and rapid clearance of the distal colon [88].

Finally, it is important to remember that constipation is a feature of some metabolic diseases, so that blood should be taken for measurement of thyroid function, as well as plasma calcium and potassium, and can be a side effect of a number of drugs, including opiates, anticholinergics, antidepressants and calcium channel blockers.

Treatment

The treatment of disturbances of defaecation in patients with diabetes is largely symptomatic. Nevertheless, the establishment of tight glycaemic control may slow, halt or even reverse the neuropathic process. There are no direct data in relation to anorectal dysfunction but, as discussed in Chapter 4, stringent control of blood glucose concentration for 4 weeks has been reported to rectify the disturbances in electrical control activity of gastric motility in diabetic patients [89]. It should be recognised that this level of glycaemic control is not achievable without an increased risk of hypoglycaemia, which may go undetected, particularly in patients with long-standing type 1 diabetes.

While a number of agents, including aldose reductase inhibitors, may be effective in the treatment of diabetic autonomic and peripheral neuropathy [90], there is no information about their effects on anorectal function.

Treatment of incontinence

Patients with faecal incontinence may only rarely be 'cured'—the major aim of treatment is to improve symptoms to a level where there is minimal impact on lifestyle. Many patients, unfortunately, wrongly consider that incontinence is the 'natural' result of childbirth and/or 'getting old' and that little can be done.

When diarrhoea is complicated by faecal incontinence, the first priority is to bring the diarrhoea under control and subsequently ascertain whether the patient has a treatable cause for incontinence. The first line of treatment for diarrhoea is the use of opiate-like antidiarrhoeal agents (e.g. loperamide, lomotil, diphenoxylate and codeine phosphate). These inhibit the local nervous reflexes responsible for both intestinal propulsion and secretion and increase the tone of the IAS [91]. Loperamide is the most potent of these and, unlike codeine phosphate, does not cross the blood–brain barrier. As many as 12 tablets of loperamide (8 mg t.d.s.) may be taken each day without unwanted side effects. It is important to exclude the possibility that diarrhoea is related to intestinal stasis with bacterial overgrowth, since loperamide may potentially exacerbate this (Chapter 5).

Rapid intestinal transit sufficient to cause diarrhoea is often associated with bile acid malabsorption. Bile acids stimulate colonic secretion and propulsion and may exacerbate symptoms of urgency and faecal incontinence. We have found that the bile acid-binding agent cholestyramine is sometimes dramatically effective in diarrhoea that is associated with urgency and faecal incontinence and resistant to loperamide and opiate-like antidiarrhoeal agents. Bile acids are released in association with a meal, and therefore it is essential that the patient is instructed to take cholestyramine half an hour before meals and that the dose is titrated with the size of the meal. We usually commence with a small dose of two sachets (8 g) before dinner in the evening and one (4 g) before lunch, but the clinician should enlist the patient's collaboration in finding the most appropriate dose according to his/her pattern of eating and the response to treatment.

Since there is evidence that diabetic diarrhoea and nocturnal incontinence may be related to sympathetic neuropathy, it is not surprising that α2-adrenergic agonists, such as clonidine, have been advocated and shown to be effective in the management of diabetic diarrhoea [92] associated with evidence of neuropathy. Clonidine artificially restores sympathetic tone, enhancing salt and water absorption and reducing propulsive contractions [93]. Clonidine also modulates colonic motor and sensory function in healthy subjects [94]. It also seems probable that clonidine may help to restore IAS stability and tone, although this has yet to be tested. Clonidine should always be considered in the management of patients with nocturnal incontinence. The doses used are comparable to those employed in the treatment of hypertension; considerable caution should be employed in treating neuropathic patients with postural hypotension.

If the patient has faecal incontinence, even in the presence of a normal or near-normal bowel action, further investigation and treatment for anorectal dysfunction is required. Loperamide should always be tried in such patients, since it reduces rectal sensitivity and reflex activity, enhances sphincter tone and has been shown to reduce urgency and incontinence, even in patients who do not have frank diarrhoea [91].

As discussed, obstetric causes for faecal incontinence may well be more common in patients with diabetes and can be treated by surgery. Defects in the sphincter ring caused by previously undetected tears can respond to an overlap sphincter repair. It may well be important to ascertain that the remaining muscle is active by carrying out measurements of myoelectrical activity before surgery. As discussed, obstetric trauma also weakens the pelvic floor and causes perineal descent and pudendal neuropathy. The progression of this may be halted, and the mechanical function of the pelvic floor improved, by a surgical procedure known as post-anal repair, in which the pelvic floor is strengthened with a darn or a graft. This procedure may also be beneficial in the management of urinary incontinence. When perineal descent has resulted in severe neuropathic weakness of the sphincter or the pudendal neuropathy caused by compression and tension is exacerbated by diabetic microangiopathy, the results of post-anal repair are often poor. Alternative procedures, such as the use of the gracilis or gluteus muscle to construct a new sphincter, the more experimental artificial sphincter devices and spinal sacral nerve stimulation have been tried, but their efficacy is uncertain [95]. When a patient is suffering from continuous soiling that does not respond to treatment, a permanent colostomy may prove to be the only reasonable solution.

Faecal impaction with overflow is usually treated by evacuation using digital extraction and enemas, followed by a regular regime of bulk laxatives and toilet training [96].

Biofeedback training (operant reconditioning) is a useful method for treating incontinence of all types. Its efficacy is thought to relate to enhancement of rectal sensitivity and improvement of the coordination between rectal perception and external sphincter contraction. The sphincter activity during conscious contraction of the external sphincter is displayed to the patient visually, who is encouraged to improve in both the strength and duration of the response. Coordination between rectal perception and pelvic floor contraction is improved by training the patient to recognise and react promptly to progressively smaller volumes of air introduced into a rectal balloon by contracting the external sphincter. Studies have shown impressive responses to biofeedback training in patients with idiopathic faecal incontinence, but when attempts were made to control for the 'active principle' by not offering any feedback, patients still did well [97]. Thus, one might conclude that the beneficial effects of biofeedback are, at least in part, related to the establishment of confidence through the nature of the relationship between the patient and the therapist.

Treatment of constipation

The first line of treatment for constipation is dietary supplementation with fibre and/or bulking agents, such as ispagula husk (e.g. Fybogel and Regulan) [98]. In our laboratory, we routinely commence all patients referred for assessment of constipation on a regime consisting of three times daily 15 ispagula husk, an extra litre of water a day and regular exercise. About 25% of patients respond to that regime, even though their constipation has been resistant to all forms of treatment for years. Bulking agents are viscous polysaccharides. They not only increase the volume of faeces but, as discussed in Chapter 4, can also improve glycaemic control in diabetes by slowing the delivery of carbohydrate from the stomach into the small intestine and small intestinal carbohydrate absorption [98]. Unfortunately, those polysaccharides that are particularly effective in reducing postprandial hyperglycaemia, such as guar gum and pectin, are completely fermented by colonic bacteria and are less effective as bulk laxatives than ispagula husk [99].

More resistant constipation may be treated with osmotic laxatives, such as lactulose, and irritant laxatives such as bisocodyl. 'Prokinetic' agents, such as cisapride, have been advocated for treatment of chronic constipation. As discussed in Chapter 4, these drugs enhance synaptic transmission by increasing the release of acetylcholine [100]. They may, therefore, be useful in offsetting the effects of neuropathy affecting the parasympathetic nerves. Unfortunately, there is no evidence to suggest that these agents are particularly effective in diabetic patients who are constipated, and their efficacy in other forms of constipation is at best controversial.

Biofeedback training is effective in about 80% of cases of severe constipation referred to our unit. Biofeedback attempts to restore the dynamics of defaecation, by training the patient to recognise the presence of stool in the rectum and to relax the external sphincter during attempts to defaecate instead of contracting it. In our laboratory, we insert the silicone rubber 'mouse' into the rectum and pull back on the tail so that it sits snugly above the sphincter. Then, with a wire electrode in the EAS and connected to an audio output, we instruct the patient to attempt to defaecate while maintaining the activity of the EAS at as low a level as possible. This procedure is preceded by abdominal massage with aromatic oils, specifically rosemary, which has the reputation of being 'good for constipation'. Massage commences with a circular motion, starting in the right iliac fossa and moving slowly along the line of the colon, up, across and down. This not only relaxes the patient, but provides the sensation of faeces moving around the colon and into the rectum ready for evacuation. It is reinforced by the suggestion that the blockage is being relieved. It was originally thought that biofeedback would only work for patients who demonstrated paradoxical contraction of the EAS and puborectalis muscles during attempts to defaecate. The observation that it can help constipated patients who have no detectable disturbance in defaecation dynamics suggests that it might work through non-specific psychological mechanisms associated with the relationship between the patient and the therapist [101]. It is essential for this type of therapy that the therapist is relaxed, unrushed, sympathetic and reassuring, inspiring confidence and belief in the efficacy of the method. Others have used the focused suggestions of hypnotherapy to alter bowel function, particularly in patients with functional bowel disorders [102]. After inducing a state of deep relaxation by progressive muscle relaxation and other suggestions, Peter Whorwell and his colleagues instruct patients to imagine that their bowel is like a river. If they are constipated, the river is stagnant and turbid and obstructed and Whorwell 'speeds it up'. This technique can be remarkably effective. When one of us (NWR) learnt the technique and tried it out on a lady who had been severely constipated for years, he implanted the suggestion that her river was a clear stream flowing merrily over pebbles in the bright sunlight. Two weeks later, the patient returned with a merry little attack of diarrhoea and he had to slow the river down!

The role of emotions in the pathogenesis of bowel disorders should always be acknowledged in the treatment plan for diarrhoea or constipation, whatever the cause. Our experience with functional disorders causing severe bowel dysfunction suggests that there is a link between emotional expression and the nature of the bowel disturbance. Patients with diarrhoea, urgency and incontinence often have considerable difficulty in containing their emotions, while those with constipation can be quite literally uptight and defensive. Psychotherapy can be remarkably effective for these patients [103]. One of us was referred a patient, a young lady called Sandra, who had been constipated for 14 years ever since her brief marriage had broken down. She lived alone and worked in the local library. During the course of therapy, she was silent and responded by looking up shyly from under her fringe in a manner reminiscent of the late Princess Diana. This restricted the therapeutic engagement somewhat, so the therapist stopped talking and, as it was summer, fell into a deep reverie on the state of English cricket. When the time came for the session to end, he merely said, 'It's time to go now, Sandra'. She looked alarmed and ran out of the rooms and the therapist doubted that he would see her again. The following week, she was quite different. Without pausing to take off her coat, she told him how she had not travelled half way across the country for him to sit there and do nothing, she had felt furious, and she had suffered with diarrhoea all week! This seemed to unlock the therapy. By the end, she was passing motions regularly, she went on holiday to New York, changed her job, met a bookish young man and continued to enjoy a regular bowel action. You could say that she had an earth-moving experience! Of course, it is difficult to provide the evidence to support such anecdotes. Nevertheless, psychotherapy has been proven to be effective in relieving the symptoms of patients with irritable bowel syndrome resistant to medical treatment [103].

It is clearly inappropriate to suggest that psychotherapeutic techniques would be useful for patients with an inert distended megacolon caused by severe neuropathy. Such patients can probably only be treated by surgical resection of the colon and a permanent ileostomy [104]. However, most patients with diabetes who have constipation are not like that. They may have a degree of neuropathy, but their medical condition may be complicated by emotional situations that may be difficult to express. People with diabetes have emotional problems like anybody else and there is evidence that this prevalence is higher [105]. For example, living with a severe life-threatening illness and keeping oneself alive day in and day out with injections, knowing that their sight is gradually deteriorating, they are losing the sense of feeling in their feet and hands, and they can no longer enjoy normal sexual activity, must put enormous strain on the patient with diabetes and his/her relationship with other people. People cope with this in different ways. Some despair. Others, perhaps the majority, adopt a stoical, stiff-upper-lip attitude and keep their diabetes and their emotions in reasonably tight control. In other words they become emotionally (and perhaps physically) constipated. The art of the physician is not only to recognise the disease, but also to understand the sort of person who gets the disease. Successful management treats both.

References

1. Feldman M, Schiller LR. Disorders of gastrointestinal motility associated with diabetes mellitus. *Ann Intern Med* 1983; **98**: 378–84.
2. Goyal RK, Spiro HM. Gastrointestinal manifestations of diabetes mellitus. *Med Clin North Am* 1971; **55**: 1031–44.
3. Camilleri M. Gastrointestinal problems in diabetes. *Endocrinol Metab Clin North Am* 1996; **25**: 361–78.
4. Rundles R. Diabetic neuropathy; general review with report of 125 cases. *Medicine* 1945; **24**: 111–160.
5. Horowitz M, Maddox AF, Wishart JM, Harding PE *et al*. Relationships between oesophageal transit and solid and liquid gastric emptying in diabetes mellitus. *Eur J Nucl Med* 1991; **18**: 229–234.
6. Enck P, Rathmann W, Spiekermann M, Czerner D *et al*. Prevalence of gastrointestinal symptoms in diabetic patients and non-diabetic subjects. *Z Gastroenterol* 1994; **32**: 637–41.

7. Martin M. Diabetic neuropathy: a clinical study of 150 cases. *Brain* 1958; **76**: 594–624.
8. Maxton DG, Whorwell PJ. Functional bowel symptoms in diabetes—the role of autonomic neuropathy. *Postgrad Med J* 1991; **67**: 991–3.
9. Drossman DA, Li Z, Andruzzi E, Temple RD *et al.* U.S. householder survey of function gastrointestinal disorders. Prevalence, sociodemography, and health impact. *Dig Dis Sci* 1993; **38**: 1569–80.
10. Thompson WG, Heaton KW. Functional bowel disorders in apparently healthy people. *Gastroenterology* 1980; **79**: 283–8.
11. Talley NJ, O'Keefe EA, Zinsmeister AR, Melton LJ. Prevalence of gastrointestinal symptoms in the elderly: a population-based study. *Gastroenterology* 1992; **102**: 895–901.
12. Read NW. The relationship between colonic motility and secretion. *Scand J Gastroenterol* 1984; **19** (suppl 84): 45–63.
13. Ritchie J. Colonic motor activity and bowel function. Part I. Normal movement of contents. *Gut* 1968; **27**: 442–456.
14. Baker WNW, Mann CV. The rectosigmoid junction zone: another sphincter. In Thomas PA, Mann CV (eds), *Alimentary Sphincters and their Disorders*. Macmillan: London, 1981, 201–11.
15. Ritchie J. Colonic motor activity and bowel function. II. Distribution and incidence of motor activity at rest and after food and carbachol. *Gut* 1968; **9**: 502–11.
16. Holdstock DS, Misiewicz JJ, Smith T, Rowlands EN. Propulsion (mass movements) in the human colon and its relationship to meals and somatic activity *Gut* 1970; **11**: 91–99.
17. Narducci F, Bassotti G, Gaburri M, Morelli A. Circadian rhythms of human colonic motility. *Dig Dis Sci* 1985; **30**: 784.
18. Karaus M, Sarna SK. Giant migrating contractions in the dog colon *Gastroenterology* 1987; **92**: 925–33.
19. Sun WM, Read NW, Prior A, Daly JA *et al.* Sensory and motor responses to rectal distention vary according to rate and pattern of balloon inflation. *Gastroenterology* 1990; **99**: 1008–15.
20. Rao SSC, Read NW, Davison PA, Bannister JJ, Holdsworth CD. Anorectal sensitivity and responses to rectal distention in patients with ulcerative colitis. *Gastroenterology* 1987; **93**: 1270–75.
21. Penttila O, Kyosola K, Klinge E, Ahonen A, Tallqvist G. Studies of rectal mucosal catecholamines in ulcerative colitis. *Ann Clin Res* 1975; **7**: 32–36.
22. Read NW, Sun WM. Anorectal manometry. In Henry M, Swash M (eds), *Coloproctology and Pelvic Floor*, 2nd edn. Butterworth: London, 1992: 119–45.
23. Sun WM, MacDonagh R, Thomas DG, Read NW. Anorectal function in patients with complete spinal transection before and after sacral posterior rhizotomy. *Gastroenterology* 1995; **108**: 990–98.
24. Duthie HL, Gairns FW. Sensory nerve endings and sensation in the anal region of man. *Br J Surg* 1960; **47**: 585–95.
25. Duthie HL. The relation of sensation in the anal canal to the functional anal sphincter: a possible factor in anal continence. *Gut* 1963; **4**: 179–82.
26. Duthie H. Dynamic of rectum and anus. *Clin Gastroenterol* 1975; **405**: 527–9.
27. Burleigh DE, DeMello A, Parks AG. Responses of isolated human internal anal sphincter to drugs and electric field stimulation. *Gastroenterology* 1979; **77**: 484.
28. Bouvier M, Gonella J. Nervous control of the internal anal sphincter of the cat. *J Physiol (Lond)* 1981; **310**: 457–69.
29. Burleigh DE. Neural and pharmacologic factors affecting motility of the internal anal sphincter. *Gastroenterology* 1983; **84**: 409–17.

30. Floyd WF, Walls EW. Electromyography of the sphincter ani externus in man. *J Physiol* 1953; **122**: 599–609.

31. Parks AG, Porter NH, Melzak J. Experimental study of the reflex mechanism controlling the muscles of the pelvic floor. *Dis Colon Rectum* 1962; **5**: 407–14.

32. Parks AG, Swash M, Urich H. Sphincter denervation in anorectal incontinence and rectal prolapse. *Gut* 1977; **18**: 656–65.

33. Gibbons CP, Bannister JJ, Trowbridge EA, Read NW. Role of anal cushions in maintaining continence. *Lancet* 1986; **i**: 886–9.

34. Gibbons CP, Bannister JJ, Trowbridge GA, Read NW. An analysis of anal sphincter pressure and anal compliance in normal subjects. *Int J Colorectal Dis* 1986; **1**: 231–7.

35. Gibbons CP, Trowbridge GA, Bannister JJ, Read NW. The mechanics of the anal sphincter complex. *J Biomech* 1988; **21**: 601–4.

36. Read MG, Read NW, Haynes WG, Donnelly TC, Johnson AG. A prospective study of the effect of haemorrhoidectomy on sphincter function and faecal continence. *Br J Surg* 1982; **69**: 396–8.

37. Narducci F, Bassotti G, Gaburri M, Morelli A. Twenty-four hour manometric recording of colonic motor activity in healthy man. *Gut* 1987; **28**: 17–25.

38. Whitehead W, Orr W, Engel B, Schuster M. External anal sphincter response to rectal distention: learned response or reflex? *Psychophysiology* 1982; **19**: 57–67.

39. Kerrigan DD, Lucas MG, Sun WM, Donnelly TC, Read NW. Idiopathic constipation associated with impaired urethrovesical and sacral reflex function. *Br J Surg* 1989; **76**: 748–51.

40. Sun WM, Read NW. Occult spinal lesions: a common undetected cause of faecal incontinence. *Lancet* 1990; **i**: 166.

41. Schmidt RE, Beaudet LN, Plurad SB, Dorsey DA. Axonal cytoskeletal pathology in aged and diabetic human sympathetic autonomic ganglia. *Brain Res* 1997; **769**: 375–83.

42. Flynn MD, O'Brien IA, Corrall RJ. The prevalence of autonomic and peripheral neuropathy in insulin-treated diabetic subjects. *Diabet Med* 1995; **12**: 310–13.

43. Tesfaye S, Stevens LK, Stephenson JM, Fuller JH *et al.* Prevalence of diabetic peripheral neuropathy and its relation to glycaemic control and potential risk (in press).

44. Horowitz M, Harding PE, Maddox A, Maddern GJ *et al.* Gastric and oesophageal emptying in insulin-dependent diabetes mellitus. *J Gastroenterol Hepatol* 1986; **1**: 97–113.

45. Fraser R, Horowitz M, Maddox A, Harding P *et al.* Hyperglycaemia slows gastric emptying in type 1 (insulin-dependent) diabetes mellitus. *Diabetologia* 1990; **30**: 675–80.

46. Rayner CK, Samsom M, Jones K, Horowitz M. Relationships of upper gastrointestinal motor and sensory function with glycemic control. *Diabetes Care* 2001; **24**: 371–81.

47. Russo A, Sun WM, Sattawatthamrong Y, Fraser R *et al.* Acute hyperglycaemia effects anorectal motor and sensory function in normal subjects. *Gut* 1997; **41**: 494–9.

48. Chey WD, Kim M, Hasler WI, Owyang C. Hyperglycemia alters perception of rectal distension and blunts the rectoanal inhibitory reflex in healthy volunteers. *Gastroenterology* 1998; **108**: 1700–1708.

49. Azvar E, Ersoz O, Karisik E *et al.* Hyperglycemia-induced attenuation of rectal perception depends on pattern of rectal balloon inflation. *Dig Dis Sci* 1997; **42**: 2206–12.

50. Russo A, Smout AJPM, Kositchaiwat C, Rayner C *et al.* The effect of hyperglycaemia on cerebral potentials evoked by rapid rectal distension in healthy humans. *Eur J Clin Invest* 1999; **29**: 512–18.

51. Sims MA, Hasler WL, Chey WD, Kim MS, Owyang C. Hyperglycemia inhibits mechanoreceptor-mediated gastrocolonic responses and colonic peristaltic reflexes in healthy humans. *Gastroenterology* 1995; **108**: 350–59.

52. Allen C, Shen G, Palta M, Lotz B *et al*. Long-term hyperglycemia is related to periph-eral nerve changes at a diabetes duration of 4 years. The Wisconsin Diabetes Registry. *Diabetes Care* 1997; **20**: 1154–8.

53. Greene D. A sodium-pump defect in diabetic peripheral nerve corrected by sorbinil administration: relationship to myoinositol metabolism and nerve conduction slowing. *Metab Clin Exp* 1986; **35**(4, suppl 1): 60–65.

54. Clouse RE, Lustman PJ. Gastrointestinal symptoms in diabetic patients: lack of asso-ciation with neuropathy. *Am J Gastroenterol* 1989; **84**: 868–72.

55. Sun WM, Katsinelos P, Horowitz M, Read NW. Disturbances in anorectal function in patients with diabetes mellitus and faecal incontinence. *Eur J Gastroenterol Hepatol* 1996; **8**: 1007–12.

56. Speakman CTM, Hoyle CHV, Kamm MA, Henry MM *et al*. Adrenergic control of the internal anal sphincter is abnormal in patients with idiopathic faecal incontinence. *Br J Surg* 1990; **77**: 134–44.

57. Ejskjaer NT, Bradley JL, Buxton-Thomas MS, Edmonds ME *et al*. Novel surgical treat-ment and gastric pathology in diabetic gastroparesis. *Diabet Med* 1999; **16**: 488–95.

58. Rogers J, Levy DM, Henry MM, Misiewicz JJ. Pelvic floor neuropathy: a comparative study of diabetes mellitus and idiopathic faecal incontinence. *Gut* 1988; **29**: 756–61.

59. Schiller LR, Santa-Ana CA, Schmulen AC, Hendler RS *et al*. Pathogenesis of fecal incontinence in diabetes mellitus: evidence for internal-anal-sphincter dysfunction. *N Engl J Med* 1982; **307**: 1666–71.

60. Wald A, Tunuguntla AK. Anorectal sensorimotor dysfunction in fecal incontinence and diabetes mellitus. Modification with biofeedback therapy. *N Engl J Med* 1984; **310**: 1282–7.

61. Rogers J, Henry MM, Misiewicz JJ. Combined sensory and motor deficit in primary neuropathic faecal incontinence. *Gut* 1988; **29**: 5–9.

62. Aitchison M, Fisher BM, Carter K, McKee R *et al*. Impaired anal sensation and early diabetic faecal incontinence. *Diabet Med* 1991; **8**: 960–63.

63. Nakanishi N, Tatara K, Naramura H, Fujiwara H *et al*. Urinary and fecal incontinence in a community-residing older population in Japan. *J Am Geriat Soc* 1997; **45**: 215–19.

64. Pinna-Pintor M, Zara GP, Falletto E, Monge L *et al*. Pudendal neuropathy in diabetic patients with faecal incontinence. *Int J Colorectal Dis* 1994; **9**: 105–9.

65. Sultan AH, Kamm MA, Hudson CN. Pudendal nerve damage during labour: prospec-tive study before and after childbirth. *Br J Obset Gynaecol* 1994; **101**: 22–28.

66. Sultan AH, Kamm MA, Hudson CN, Bartram CI. Anal sphincter disruption during vaginal delivery. *N Eng J Med* 1993; **329**: 1905–11.

67. Kuhl C, Hornness PJ, Anderson O. Etiology and pathophysiology of gestational dia-betes mellitus. *Diabetes* 1985; **34**: 66–70.

68. Read NW, Abouzekry L. Why do patients with faecal impaction have faecal inconti-nence: *Gut* 1986; **27**: 283–7.

69. Geib D, Jones JD. Unprecedented causes of constipation. *J Am Med Assoc* 1902; **38**: 1305–6.

70. Read NW, Timms JM, Barfield LJ, Donnelly TC, Bannister JJ. Impairment of defeca-tion in young women with severe constipation. *Gastroenterology* 1986; **90**: 53–60.

71. Preston DM, Lennard-Jones JE. Anismus in chronic constipation. *Dig Dis Sci* 1985; **30**: 413–18.

72. Read NW, Sun WM. Haemorrhoids, constipation, and hypertensive anal cushions. *Lan-cet* 1989; **i**: 610.

73. Battle WM, Snape WJ Jr, Alavi A, Cohen S *et al.* Colonic dysfunction in diabetes mellitus. *Gastroenterology* 1980; **79**: 1217–21.

74. Sarna S, Erasmus LP, Haslbeck M, Holzl R. Visceral perception and gut changes in diabetes mellitus. *Neurogastroenterol Motil* 1994; **6**: 85–94.

75. Bannister JJ, Timms JM, Barfield L, Read NW. Physiological studies in young women with chronic constipation. *Int J Colorectal Dis* 1986; **1**: 175–82.

76. Brocklehurst JC. Constipation in the elderly. In *Constipation*, Camm M, Jones JL (eds). Wrightson Biomedical: Petersfield, Hants, 1994; 34.

77. Read NW, Abouzekry L, Read MG, Howell P *et al.* Anorectal function in elderly patients with faecal impaction. *Gastroenterology* 1985; **89**: 959–66.

78. Hancock BD. The internal anal sphincter and anal fissure. *Br J Surg* 1977; **64**: 92–5.

79. Sun WM, Donnelly TC, Read NW, Johnson A. The hypertensive anal cushion as a cause of the high anal pressures in patients with haemorrhoids. *Br J Surg* 1990; **77**: 458–62.

80. Read NW, Sun WM. Reflex anal dilatation: the effect of parting the buttocks on anal function in normal subjects and patients with anorectal and spinal diseases. *Gut* 1991; **32**: 670–73.

81. Rao SSC, Sun WM. Current techniques of assessing defecation dynamics. *Dig Dis Sci* 1997; **15**(suppl 1): 64–77.

82. Sun WM, Rao SS. Manometric assessment of anorectal function. *Gastroenterol Clin N Am* 2001; **30**: 15–32.

83. Mahieu P. Defecography. I. Description of a new procedure and results in normal patients. *Gastrointest Radiol* 1984; **9**: 247–51.

84. Kiff ES, Swash M. Slowed conduction in the pudendal nerves in idiopathic (neurogenic) faecal incontinence. *Br J Surg* 1984; **71**: 614–16.

85. Bannister JJ, Davison P, Timms JM, Gibbons C, Read NW. Effect of stool size and consistency on defaecation. *Gut* 1987; **28**: 1246–50.

86. Metcalf AM, Phillips SF, Zinsmeister AR. Simplified assessment of segmental colonic transit. *Gastroenterology* 1987; **92**: 40–47.

87. Metcalf AM, Phillips SF, Zinsmeister AR. Simplified assessment of segmental colonic transit. *Gastroenterology* 1987; **92**: 40–47.

88. O'Brien MD, Phillips SF. Colonic motility in health and disease. *Gastroenterol Cli N Am* 1996; **25**: 147–62.

89. Kawagishi T, Nishizawa Y, Emoto M, Maekawa K *et al.* Gastric myoelectrical activity in patients with diabetes. Role of glucose control and autonomic nerve function. *Diabetes Care* 1997; **20**: 848–54.

90. Giugliano D, Marfella R, Quatraro A, De-Rosa N *et al.* Tolrestat for mild diabetic neuropathy. A 52-week, randomized, placebo-controlled trial. *Ann Intern Med* 1993; **118**: 7–11.

91. Sun WM, Read NW, Verlinden M. Effects of loperamide oxide on gastrointestinal transit time and anorectal function in patients with chronic diarrhoea and faecal incontinence. *Scand J Gastroenterol* 1997; **32**: 34–8.

92. Schiller LR, Santa Ana CA, Morawski SG, Fordtran JS. Studies of the antidiarrhoeal action of clonidine. *Gastroenterology* 1985; **89**: 982–8.

93. Fedorak R, Field M, Chang E. Treatment of diabetic diarrhoea with clonidine. *Ann Intern Med* 1985; **102**: 197–9.

94. Bharucha AE, Camilleri M, Zinsmeister AR, Hanson RB. Adrenergic modulation of human colonic motor and sensory function. *Am J Physiol* 1997; **273**: G997–1006.

95. Williams NS, Hallan RI, Koeze TH, Watkins ES. Construction of a neoanal sphincter by transposition of the gracilis muscle and prolonged neuromuscular stimulation for the treatment of faecal incontinence. *Ann R Coll Surg* 1990; **72**: 108–13.

96. Bartolo DCC, Sun WM. Colorectal and anorectal motor dysfunctions. In Shearman DJ, Finlayson NC, Camilleri M (eds). *Diseases of the Gastrointestinal Tract and Liver.* 3rd edn. Churchill Livingstone: New York, 1997; 1315–41.

97. Miner PB, Donnelly TC, Read NW. Investigation of mode of action of biofeedback in treatment of fecal incontinence. *Dig Dis Sci* 1990; **35**: 1291–8.

98. Locke GR, Pemberton JH, Phillips SF. AGA Medical Position Statement: guidelines on constipation. *Gastroenterology* 2000; **119**: 1761–78.

99. Tomlin J, Read NW. The relation between bacterial degradation of viscous polysaccharides and stool output in human beings. *Br J Nutr* 1988; **60**: 467–75.

100. Briejer MR, Akkermans LM, Schuurkes JA. Gastrointestinal prokinetic benzamides: the pharmacology underlying stimulation of motility. *Pharmacol Rev* 1995; **47**: 631–51.

101. Chiotakakou-Faliakou E, Kamm MA, Roy AJ, Storrie JB. Biofeedback provides long-term benefit for patients with intractable, slow and normal transit constipation. *Gut* 1998; **42**: 517–21.

102. Whorwell PJ. Hypnotherapy for selected gastrointestinal disorders. *Dig Dis Sci* 1990; **8**: 223–5.

103. Guthrie E, Creed F, Dawson D, Tomenson B. A randomised controlled trial of psychotherapy in patients with refractory irritable bowel syndrome. *Br J Psychiat* 1993; **163**: 315–21.

104. Kamm MA, Hawley PR, Lennard-Jones JE. Outcome of colectomy for severe idiopathic constipation. *Gut* 1988; **29**: 969–73.

105. Van der Does FE, De Neeling JN, Snoek FJ *et al.*. Symptoms and well-being in relation to glycemic control in type II diabetes. *Diabetes Care* 1996; **19**: 204–10.

7

Hepato-biliary and Pancreatic Function

Ad A. M. Masclee and **Bart van Hoek**

Introduction

Alterations in the function of the liver, biliary system and exocrine pancreas are common in diabetic patients. However, in contrast to other systemic disorders with gastrointestinal involvement, symptoms originating from these organs are less prominent, apart from biliary colic due to gallstones. In this chapter the functional interactions between the liver and exocrine pancreas on the one hand, and the endocrine pancreas on the other, are discussed. Both the impact of diabetes on hepato-biliary and exocrine pancreatic function and the hepatic and exocrine pancreatic disorders that may lead to alterations in glucose metabolism, and subsequently result in diabetes mellitus, are reviewed.

The liver and diabetes

The liver plays an important role in glucose metabolism. It is, therefore, not surprising that diabetes mellitus can affect hepatic function and that glucose

Gastrointestinal Function in Diabetes Mellitus. Edited by Michael Horowitz and Melvin Samsom
© 2004 John Wiley & Sons, Ltd   ISBN: 0-471-89916-X

metabolism can be altered in liver disease. In some cases chronic liver disease and diabetes may result from the same cause [1].

Normal carbohydrate metabolism and the liver

Normal carbohydrate homeostasis involves hormones (such as insulin, glucagon, cortisol, growth hormone and catecholamines), physiological processes (exercise, fasting, stress), biochemical pathways (glycolysis, formation and breakdown of glycogen, gluconeogenesis, the Krebs cycle and lipogenesis) and substrate exchanges between organs and tissues [2].

After feeding, the liver takes up glucose and uses it for glycolysis or for the formation of glycogen. The liver releases glucose from the breakdown of glycogen and from gluconeogenesis for utilisation by peripheral tissues, mainly the brain cells and red blood cells, but also by muscle cells and adipocytes for storage. After ingestion of a meal, the liver retains at least 50% of an oral glucose load for glycogen synthesis and other metabolic functions. Via an indirect pathway, glucose is not directly taken up by the liver but is first released into the circulation and taken up by peripheral tissues, where glycolysis to gluconeogenic precursors (such as lactate and pyruvate) takes place. These precursors are then released into the circulation, taken up by the liver and converted to glycose via glyconeogenesis. The glucose produced is then incorporated into glycogen.

Glucose uptake by the hepatocyte is a non-insulin-dependent process, taking place through facilitated diffusion via hepatic glucose transporters. The glucose concentration in the hepatocyte equals that of the sinusoids. The next step is conversion of glucose to glucose-6-phosphatase by glucokinase (Figure 7.1). Under

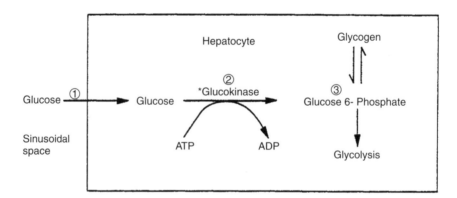

Figure 7.1 Glucose uptake by the liver. (1) Rapid diffusion of glucose from sinusoidal space into the hepatocyte via facilitated diffusion by a specific hepatic glucose transporter protein. (2) The rate-limiting enzyme for uptake of glucose by the liver. High K_m of hepatic glucokinase for glucose makes this system very sensitive to changes in the serum glucose concentration. (3) Metabolic fate of the glucose 6-phosphate is dependent on nutritional state. Asterisk indicates an enzyme that is significantly altered in diabetes. From Katbamna *et al.* [2], with permission

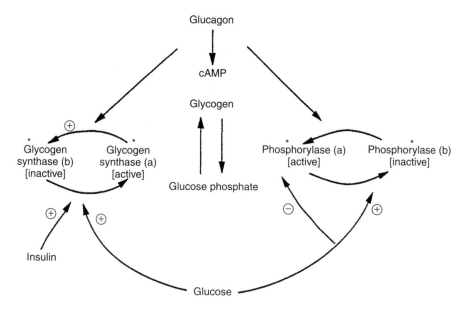

Figure 7.2   Regulation of glucogen metabolism is controlled by complex interactions that occur in the hepatocyte. Glucagon via cAMP-dependent phosphorylation–dephosphorylation exerts its influence by increasing phosphorylase activity and diminishing the activity of glucogen synthase. Glucose binds to phosphorylase [P(a)], causing an inactivation of P(a). The decrease in concentration of P(a) allows for the activation of glycogen synthase and subsequent glycogen synthesis. Asterisks represent enzymes that are significantly altered in diabetes. From Katbamna *et al.* [2], with permission

physiological conditions, this enzyme is not saturated. Therefore, the capacity of the liver to monitor the sinusoidal glucose concentration is not dependent on hormonal control under normal physiological conditions. The rate-limiting enzymes in hepatic glycogen synthesis and breakdown are glycogen synthase and glycogen phosphorylase (Figure 7.2). High sinusoidal glucose leads to inactivation of phosphorylase, which in turn activates glycogen synthase, so that glycogen is synthesised. This occurs within 2 min of an increase in glucose concentration. Glucose may also directly activate glycogen synthase. Although insulin influences the synthesis of glycogen, the intrahepatic glucose concentration is more important in regulating glycogen metabolism after meals. After a 48 h fast, when glycogen is depleted, low-dose insulin infusion inhibits degradation of newly formed glycogen and allows gluconeogenesis, with storage of the newly formed glucose as glycogen. At higher rates of insulin infusion, both glycogenolysis and gluconeogenesis are inhibited, due to the intrahepatic effect of insulin rather than to a decreased availability or extraction of gluconeogenic precursors. Portal venous insulin levels can be 10 times higher than peripheral blood insulin levels, leading to significant changes in hepatic glucose metabolism with seemingly small changes in serum insulin concentrations. Periportal hepatocytes

exhibit greater activities of the enzymes of gluconeogenesis and glycogensyn-
thesis, while the perivenous hepatocytes exhibit greater enzymatic activity for
glycolysis. The liver glycogen storage (around 70 g for an adult) is not enough
to meet the 24 h glucose requirement of the brain (145 g) and other glycolytic
tissue (35 g), mainly cellular blood components. In short-term fasting (< 24 h)
the degradation of hepatic glycogen accounts for 50–75% of hepatic glucose
output, gluconeogenesis for the remainder. As fasting continues and hepatic
glycogen is depleted, gluconeogenesis accounts for up to 98% of hepatic glucose output at 2 days. The hormonal signal that is the most important in the
initiation of glycogenolysis is the fall of the plasma insulin level to 25% of the
postprandial level during fasting. Apart from insulin, gluconeogenesis is also
controlled by glucagon, which stimulates phosphoenolpyruvate carboxykinase
(PEPCK), the rate-limiting enzyme of gluconeogenesis (Figure 7.3).

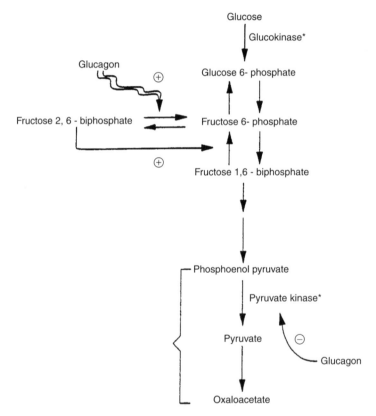

Figure 7.3 Metabolic changes that facilitate glucose production from gluconeogenesis.
Fructose 2,6-biphosphate is a potent stimulator of glycolysis and inhibitor of gluconeogenesis. In conditions such as stress, fasting or insulin deficiency, two important effects of
glucagon are to inhibit the formation of fructose 2,6-biphosphate and pyruvate kinase,
effectively shutting down glycolysis so that gluconeogenesis can proceed. Asterisks
represent enzymes that are significantly altered in diabetes. From Katbamna *et al.* [2], with
permission

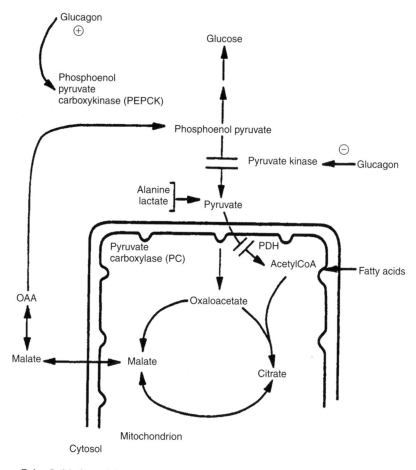

Figure 7.4 Oxidation of fatty acids to acetyl CoA results in decreased pyruvate dehydrogenase (PDH) activity and increased conversion of pyruvate to oxaloacetate (OAA) via pyruvate carboxylase. This causes pyruvate to be channelled into the gluconeogenic pathway. Alanine and glucagon (via cAMP-dependent protein phosphorylation) strongly inhibit pyruvate kinase. Glucagon also promotes phosphoenol pyruvate carboxykinase, which is the rate-limiting enzyme of gluconeogenesis. The net result of these changes is that gluconeogenesis predominates and glycolysis is greatly decreased. From Katbamna *et al.* [2], with permission

During fasting, fatty acids are released from adipose tissue and most of these are metabolised by peripheral tissues. A portion are converted to ketones for utilisation by the brain and other tissues, but most are passively cleared by the liver (Figure 7.4).

Hepatic carbohydrate metabolism in diabetes

In (insulin-dependent) type 1 diabetes mellitus the low or absent insulin level results in enhanced rate of glucose output by the liver and diminished peripheral glucose uptake. Despite an increased insulin-binding activity, hepatic extraction from portal blood is diminished and there is a loss of feedback inhibition on gluconeogenesis. Hepatic glucose output remains inappropriately high for a given glucose and insulin concentration, suggesting hepatic insulin resistance. The insulin receptor activity in the hepatocyte is diminished, and glucagon concentrations are elevated, which, together with insulin deficiency, diminishes glucose uptake by the insulin-sensitive tissues. Glucagon also stimulates glycogenolysis and gluconeogenesis, thereby further increasing hepatic glucose output. Insulin deficiency leads to low hepatic glucokinase levels, resulting in decreased glucose uptake and phosphorylation for glycolysis. So, in contrast to the normal situation, in type 1 diabetes the level of enzyme declines enough that the enzyme, rather than glucose availability, becomes rate limiting. Treatment with insulin reverses these changes and normalises uptake of glucose by the hepatocyte. Insulin deficiency decreases hepatic glycogen content. The normal inactivation of glycogen phosphorylase and activation of glycogen synthase by glucose (Figure 7.2) is defective in type 1 diabetes [2].

In (non-insulin-dependent) type 2 diabetes there is decreased peripheral glucose uptake and elevated hepatic glucose output, which leads to basal hyperinsulinaemia. The resulting hyperglycaemia exacerbates both defects. Hepatic glucose output is not suppressed by insulin in these patients. Hepatic glucose production is the major source of postprandial blood glucose levels in type 2 diabetes. In these patients, after an overnight fast 90% of total hepatic glucose is derived from gluconeogenesis, as compared to 70% in non-diabetics. Due to peripheral insulin resistance, lipolysis and release of free fatty acids occur in adipose tissue. This leads to enhanced fatty acid oxidation, which stimulates gluconeogenesis by making precursors available. In type 2 diabetics hepatic glycogen metabolism is also altered, with accumulation of glycogen during fasting and decreased total muscle glycogen despite hyperglycaemia [2].

Altered glucose metabolism due to liver disease

Increased energy expenditure, decreased glycogen storage

In cirrhosis, there is an increased energy expenditure and abnormal substrate metabolism. A smaller than normal hepatic glycogen storage capacity leads to prolonged catabolic episodes at night, with use of 'fat and protein' rather than carbohydrates, resulting in malnutrition and cachexia. A 'nibbling' pattern of food intake with a late evening meal and an early breakfast can minimise these effects (Figure 7.5) [3].

Glucose intolerance of chronic liver disease

Chronic liver disease may be implicated in the aetiology of associated ('hepatogenic') diabetes mellitus. As many as 70% of cirrhotic patients become hyperglycaemic following an oral glucose load [4]. This may reflect, at least in part, peripheral insulin resistance, for which most patients compensate with higher insulin levels [5,6]. Insulin clearance by the liver can also be reduced in cirrhosis. In some patients insulin secretion after oral glucose is blunted,

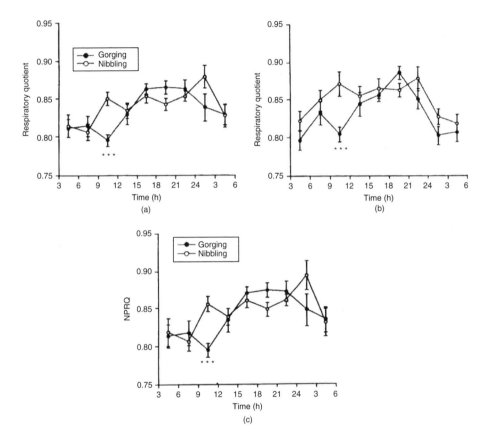

Figure 7.5   Respiratory quotient (RQ) in patients with liver cirrhosis (a) ($n = 7$) and healthy volunteers (b) ($n = 13$), and non-protein respiratory quotient (NPRQ) in cirrhotic patients (c) ($n = 7$) during 'gorging' (●) vs. 'nibbling' (○) feeding pattern. In the 'gorging' pattern the nightly catabolic episodes are longer ($* * *$, $p < 0.001$). Therefore, especially in cirrhosis, a 'nibbling' feeding pattern with a late evening meal and an early breakfast is preferable. From Verboeket-van de Venne *et al.* [3], with permission

with a delayed appearance of C-peptide, leading to delayed peripheral utilisation of glucose [7,8]. Fasting blood glucose levels are normal, which represents a major difference from genuine diabetes. Furthermore, diabetic complications do not occur.

With more severe hyposecretion of insulin, there is also continued hepatic glucose production due to lack of inhibition by insulin [9]. This then leads to overt diabetes, with fasting hyperglycaemia and more marked postprandial hyperglycaemia.

Treatment is dictated by the magnitude and aetiology of hyperglycaemia and the severity and prognosis of liver disease. When a cirrhotic patient temporarily requires high carbohydrate–low protein feeding during hepatic encephalopathy, this takes precedence over any impairment of glucose tolerance. When using oral antidiabetic medication, the shorter-acting agents, such as tolbutamide, are preferred to reduce the risk of hypoglycaemia, since hepatic metabolism of drugs may be impaired [7]. Because of the risk of lactic acidosis, biguanides such as metformin should be avoided in severe liver disease. Insulin therapy can be given as in non-cirrhotic patients, but adequate glycaemic control may prove more difficult to achieve.

Hypoglycaemia in acute liver failure

Impaired degradation of insulin, reduced caloric intake due to encephalopathy, increased peripheral utilisation of glucose, impaired hepatic metabolism and formation of glucose may all contribute to hypoglycaemia in acute liver failure and the very late stages of chronic liver failure. Infusion of 20% or even 50% glucose solutions may be necessary until a liver transplant is performed, in order to prevent hypoglycaemia [10].

Hepatic histologic changes and diseases due to diabetes

Glycogenic infiltration in type 1 diabetes

Glycogenic infiltration of the liver cell nuclei, which resembles vacuolisation, occurs in some two-thirds of type 1 diabetic patients. The amount of glycogen in the livers of poorly controlled diabetics can be increased. Hepatomegaly is present in 60% of such patients with poor control, while the liver is enlarged in only 9% of well-controlled type 1 diabetics. While liver size returns to normal when glycaemic control improves in this group, in the initial stages of treatment glycogen deposition and size may temporarily increase [11]. Very poor diabetic control is associated with an increased water content of hepatocytes, probably to keep the glycogen in solution. Usually there are no hepatic signs or symptoms from glycogenic infiltration. The liver can be enlarged. Some right upper quadrant pain or 'heaviness' can be present. Poor diabetic control can lead to a slight rise in serum bilirubin and hyperglobulinaemia, both returning to normal with improved diabetes control. Diagnosis of glycogenic infiltration is by liver biopsy, preferably with electron microscopy. In general in clinical practice, such a liver biopsy will not serve any purpose and can be omitted. Treatment is by improving diabetes control. No specific follow-up is indicated.

Non-alcoholic steatohepatitis

Non-alcoholic steatohepatitis (NASH) frequently occurs in obese type 2 diabetics, but can also occur in type 1 diabetes. It is the most important hepatic abnormality in diabetes. Alcohol abuse should be excluded. According to the definition of NASH, a man should drink a maximum of three glasses a day and women two glasses, but in any case of steatohepatitis reassessment of liver biochemistry after 3 months of abstinence is recommended to exclude alcohol as a significant cause. Since there is often a macrovesicular steatosis only, defined as fat exceeding 5% of the liver weight, 'non-alcoholic fatty liver disease' would be a more appropriate term. However, because NASH is the name in current use we will also use it, while recognising that in many cases hepatitis is minimal. Steatosis can be associated with (usually lobular) hepatitis. In some cases of NASH, fibrosis or even cirrhosis can be present [12–14]. The prevalence of progression of NASH to cirrhosis is controversial and is probably around 10% but may be up to 40%, particularly in obese women [15–17]. Of all cases of cirrhosis, 12% are due to NASH. Autopsy studies indicate that cirrhosis is twice as common in 'diabetics' as in the general population. There also is some epidemiological evidence that NASH may be the underlying disorder in some cases of cryptogenic cirrhosis [18,19]. Mallory bodies may be present in NASH despite complete abstinence from alcohol. Once present, fibrosis progresses in 40% of the patients, especially in obese women. The localisation of fibrosis is especially around the hepatic venules (zone 3) and perisinusoidal [20,21]. Patients with NASH have been found to have an increased prevalence of haemochromatosis (HFE) gene mutations, and it is likely that iron plays a role in hepatic injury and fibrosis in such patients [22,23]. Recently a system for grading and staging histology in NASH was developed [24].

Macrovesicular steatosis is most marked in zone 3. The deficiency of insulin and an increased secretion of glucagon in type 1 diabetes results in enhanced lipolysis, while glucose uptake is decreased. Thus, triglyceride uptake by adipose tissue, hepatic uptake of free fatty acids, hepatic glycogen degradation and gluconeogenesis are increased, while glucose utilisation is inhibited. Lypolysis from expanded fat depots is increased, with higher supply of fatty acids to the liver. Although obesity carries a risk of around 30% of steatosis and around 20% of steatohepatitis, the presence of type 2 diabetes is independently associated with a 2.6-fold increase in the prevalence of steatohepatitis [25].

Usually there are no hepatic signs or symptoms in NASH. The liver can be enlarged, and have a smooth edge. Some fatigue and right upper quadrant pain or 'heaviness' may be present. In type 2 diabetes, hepatomegaly is due to increased deposition of fat. Eighty per cent of patients with NASH have abnormal liver biochemistry, particularly γ-glutamyl transpeptidase, but also aminotransferases and alkaline phosphatase. There is no relationship between either liver size, symptoms or the severity of histological abnormalities and liver function tests [26]. NASH may precede the onset of glucose intolerance [27]. Sometimes a huge liver in diabetes is associated with retarded growth, obesity, florid facies and hypercholesterolaemia (Mauriac syndrome) [28]. Differential diagnosis of NASH in diabetic patients includes all other causes of macrovesicular steatosis, as mentioned in Table 7.1.

Abdominal ultrasound can confirm the presence of a 'bright' liver, indicating steatosis, without focal abnormalities. Since there is an increased incidence of gallstones in both diabetes and obesity, these are often found. Ultrasound has a sensitivity of 80% and a specificity of almost 100% for steatosis. On a

Table 7.1 Differential diagnosis of NASH in diabetic patients includes all other causes of macrovesicular steatosis

Alcohol

Drugs
  e.g. Corticosteroids, amiodarone, perhexiline maleate,
  nifedipine, diltiazem, oestrogens, tamoxifen

Nutritional
  Obesity, rapid weight loss, prolonged parenteral nutrition,
  kwashiorkor, malabsorption, coeliac disease, gastric
  partitioning operations, pancreatic disease

Small bowel bacterial overgrowth
  Small intestinal diverticulosis, jejuno–ileal bypass

Metabolic
  Wilson's disease, hyperlipidaemias and several others, such
  as galactosaemia, glycogenoses, fructose intolerance,
  tyrosinaemia, $\alpha\beta$-lipoproteinaemia, Weber–Christian
  disease, acetyl coenzyme A dehydrogenase deficiency

computed tomography (CT) scan without contrast the liver has an aspect as if contrast has been given, with a liver–spleen difference in attenuation of less than 10 HU. After CT contrast the spleen is 'brighter' than the fatty liver. A liver–spleen difference of more than 18–20 HU is diagnostic on contrast CT, while a liver attenuation higher than spleen attenuation excludes hepatic steatosis. Conventional magnetic resonance imaging (MRI) is not very useful for diagnosing steatosis. CT without contrast is the standard [29]. Only liver biopsy can assess the degree of fibrosis or cirrhosis and the severity of hepatitis. An iron stain can help in assessing increased hepatic iron as a risk factor for developing fibrosis. A liver biopsy can also help to exclude other causes of liver disease (e.g. autoimmune hepatitis). The presence of microvesicular fat is unusual in diabetes and should raise the suspicion of causes of impaired β-oxidation in the mitochondria. Mallory bodies and hepatitis were often considered a hallmark of alcoholic liver disease, but can also occur in NASH, including that associated with diabetes [17,30–33]. In patients below 40 years of age, with transaminases (ASAT) and (ALAT) less than twice the upper limit, non-obese [bodymass index (BMI) < 28] and no diabetes mellitus, a liver biopsy may be avoided, since these patients usually do not develop significant fibrosis [34]. In patients with diabetes and NASH with persistently abnormal liver biochemistry it may be wise to repeat a liver biopsy some years after the first biopsy in order to allow assessment of progression of fibrosis.

Peripheral insulin resistance is central in the development of NASH in both obese people and type 2 patients, but also in the 3% of NASH patients who are thin and do not have diabetes [35–38]. It leads to hypertriglyceridaemia and peripheral lipolysis, with increased supply of free fatty acids (FFA) to hepatocytes, increased esterification of FFAs into triglyceride and decreased export of triglyceride from the liver, leading towards steatosis. Impaired mitochondrial β-oxidation and peroxisomal oxidation of free fatty acids are present. Due to impaired mitochondrial electron transport, free radicals are formed and glutathion is depleted. The peroxisome proliferator-activated receptor (PPAR)-α and CYP2E1 and CYP4A are upregulated as part of this process [39]. PPAR-α is also induced during fasting, stimulating hepatic fatty acid oxidation [40]. The free radicals give rise to the second hit by reactive oxygen species, leading to membrane lipid peroxidation and mitochondrial DNA damage, necrosis and apoptosis of hepatocytes and attraction of an inflammatory infiltrate through cytokines. Increased sensitivity to TNF-α induced liver injury in obesity and diabetes often exists among others probably due to increased interferon-γ and decreased IL-10 concentrations and inhibition of (the protective effect of) NFαB stimulation [41,42]. IL-10 promoter region polymorphisms may increase susceptibility to more advanced stages of steatohepatitis in some patients [43]. Tumour necrosis factor α and TGF β, among others, activate stellate cells, leading to fibrogenesis and fibrosis. The severity of lipid peroxidation and fibrosis correlate with the amount of fat in the liver. Peroxidation releases malondialdehyde, which stimulates collagen production. 4-Hydroxynonenal, released by lipid peroxidation, is a strong chemo-attractant for neutrophils [44]. Increased iron storage may give rise to extra free radical formation in certain patients. The fact that central obesity is especially associated with NASH may be explained by the fact that fatty acids are more rapidly mobilised from central (visceral) than from subcutaneous fat deposits, which drain directly to the liver via the portal vein. Some drugs (e.g. methotrexate, which induces PPAR-α) can exacerbate NASH and should be avoided in NASH.

If liver biopsy shows only fatty change, the prognosis is excellent. When features of steatohepatitis or fibrosis are evident, it appears that in 10–20 years around 3% of individuals may develop cirrhotic liver failure. A larger proportion—perhaps 10%—may proceed to (sometimes asymptomatic) cirrhosis [16,45].

Treatment of NASH is aimed at both decreasing insulin resistance and reducing the effects of free radicals. The first is achieved by steady, slow weight loss through diet and exercise. Diabetes control also can lead to improvement in fatty change and return of liver function tests to normal. In contrast, severe sudden weight loss may aggravate steatohepatitis; acute hepatic failure from too rapid weight loss in NASH has been described. Metformin can reduce glucose production by the liver and sensitise target tissues (skeletal muscle, adipose tissue and the liver) to insulin, but should be avoided in severe liver disease. Recently, a new class of drugs, the thiazolidinediones (also known as glitazones) have become available, with direct insulin-sensitising actions [46]. Troglitazone was the first of these new drugs, but it was withdrawn after more than 60 deaths due to hepatic failure from it were described. Rosiglitazone and piaglitazone are other members of this family of drugs, and their use in Europe is now allowed, in combination with metformin, for obese patients with insufficient glycaemic control and in combination with sulphonylureas if metformin is either not tolerated or contraindicated. Substantial reductions in blood glucose concentrations have been achieved with these combinations. Reductions in insulin doses have been reported when thiazolidinediones were used in combination with insulin, but only piaglitazone is currently approved for this combination in the USA, since the combination of insulin and rosiglitazone was associated with an increased incidence of cardiac failure in trials. Although there is little evidence that hepatic impairment can occur from rosiglitazone and piaglitazone, more experience is needed, and currently aminotransferases over 2.5 times above the upper limit of normal have been considered as a contraindication to the use of these drugs, as is cardiac failure.

Reduction of the effect of free radicals is the second target of therapy, but this therapy is even more in the developmental stage. A diet that is too rich in polyunsaturated fat appears to increase free radical formation and probably should be avoided in NASH [47]. On the other hand, a diet with too much saturated fat will increase the already elevated cardiovascular risk in diabetes. In patients on parenteral nutrition, the composition of the nutrition may aggravate NASH and should be carefully chosen [47–49]. Administration of ursodeoxycholic acid may lead to improvement of liver tests and fatigue, according to a non-randomised study [50]. Recently a small study suggested that α-tocopherol (vitamin E) might reduce inflammation in NASH—possibly by modulation of cytokines [51]. Abstinence from alcohol for NASH patients seems wise. Other interventions, e.g. phosphatidylcholine, lecithin, selenium, betanaine, *S*-adenosyl-methionine, anti-cytokine therapy and antifibrotic drugs, clearly warrant further investigation. Since only a minority of NASH patients will develop liver failure and cirrhosis, defining whom to treat is another challenge for future trials.

Focal fatty liver

This diagnosis is usually made on ultrasound. A dual-energy CT scan helps to differentiate these lesions from other low-density lesions. The focal accumulations of macrovesicular fat can resolve with time, and may recur. They occur frequently in diabetes, alcoholics, the obese, during hyperalimentation and in Cushing's syndrome. A needle biopsy is only warranted if non-invasive imaging cannot establish the diagnosis.

Drug-induced liver disease

Sulphonylurea therapy can be complicated by cholestatic or granulomatous liver disease. Obviously, many other drugs given to a diabetic patient can lead to liver disease. Unlike other sulphonylureas, the pharmacokinetics of glimepiride are essentially unaltered in liver disease [52].

Pyogenic liver abscess

If no specific cause for a pyogenic liver abscess can be found—as occurs in half of the cases—diabetes, often with gas-forming organisms (e.g. *Klebsiella*), must be considered [53]. Due to immunological abnormalities, diabetics are at increased risk for developing pyogenic liver abscesses.

Causes of both diabetes and liver disease

Diabetes and chronic liver disease can have a common cause (Table 7.2). We discuss the most important causes.

Table 7.2   Liver disease associated with diabetes mellitus

Hepatic abnormalities due to diabetes
   Glycogenic infiltration of the liver cell nuclei
Non-alcoholic fatty liver disease
     Macrovesicular steatosis
     Non-alcoholic steatohepatitis
     Fibrosis/cirrhosis
     Focal fatty liver
   Drug-induced liver disease
   Pyogenic liver abscess

Altered glucose metabolism in liver disease
   Increased energy expenditure, decreased glycogen storage
   Glucose intolerance of cirrhosis
   Hypoglycaemia in acute liver failure

Diabetes and chronic liver disease owing to common causes
   Alcoholism
   Genetic haemochromatosis
   Viral hepatitis C and B
   Autoimmune hepatitis, primary biliary cirrhosis

Cirrhosis and diabetes in alcoholism

While alcohol is a common cause of both liver cirrhosis and pancreatitis, most patients have either one or the other. Pancreatitis is usually initially associated with exocrine insufficiency but diabetes may occur, especially after pancreatic surgery. In the case of cirrhosis, the diabetes may be 'hepatogenic'.

Hereditary haemochromatosis

Diabetes mellitus is present in about one-third of patients with genetic haemochromatosis [54,55]. In the study by Niederau of 112 patients with cirrhosis, 79 had overt diabetes [55]. Of these subjects, 61% were insulin-dependent, and 39% were non-insulin-dependent. Twenty per cent of non-cirrhotic patients are clinically diabetic, 6 out of 10 non-insulin-dependent. Hyperglycaemia may be easy to control or resistant to large doses of insulin. It can be related to damage to the pancreas by iron deposition, to impaired glucose tolerance in cirrhosis or to a family history of diabetes. There is a greater prevalence of diabetes mellitus in first-degree relatives of diabetic patients with genetic haemochromatosis than in those patients with haemochromatosis who do not have diabetes [56]. The overall prevalence of glucose intolerance (clinical and biochemical) is 79% in cirrhosis and 33% in non-cirrhotic individuals with genetic haemochromatosis. Although this seems to support an important role for cirrhosis, it may also reflect parallelism between selective islet cell damage and liver damage in untreated haemochromatosis.

The classical picture is that of the 'diabete bronzé', often a male with increased pigmentation, hepatomegaly, diminished sexual activity and loss of body hair.

Overt haemochromatosis is 10 times more common in men than in women, who lose iron with menstruation and pregnancy. The peak incidence of diagnosis is age 40–60 years. Children often present with a more acute course, with skin pigmentation, endocrine changes and cardiac disease. Increasingly, genetic haemochromatosis is diagnosed before liver cirrhosis is present. Diagnosis is suspected by a transferrin saturation above 50% or an increased serum ferritin or increased liver iron seen on MRI [57,58] and confirmed by a hepatic iron index (HII; μmol iron/g dry liver tissue, divided by age in years) above 1.9—a HII below 1.5 is normal—or by presence of the Cys282Tyr mutation on chromosome 6 [59–64]. A second mutation (C187G, causing a H63D protein change) also occurs in patients with hereditary haemochromatosis (HHC) in 74% of iron-overloaded patients who are heterozygous for the C282Y mutation, compared to 10% of controls [65]. These compound heterozygotes usually have less marked iron overload, as in patients with the recently described syndrome of hepatic iron overload with normal serum transferrin saturation. These patients have hyper-ferritinaemia but lower hepatic iron concentrations than patients with typical (homozygous C282Y) HHC. They are also older and often have obesity, hyperlipidaemia, glucose intolerance and/or systemic arterial hypertension [66]. Treatment is usually by regular phlebotomy. There is an increased incidence of hepatocellular carcinoma in HHC. Earlier diagnosis of haemochromatosis is associated with an improved prognosis, since early treatment can prevent cirrhosis and other complications of haemochromatosis. Paradoxically, due to this improved prognosis, vascular complications (retinopathy, nephropathy, neuropathy, peripheral vascular disease), initially deemed rare in diabetes of haemochromatosis, are now recognised with a frequency equal to that in other patients with diabetes mellitus unrelated to haemochromatosis [56,67].

Viral hepatitis

Viral hepatitis B and C (HBV and HCV) occur more frequently in diabetes than in the general population [68]. This may reflect the frequent parenteral exposure of diabetics. Conversely, diabetes has been considered to be one of the many extrahepatic manifestations of hepatitis C. Furthermore, therapy with interferon can induce diabetes [69,70]. Interferon-α may also improve glucose tolerance in both non-diabetic and diabetic HCV-infected patients [71]. A recent paper suggests that HCV infection itself, especially with genotype 2a, can also cause diabetes [72]. Indeed, the prevalence of HCV infection appears to be higher in diabetics compared with an appropriate control group of hospital patients. Replication of HCV in extrahepatic organs might be the mechanism, either through a direct cytopathic effect, or due to induction of immunological tissue damage. Alternatively virus-associated autoimmunity could be the cause of diabetes in HCV infection, triggering latent autoimmunity or causing *de novo* autoimmune disease through molecular mimicry (there is regional amino acid homology with glutamic acid decarboxylase, an islet cell antigen) or immune dysregulation (supported by other autoimmune associations as thyroiditis, thrombocytopenia and lichen planus) [73,74]. An argument against the mimicry theory is that most patients with HCV and diabetes have type 2 diabetes and no islet cell antibodies.

Autoimmune hepatitis and primary biliary cirrhosis

There seems to be a slightly increased incidence of autoimmune hepatitis (AIH) in patients with diabetes mellitus, and vice versa. Obviously, treatment of AIH with corticosteroids can lead to impaired glucose tolerance and overt diabetes. Immune dysregulation may also play a role, since a cross-reactive immune response to carboxypeptidase H, an autoantigen in type 1 diabetes mellitus, has been demonstrated in a patient with both AIH and type 1 diabetes [75]. Type 1 diabetes mellitus has also been seen in association with primary biliary cirrhosis (PBC) [76,77]. Certain vitamin D_3 receptor polymorphisms may be associated with both diseases [78]. Furthermore, the combination of diabetes and AIH or PBC has been described in patients with autoimmune polyglandular syndromes [79–81]. Since many patients with AIH or PBC already have cirrhosis when the disease is diagnosed, part of the association may be due to 'hepatogenic diabetes' rather than autoimmunity.

Biliary system

Gallstones and diabetes

It is widely believed that gallstones occur more frequently in patients with type 1 and 2 diabetes mellitus than in the general population. However, evidence to support this concept is limited. Autopsy- and population-based studies have demonstrated an association [82,83] but others have not [84,85]. Feldman et al. [85], in an autopsy study of 1319 subjects, found only a slight, and non-significant, difference in the prevalence of gallstones between diabetic and non-diabetic subjects (25% vs. 23%, respectively).

A number of studies have evaluated the prevalence of gallstones in a diabetic population and showed a significant association [83–86], but this has not been a consistent observation [87]. In Western countries the majority of gallstones are composed of cholesterol. The aetiology of cholesterol gallstones is multifactorial and a number of risk factors have been identified, including age, sex, genetic factors, obesity, hyperlipidaemia, diet, drugs, etc. Several of these risk factors also apply to diabetes mellitus. Recently, Chapman et al. [82], when screening a large population of diabetic patients, found a higher prevalence of gallstone disease in diabetics than controls (33% vs. 21%; $p < 0.001$). As expected, the prevalence of gallstones was higher in females than in males. In both sexes the prevalence of gallstones was higher in patients, with type 2 than type 1 diabetes mellitus: for males, controls 18%, type 2 diabetes 33% ($p < 0.05$), type 1 diabetes 16%; for females, controls 23%, type 2 diabetes 49% ($p < 0.001$), type 1 diabetes 36% ($p < 0.05$). Hayes *et al.* [84] found no differences in glycaemic control (glycated haemoglobin) between diabetics with and without gallstones. Although hyperglycaemia influences gallbladder motility and bile secretion (to be discussed), there is no evidence supporting the concept that the prevalence of gallstones is related to chronic glycaemic control.

Thus, it seems that the prevalence of gallstones is related to the type of diabetes. Patients with type 2 diabetes have elevated plasma insulin levels usually in the presence of obesity. An elevated plasma insulin has been associated with an increased prevalence of gallstone disease [88] and may account for the strong association between type 2 diabetes and gallstones. Type 2 diabetes is usually found in obese subjects and it has been clearly shown that obesity is a risk factor for gallstone formation. Ruhl *et al.* have demonstrated in a recent study that both hyperinsulinaemia and diabetes (i.e. increased fasting blood glucose levels) are independent risk factors for gallbladder disease and gallstones in women, and that only diabetes is a risk factor for men [89]. An association between altered carbohydrate metabolism and gallstones has been hypothesised. Recently, De Santis *et al.* [83] performed oral glucose tolerance tests in subjects with and without gallstones and concluded that the prevalence of diabetes was higher in subjects affected by gallstone disease than in controls (11.6% vs. 4.8%; odds ratio, 2.55; 95% confidence interval, 1.39–4.67).

Gallstone formation

The majority of gallstones in patients with diabetes are composed of cholesterol. The pathogenesis of cholesterol gallstone formation is complex and many factors are involved, such as changes in bile composition (cholesterol, bile acids, phospholipids), changes in gallbladder motility and the presence of nucleation-promoting factors. Which of these factors contribute to gallstone formation in diabetics? First, diabetics have abnormal serum lipid profiles and increased biliary cholesterol secretion, resulting in increased cholesterol saturation of bile [83,88]. Second, gallbladder motor function may be abnormal in patients with diabetes mellitus. Increased fasting and postprandial gallbladder volumes have been reported, suggesting a hypotonic gallbladder. Using ultrasonography, several authors have indeed reported larger fasting gallbladder volumes [90–92] but others have not [93,94]. Fasting volume is dependent on vagal cholinergic tone and on the gastrointestinal hormone, CCK. When analysing studies on gallbladder motility in detail, it is obvious that larger fasting volumes are observed, especially in diabetic patients with autonomic neuropathy [92,93]. In these studies autonomic neuropathy was assessed by cardiovascular reflex tests. Larger fasting gallbladder volumes were present in both type 1 and type 2 diabetics with cardiac autonomic neuropathy [92]. Basal plasma CCK levels in diabetics do not differ from healthy controls [92,95].

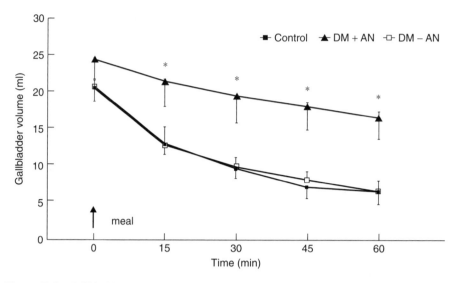

Figure 7.6   Gallbladder volume before and after ingestion of a 400 kCal meal in type 1 diabetic patients with autonomic neuropathy ($n = 12$, triangles) and without autonomic neuropathy ($n = 8$, large squares) and healthy controls ($n = 8$, small squares). Asterisks denote significant differences between diabetics with autonomic neuropathy and those without autonomic neuropathy and controls. From Dymock *et al.* [56], with permission

The gallbladder contraction after a meal is also reduced in diabetic patients, especially in those patients with autonomic neuropathy [90,92,96,97] (Figure 7.6). Impaired gallbladder emptying with larger residual gallbladder volumes may promote stasis of gallbladder bile and subsequent crystal and stone formation when the bile is supersaturated with cholesterol. CCK is the major humoral factor for gallbladder contraction. Impaired postprandial gallbladder contraction may result from either reduced CCK release, impaired CCK secretory capacity in the jejunum or reduced sensitivity of the gallbladder to CCK. Whereas some studies [92,95] have shown that postprandial CCK release is reduced in diabetics, others have failed to observe any difference in CCK release between diabetics and controls or have even observed higher postprandial plasma CCK levels [98,99]. Differences in postprandial CCK secretion may result from disordered, particularly delayed, gastric emptying, which occurs frequently in diabetic patients (Chapter 4). Stone *et al.* [96] have observed impaired responsiveness of the gallbladder to CCK in diabetics. Others have not been able to reproduce this finding. In fact, most authors agree that the sensitivity of the gallbladder to CCK is no different in diabetics from controls [92,93,100]. Unfortunately, none of the studies evaluating gallbladder motility and CCK secretion in diabetics has taken into account the blood glucose concentration.

A number of factors may contribute to impaired postprandial gallbladder contraction in diabetes. First, the presence of autonomic neuropathy is relevant. Gallbladder emptying differs between diabetics with and without autonomic neuropathy. A close correlation between clinical autonomic neuropathy and chronic glycaemic control is well established. Apart from chronic hyperglycaemia, acute changes in the blood glucose concentration influence gallbladder motor function. During acute hyperglycaemia, gallbladder motor function is dose-dependently impaired in both healthy subjects and patients with type 1 diabetes [100,101]. At blood glucose concentrations of 15 mmol/l gallbladder emptying is significantly reduced, both in type 1 diabetics and in healthy subjects made hyperglycaemic by intravenous glucose infusion. It has been shown that already at glucose levels in the physiological range of 8 mmol/l gallbladder emptying in response to CCK infusion or meal ingestion is impaired [100,101]. The aetiology of cholesterol gallstones is multifactorial. Other factors, apart from gallbladder motility, are important in the pathogenesis of cholesterol gallstone formation. These factors include cholesterol supersaturated bile, and nucleation-promoting factors.

Symptomatic gallstones and therapy

When gallstones have developed, is the clinical picture in diabetics different from controls and is the risk for cholecystitis increased? Recent studies have shown that the prevalence of symptomatic gallstone disease is not much higher in type 1 and 2 diabetes than in controls [83,102]. Follow-up studies of asymptomatic gallstone patients have shown that only few patients become symptomatic over time [102]. In that study, during a 5 year follow-up, 15% developed symptoms of biliary-type pain. Previously diabetics have been considered to have a higher chance for complications from gallstones and in some cases prophylactic cholecystectomy has been performed. This policy has been challenged because the risk of complications, such as biliary sepsis, perforation or gangrenous cholecystitis, appears to be only moderately increased [103] and despite this, the risk of cholecystectomy in diabetics is similar to that in non-diabetics [102–105]. In diabetic patients with acute cholecystitis, early cholecystectomy is indicated.

Combined kidney and pancreas transplantation is now frequently performed in type 1 diabetic patients with end-stage renal disease. Recent studies indicate that the incidence of gallstones in these patients is very high [106]; in over 30% of pancreas recipients gallstones develop within 12 months (Figure 7.7). The incidence of gallstones in kidney transplant recipients with diabetes is also high (27%) and significantly greater than in non-diabetic kidney transplant recipients (12%). Thus, diabetic patients are especially at risk of developing gallstones after transplantation. An interaction between diabetes mellitus-induced gallbladder dysmotility and cyclosporine-induced cholestasis represents a potential mechanism. In patients on immunosuppression, acute cholecystitis is a serious and potentially life-threatening complication. Therefore, in these patients serial ultrasonography of the gallbladder should be performed during follow-up after

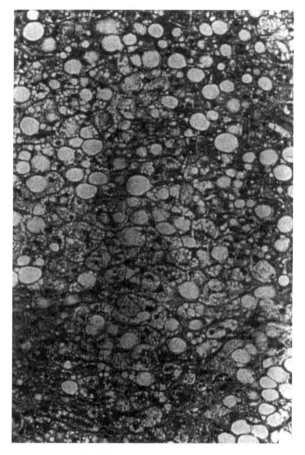

Figure 7.7 Multiple cholesterol gallstones from a type 1 diabetic patient who underwent cholecystectomy for symptomatic gallstone disease 18 months after combined kidney–pancreas transplantation

transplantation, and cholecystectomy considered when gallstones develop, even in the absence of symptoms. Some clinicians even feel that prophylactic cholecystectomy during kidney–pancreas transplantation is justified because of the high risk of gallstones and subsequent biliary infectious complications while on immunosuppression.

There is no evidence of an increased incidence of acute or complicated cholecystitis in diabetics. Studies of the surgical therapy of acute cholecystitis differ from early reports and suggest that there may be no difference in rates of mortality or serious complications in diabetics undergoing biliary surgery when compared with appropriate controls. Using the available data, decision analysis model have shown that, as in non-diabetics, prophylactic cholecystectomy is without benefit and should not be recommended for diabetics with asymptomatic gallstones [105]. Screening for asymptomatic gallstones in diabetics in not recommended, apart from subgroups such as patients after combined kidney and pancreas transplant. Cholecystectomy should only be performed in cases of symptomatic cholelithiasis, preferably by laparoscopy, as is the case in the general population. The outcome of (laparoscopic) biliary surgery in diabetics is not different from non-diabetics. However, the 'conversion rate', i.e. converting from laparoscopic surgery to a traditional cholecystectomy because of technical considerations, is significantly higher than reported in the general population [107]. In the case of bile duct stones in older diabetic patients, endoscopic retrograde cholangio-pancreaticography (ERCP) with sphincterotomy and stone extraction is the therapy of choice, as in non-diabetics.

Pancreas

Exocrine–endocrine interaction

For many years the pancreas has been considered to consist of two discrete organ systems, the exocrine pancreas and the endocrine pancreas. It is now recognised that the pancreas is an integrated organ that is involved in the digestion and metabolic processing of nutrients. Anatomical and functional interactions between the exocrine and endocrine pancreas have been described. In mammals the islets of Langerhans are distributed throughout the pancreas. Such an arrangement, with close cell to cell contact between exocrine and endocrine tissue, may provide metabolic advantages. Vascular anastomoses between the islets and interacinar capillaries have been demonstrated, whereby the exocrine pancreas receives a significant proportion of its blood supply via the islets [108]. Thus, acinar cells are exposed to high concentrations of islet hormones.

Animal studies have shown that insulin exerts direct effects on pancreatic acinar cells. In rats rendered diabetic by streptozotocin, pancreatic amylase output is markedly reduced [109]. This effect can be reversed by giving insulin. The hypothesis that insulin contributes to the regulation of acinar cell function is supported by the presence of insulin receptors on acinar cells [110]. The physiological role of insulin on stimulated pancreatic exocrine secretion has been demonstrated by Lee *et al.* using insulin antiserum [111]. Both meal- and CCK-stimulated exocrine pancreatic secretion are inhibited during infusion of anti-insulin serum. Most of the work on the interaction between islets and acini has been derived from animal studies. The role of insulin in regulating human exocrine pancreatic secretion is less clear. During euglycaemic hyperinsulinaemia the basal pancreatic enzyme output is reduced [112], indicating an inhibitory effect of insulin, as has also been demonstrated on gastrointestinal motility [113]. When pancreatic exocrine secretion was stimulated by exogenous CCK, exocrine output was not reduced but, on the contrary, even significantly increased [112] (Figure 7.8). These results point to a potentiating effect of insulin on CCK-stimulated pancreatic enzyme secretion in man.

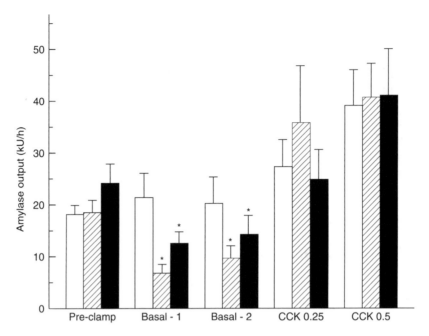

Figure 7.8   Amylase output (KU/h, mean ± SEM) in nine healthy volunteers during the pre-clamp period, during hyperglycaemia at 15 mmol/l (black bars) or during euglycaemia hyperinsulinaemia (glucose 5 mmol/l, insulin 150–200 mU/L; striped bars) compared to saline infusion (control, grey bars) during the first hour (Basal-1) and second hour (Basal-2) under basal conditions and in response to graded continuous infusion of CCK (0.25 and 0.50 Ivy Dog Units/kg/h). Asterisks denote significant ($p < 0.05$) differences compared to control

Because of the close anatomical and functional relations between the endocrine and the exocrine pancreas, a disturbance or disease in one system will inevitably affect the other. Evidence for this interaction is derived from studies demonstrating that diabetes mellitus frequently occurs in the course of chronic pancreatitis, and that abnormal exocrine pancreatic function occurs frequently in patients with diabetes mellitus.

Exocrine pancreatic function in diabetes

Much of the information about exocrine function in diabetes is derived from animal studies. In diabetic rats, amylase secretion is markedly reduced and does not increase after a meal. The duration and severity of diabetes show negative correlations with amylase secretion [113]. Several studies have assessed exocrine pancreatic function in diabetic patients [114–118]. It has been clearly demonstrated that a significant number of type 1 diabetics have impaired exocrine pancreatic function, as shown by a reduced duodenal output of enzymes in response to endogenous (meal, intraduodenal nutrients) and exogenous stimuli (secretin + cholecystokinin infusion). Chey *et al.* [114] reported that exocrine function was impaired in 77% of type 1 patients. Blood glucose levels were not taken into account in these studies. Several theories have been postulated to explain these findings. Atrophy of exocrine tissue may be due to a lack of tropic insulin action; pancreatic fibrosis could be the result of angiopathy and neuropathy and lead to impaired exocrine function. Apart from direct pancreatic function tests, indirect tests, such as urinary (PABA) recovery, or faecal tests such as fat excretion, chymotrypsin and elastase-1 concentrations, are abnormal in a substantial proportion of diabetics [118,119]. Despite the high frequency of reduced exocrine function in diabetics, few patients develop overt exocrine pancreatic insufficiency, because of the large functional reserve capacity of the exocrine pancreas. Pancreatic exocrine insufficiency becomes clinically manifest only when less than 10% of the secretory capacity is preserved. In contrast to type 1 diabetes, abnormalities of exocrine function are observed less frequently in type 2 diabetes [119]. These observations are consistent with the concept that insulin plays a role in the maintenance of normal exocrine pancreatic function.

Patients with juvenile-onset type 1 diabetes mellitus appear to be more prone to a reduced pancreatic enzyme output than patients with maturity-onset type 1 diabetes [115]. Frier *et al.* [120] reported that there is a significant correlation between residual capacity of C-peptide secretion and pancreatic exocrine secretory function in juvenile-onset diabetics. The authors have suggested that a progressive deterioration of exocrine pancreatic function in juvenile-onset diabetes exists, but that this is not the case in maturity-onset diabetes, due to a disruption of the endocrine–exocrine interaction. In the maturity-onset form the partial preservation of endogenous insulin secretion may be sufficient to maintain normal exocrine function.

For screening of exocrine insufficiency in patients with diabetes mellitus, faecal fat excretion is advised but steatorrhoea becomes manifest with severely impaired exocrine function. In a recent study it was recommended to screen patients with type 1 and type 2 diabetes mellitus for exocrine insufficiency using the faecal elastase-1 test [119]. In that study reduced faecal elastase-1 concentrations were observed in 50% of type 1 patients and 35% of type 2 patients. These data have to be confirmed by others but at least suggest that exocrine dysfunction is not uncommon in type 1 and type 2 diabetics. When exocrine insufficiency is diagnosed, supplementation with pancreatic enzymes should be started. Doses containing at least 10 000 (FIP) units of lipase, ingested before the meal, are recommended. Enzyme replacement improves nutrient digestion and absorption and may affect glycaemic control. Therefore the diabetes should be closely monitored when enzyme replacement is initiated.

Mechanism of exocrine dysfunction in diabetes

Several factors have been implicated in the reduced pancreatic enzyme output observed in diabetics (Table 7.3). First, postprandial CCK secretion was found

Table 7.3   Pathophysiology of pancreatic exocrine dysfunction in diabetes mellitus

Deficiency of insulin as a trophic factor for acinar cells
High glucagon levels
Impaired CCK secretion or altered sensitivity of acinar cells for CCK
Influence of other gut peptides: somatostatin, pancreatic polypeptide, peptide YY
Autonomic neuropathy
Autoimmune process: islet cell antibodies, pancreatic cytokeratin autoantibodies
Diabetic microangiopathy, fibrosis
Pancreatic atrophy
Actual glucose levels (hyperglycaemia)

to be impaired in some studies [92,95] but others have not found a reduction in CCK secretion in diabetics vs. controls [98,99]. Gastric emptying and delivery of nutrients to the duodenum frequently is delayed and may give rise to impaired postprandial CCK secretion. It is not known whether the ileal or colonic brake, as a feedback mechanism of the distal gut regulating proximal gut function, is activated in diabetics. Peptide YY (PYY), as an ileal brake hormone, may inhibit exocrine pancreatic secretion. Second, autonomic neuropathy may contribute to impaired exocrine pancreatic function. Recent studies with CCK receptor antagonists indicate that over 70% of meal-stimulated exocrine secretion is dependent on neural mechanisms [121]. Neural mechanisms are more relevant than hormonal mechanisms in the regulation of pancreatic secretion. This is especially important when studying diabetic patients, since in these patients neuropathy may play a crucial role in the pathogenesis of gastrointestinal complications. In contrast to animal studies, no association between exocrine function with the duration of diabetes, presence or absence of neuropathy, microangiopathy or metabolic control was found in humans [116,117]. This is surprising, since pancreatic exocrine secretion is regulated to a large extent by neural factors, especially local or intrinsic neural mechanisms.

It has been clearly established that, as with other regions of the gastrointestinal tract, blood glucose levels influence exocrine pancreatic secretion [100,101,112, 122]. During acute hyperglycaemia (blood glucose ~ 15 mmol/l), pancreatic enzyme output is impaired, at least in healthy volunteers. The effect of actual blood glucose levels on pancreatic secretion in type 1 and type 2 diabetes has not been evaluated. A hormonal imbalance may also contribute to impairment of exocrine function. Alterations in insulin, glucagon or somatostatin secretion in diabetics may directly influence the exocrine pancreas. In type 1 diabetics, pancreatic enzyme output is reduced. However, insulin administration does not reverse the reduction in exocrine function.

In animal experiments, atrophy of the exocrine pancreas has been observed following chronic glucagon administration [123]. In humans glucagon exerts an inhibitory effect on pancreatic exocrine secretion [124]. Patients with diabetes have α-cell hyperfunction with elevated plasma glucagon levels. Because glucose penetration into α-cells is disturbed in insulin-deficient islets, glucagon release by α-cells in response to hyperglycaemia is not impaired. Pancreatic polypeptide (PP) and somatostatin may contribute to the regulation of acinar cell function. Infusion of exogenous PP to plasma levels comparable to those observed after a meal inhibits pancreatic secretion [125]. Therefore, a role for this peptide in the physiological control of exocrine pancreatic secretion has been postulated. In general, PP levels are either in the normal range of slightly increased in diabetic patients [99,118]. In cases of chronic pancreatitis with exocrine insufficiency, plasma PP levels are reduced and an impaired postprandial PP response is considered to be indicative of loss of 'functional pancreatic cell mass' [126]. PP secretion is influenced by blood glucose concentrations. During hyperglycaemia PP levels are dose-dependently reduced, whereas PP secretion increases significantly in response to hypoglycaemia [101,127].

Pancreatic atrophy has been documented in diabetics. Autopsy studies of patients with juvenile-onset diabetes have revealed lower weight and volume of the pancreas with intra- and peri-insular inflammatory infiltrates, sclerosis and mild atrophy of the acini. No correlation was found between duration of diabetes, or age at onset of diabetes, with the morphological changes [128]. More recent studies employing ultrasonography are in agreement with the autopsy findings of markedly smaller pancreases in patients with type 1 diabetes [129]. Atrophy of the pancreas may well contribute to reduced enzyme output in type 1 diabetics.

It has been suggested that in patients with type 1 diabetes the endocrine and exocrine pancreas are affected by a common autoimmune process. In patients with type 1 diabetes with islet-cell antibodies, but not in patients without these antibodies, atrophic exocrine glands and lymphocytic infiltration of exocrine tissue has been observed [130]. Antibodies against the cytokeratin of pancreatic acinar cells have been found in newly diagnosed type 1 diabetes patients [131]. These antibodies have a strong positive association with islet-cell antibody activity. A close association between lymphocytic infiltration around acinar cells and atrophy of the exocrine gland has been documented, suggesting a primary involvement of the exocrine pancreas in the immunological events of type 1 diabetes. In experimental models of virus-induced diabetes mellitus, inflammatory lesions of the exocrine pancreas are present. It has therefore been suggested that viral infection may be the common cause of the multiglandular damage by triggering autoimmune events [132]. In a prospective study of patients with diabetes mellitus in which pancreatic morphology was evaluated in detail by ERCP, it was found that abnormal pancreatic ductograms were present, not only in a high percentage of type 1 patients but also in type 2 patients with islet cell antibodies [133]. However, in type 2 patients without islet cell antibodies, ductograms were normal. Because abnormal ductograms were frequently present in type 2 patients with sufficient residual β-cell function, these findings contradict the islet–acinar concept, in which lack of insulin is held responsible for exocrine pancreatic atrophy. In fact, these studies suggest that a common immunological process may involve both the exocrine and endocrine pancreas in type 1 diabetics.

Pancreatic enzyme output to the duodenum, especially that of amylase, is frequently impaired in diabetics. This does not automatically result in maldigestion of fat and carbohydrates. Steatorrhoea occurs when lipase secretory capacity of the pancreas is reduced to below 10%. Steatorrhoea in diabetic patients may result from other causes, such as rapid intestinal transit, motility disorders, coeliac disease or small intestinal bacterial overgrowth. Most patients with diabetes mellitus do not have symptoms of overt exocrine pancreatic insufficiency, i.e. steatorrhoea or weight loss [114]. This can be explained by the fact that digestive enzymes are secreted in excess by the pancreas. For starch digestion other enzymes can compensate for reduced amylase output, including salivary iso-amylases and oligosaccharidases of the small intestine. Gastric lipase may partially compensate for loss of pancreatic lipase activity.

Diabetes as a sequela of pancreatic disease

In patients with chronic pancreatitis, impaired secretion of insulin from β-cells of the pancreatic islets leads to the development of secondary diabetes. In these patients β-cell function decreases in parallel with exocrine function, but usually a decline in exocrine function precedes that of endocrine function. Patients with chronic pancreatitis may present with diabetes as the first sign or symptom of their disease. In general, β-cell function is preserved better in these patients than in those with type 1 diabetes mellitus [134]. In patients with 'pancreatic diabetes', glucose metabolism abnormalities occur as result of both impaired insulin production and insulin resistance. These patients have impaired glucagon levels, blunted epinephrine response to insulin induced hypoglycaemia and an increased risk of hypoglycaemia while on insulin therapy [135]. Among unselected patients with chronic pancreatitis, one-third have insulin-dependent diabetes, one-third have non-insulin-dependent diabetes or impaired glucose tolerance, and one-third have normal glucose tolerance [134]. When gross morphological abnormalities, such as pancreatic calcifications, are present, insulin-dependent diabetes is seen in up to 70% of patients (Table 7.4). The prevalence and severity of the microvascular complications in pancreatic diabetes are comparable to type 1 diabetics. Therefore, optimisation of glycaemic control should be a major focus of the management of these patients.

The clinician should be aware of the possibility of impaired exocrine function in patients with diabetes mellitus, particularly when weight loss occurs despite an apparently adequate caloric intake. Results of indirect pancreatic function tests are difficult to interpret because of suboptimal sensitivity and specificity. Accelerated intestinal transit and small intestinal bacterial overgrowth, which both occur in diabetic patients, may lead to false-positive results with indirect pancreatic function tests. When pancreatic enzyme supplementation is initiated in

Table 7.4 Diabetes mellitus as a consequence of pancreatic disease

Pancreatitis	
Acute	1–5%
Chronic non-calcifying	10–30%
Chronic calcifying	50–70%
Pancreatic carcinoma	50%
Pancreatic surgery	
Pancreatic head resection	20–30%
Distal pancreatectomy	40%
Total pancreatectomy	100%
Haemochromatosis	
Primary	70%
Secondary	15%
Cystic fibrosis	20%

diabetics with exocrine pancreatic insufficiency, improvement in nutrient utilisation may modify glycaemic control, so that the insulin regimen has to be altered. During high plasma glucose levels, pancreatic function is impaired. One should therefore aim at optimal glucose control in these patients.

Pancreatic carcinoma

Several studies have provided evidence that the risk of pancreatic cancer is increased in patients with type 1 and type 2 diabetes mellitus [136,137]. In fact, diabetes has been associated with an increased risk of several cancers, including those of the pancreas, liver, endometrium and kidney [136]. The pooled relative risk of pancreatic cancer for diabetics vs. non-diabetics in a meta-analysis was 2.1 (95% confidence interval 1.6–2.8). Patients presenting with diabetes mellitus within a period of 12 months of the diagnosis of pancreatic cancer were excluded because in these cases diabetes may be an early presenting sign of pancreatic cancer rather than a risk factor [137]. In a recently published population-based case-control study of pancreatic cancer conducted in the USA, a significant positive trend in risk for pancreatic cancer increasing with years of diabetes prior to diagnosis of pancreatic cancer was apparent. Diabetics diagnosed at least 10 years prior to diagnosis had a significant, 50% increased risk [138]. Those treated with insulin had risks similar to those not treated with insulin (odds ratios 1.6 and 1.5, respectively).

The diabetes mellitus that occurs in patients with pancreatic cancer is characterised by marked insulin resistance that improves after tumour resection. Islet amyloid polypeptide (IAPP), a hormonal factor secreted from pancreatic beta cells, decreases insulin sensitivity and plasma levels of IAPP are elevated in pancreatic cancer patients who have diabetes [139]. IAPP overproduction may well contribute to the diabetes that occurs in these patients. Others have not been able to confirm that pancreatic cancer is more frequent among patients with long-standing diabetes [140]. The increased incidence of pancreatic cancer in diabetics probably is the result of diabetes as an early presenting sign. Evidence that diabetes mellitus predisposes to pancreatic cancer exists, but the association is weak.

Acute pancreatitis

Acute pancreatitis is characterised by an acute inflammatory response of the pancreatic tissue, which is usually followed by complete clinical and functional restitution of the pancreas. Glucose intolerance and hyperglycaemia may be present during the acute phase and, if so, are of prognostic relevance, i.e. both the severity and the duration of the disturbance in carbohydrate metabolism are related to the extent of tissue damage [141,142]. In patients with acute pancreatitis, plasma insulin concentrations are lower than in healthy individuals with a comparable degree of stress. In the acute phase plasma glucagon is increased. The combination of hyperglucagonaemia and hypoinsulinaemia is sufficient to account for the development of ketoacidosis [143]. Hyperglycaemia usually subsides within 4–6 weeks, so that overt diabetes develops in only 1–5% of patients after a single episode of acute pancreatitis.

The potential role of diabetes in the aetiology of acute pancreatitis is poorly defined. An association might be expected, as both gallstones and hypertriglyceridaemia are risk factors for acute pancreatitis and are more common in diabetes. In several series of patients with acute pancreatitis there have been more diabetic subjects than expected [141,144], but case control studies have not been performed and thus the aetiological link has not been firmly established. In a recent multicentre retrospective study it was shown that hypertriglyceridaemia was the cause in up to 4% of cases of acute pancreatitis [145]. The most common presentations of patients with acute pancreatitis resulting from hypertriglyceridaemia were that of a poorly controlled diabetics or alcoholics with hypertriglyceridaemia. It is likely that diabetes is much less important than other factors, or even has no role at all, in the pathogenesis of acute pancreatitis. It should be kept in mind that when acute pancreatitis occurs in a diabetic patient, ketoacidosis may be severe and morbidity and mortality are high.

Gastrointestinal and pancreatic hormones

Gastrointestinal hormones play an important role in the regulation of gallbladder motility and exocrine pancreatic function. CCK is the major hormonal regulator of gallbladder contraction and is also involved in postprandial pancreatic enzyme secretion. Animal studies have shown that PP, when infused to postprandial plasma levels, inhibits pancreatic secretion. Several studies have evaluated CCK and PP secretion in diabetic patients. Fasting plasma CCK levels were not different between diabetics and controls, but postprandially normal, reduced and also increased plasma CCK levels have been observed [92,95,98,99]. The reason for this discrepancy in results is not obvious, but the composition of the meal, the rate of gastric emptying of the meal, and the presence of autonomic neuropathy, may have influenced the results. It is unlikely that changes in gallbladder motility in diabetics result from differences in CCK secretion. Plasma PP concentrations are increased in patients with diabetes mellitus [100,126]. There is a positive correlation between PP concentrations and the severity of the diabetes. On the other hand, the PP secretion in response to vagal cholinergic stimuli, such as sham feeding, is significantly reduced in diabetics with autonomic neuropathy [93]. Plasma PP concentrations parallel exocrine pancreatic secretion in response to a meal or to hormonal stimulation. Therefore, PP responsiveness can be considered a direct correlate of exocrine secretion. During hyperglycaemia, postprandial hormone secretion is reduced (CCK, gastrin, PP), at least in healthy volunteers [101,112,146]. The influence of hyperglycaemia on plasma hormone levels in diabetics is less clear. However, during hyperglycaemia PP secretion is reduced in diabetics [147]. We have demonstrated that fasting CCK levels are not affected in type I diabetics during hyperglycaemic conditions [100].

Kidney–pancreas transplantation

Combined kidney and pancreas transplantation is considered an effective therapy for type I diabetes patients with end-stage renal failure and significantly prolongs survival [148,149]. This combined procedure results in euglycaemia at the expense of chronic immunosuppression, hyperinsulinaemia and dyslipidaemia. As discussed, these patients are predisposed to the development of cholesterol gallstones [106].

The incidence of cholelithiasis is also increased in kidney transplants with diabetes mellitus, but not to the same magnitude as seen after combined kidney–pancreas transplantation in diabetes. Whether the predisposition is related to diabetes, hyperlipidaemia, altered pancreatic hormone secretion or immunosuppression (cyclosporine) remains unclear. It is not known whether gallbladder motility changes after pancreas–kidney transplantation. For gastric emptying, a significant improvement correlating with symptoms has been observed after successful combined pancreas–kidney transplantation [150]. Screening for cholelithiasis in pancreas and pancreas–kidney transplants is warranted and cholecystotectomy recommended because acute cholecystitis is a serious and potentially life-threatening complication in immunocompromised patients.

When pancreatic transplantation is performed, the pancreatic duct can be drained via the urinary bladder or a small intestinal anastomosis (enterostomy). A duodenocystostomy offers the advantage that pancreatic graft function can be monitored by exocrine secretion into the urinary bladder. During episodes of rejection pancreatitis occurs and the output of enzymes to the bladder may be increased. However, recent studies have found only a weak correlation between endocrine and exocrine function in the transplanted pancreas, indicating that urinary amylase output is not a sensitive parameter of graft rejection [151].

Conclusions

There is a close functional interaction between the liver and endocrine pancreas in relation to glucose homeostasis. In patients with diabetes mellitus, hepatic abnormalities occur frequently, especially non-alcoholic steatohepatitis. Patients with liver cirrhosis have an increased energy expenditure and abnormal substrate and glucose metabolism. Because of the smaller glycogen storage capacity, these patients are more prone to hypoglycaemia and catabolic episodes. Adequate dietary supplementation, including a late evening meal, may prevent nocturnal catabolic episodes. Diabetes and chronic liver disease may have common causes, such as haemochromatosis, autoimmune hepatitis and primary biliary cirrhosis.

Although gallstones are more prevalent in diabetics, the number of patients with gallstones that eventually become symptomatic does not appear to be increased and prophylactic cholecystectomy is not recommended. The risk for infectious or postoperative biliary complications is also not increased in diabetics.

Close anatomical and functional interaction exists between the exocrine and endocrine pancreas. In diabetic patients exocrine insufficiency is not uncommon and frequently unrecognised. Weight loss due to maldigestion may be a presenting symptom. On the other hand, diabetes may be a consequence of pancreatic disease, such as chronic pancreatitis.

References

1. Petrides AS. Liver disease and diabetes mellitus. *Diabetes Rev* 1994; **2**: 2–18.
2. Katbamna BH, Petrelli M, McCullough AJ. The liver in diabetes mellitus and hyper-lipidaemia. In Zakim D, Boyer TD (eds), *Hepatology. A Textbook of Liver Disease*, 2nd edn. W.B. Saunders: Philadelphia, PA, 1990: 73–84.
3. Verboeket-van de Venne WPHG, Westerterp KR, van Hoek B, Swart GR. Energy expenditure and substrate metabolism in patients with cirrhosis of the liver: effects of the pattern of food intake. *Gut* 1995; **36**: 110–16.
4. Megyesi C, Samols E, Marks V. Glucose tolerance and diabetes in chronic liver disease. *Lancet* 1967; **ii**: 1051.
5. Taylor R, Heine RJ, Collins J *et al*. Insulin action in cirrhosis. *Hepatology* 1985; **5**: 64.
6. Nolte W, Hartmann H, Ramadori G. Glucose metabolism and liver cirrhosis. *Exp Clin Endocrinol Diabetes* 1995; **103**: 63–74.
7. Kruszynska YT. Glucose control in liver disease. *Curr Med Lit Gastroenterol* 1992; **11**: 9.
8. Kruszynska YT. Relationship between insulin sensitivity, insulin secretion and glucose tolerance in cirrhosis. *Hepatology* 1991; **14**: 103.
9. Petrides AS, Vogt C, Schultze-Berge D *et al*. The pathogenesis of glucose intolerance and diabetes mellitus in cirrhosis. *Hepatology* 1994; **19**: 616.
10. Mann FC, Magath TB. Studies on the physiology of the liver. II. The effect of the removal of the liver on the blood sugar level. *Arch Intern Med* 1992; **30**: 73.

11. Goodman JI. Hepatomegaly and diabetes mellitus. *Ann Intern Med* 1953; **39**: 1077.

12. Schaffner F, Thaier H. Non-alcoholic fatty liver disease. In Popper H, Schaffner F (eds), *Progress in liver diseases*, vol. VIII. Grune and Stratton: Orlando, FL, 1987; 283–98.

13. Ludwig J, Viggiano TR, McGill DB, Ott BJ. Non-alcoholic steatohepatitis. Mayo Clinic experience with a hitherto unnamed disease. *Mayo Clin Proc* 1980; **55**: 434–8.

14. Ludwig J, McGill DB, Lindor KD. Review: non-alcoholic steatohepatitis. *J Gastroenterol Hepatol* 1997; **12**: 398–403.

15. Bacon BR, Farahvash MJ, Janney CG, Neuschwander-Tetri BA. Non-alcoholic steatohepatitis: an expanded clinical entity. *Gastroenterology* 1994; **107**: 1103–9.

16. Teli MR, James OFW, Burt AD, Bennett MK, Day CP. The natural history of non-alcoholic fatty liver: a follow-up study. *Hepatology* 1995; **22**: 1714–19.

17. Baldridge AD, Perez-Atayde AR, Graeme-Cook F, Higgins L, Lavine JE. Idiopathic steatohepatitis in childhood: a multicenter retrospective study. *J Paediat* 1995; **127**: 700–704.

18. Caldwell SH, Oelsner DH, Lezzoni JC, Hespenheide EE *et al*. Cryptogenic cirrhosis: clinical characterization and risk factors for underlying disease. *Hepatology* 1999; **29**: 664–9.

19. Poonawala A, Nair SP, Thuluvath PJ. Prevalence of obesity and diabetes in patients with cryptogenic cirrhosis: a case-control study. *Hepatology* 2000; **32**: 689–92.

20. Falchuk KR, Fiske SC, Haggit RC *et al*. Pericentral hepatic fibrosis and intracellular hyaline in diabetes mellitus. *Gastroenterology* 1980; **78**: 535.

21. Latry P, Bioulac-Sage P, Echinard E *et al*. Peri-sinusoidal fibrosis and basement membrane-like material in the livers of diabetic patients. *Hum Pathol* 1987; **18**: 775.

22. George DK, Goldwurm S, MacDonald GA *et al*. Increased hepatic iron concentration in non-alcoholic steatohepatitis is associated with increased fibrosis. *Gastroenterology* 1998; **114**: 311–18.

23. George DK, Goldwurm S, MacDonald GA, Cowley LL *et al*. Increased hepatic iron concentration in non-alcoholic steatohepatitis is associated with increased fibrosis. *Gastroenterology* 1998; **114**: 311–18.

24. Brunt EM, Janney CG, DiBisceglie AM, Neuschwander-Tetri BA, Bacon BR. Non-alcoholic steatohepatitis: a proposal for grading and staging the histological lesions. *Am J Gastroenterol* 1999; **94**: 2467–74.

25. Wanless IR, Lentz JS. Fatty liver hepatitis (steatohepatitis) and obesity: an autopsy study with analysis of risk factors. *Hepatology* 1990; **12**: 1106–10.

26. Powell EE, Cooksley WGE, Hanson R, Searle J *et al*. The natural history of non-alcoholic steatohepatitis. *Hepatology* 1990; **11**: 74–80.

27. Batman PA, Scheuer PJ. Diabetic hepatitis preceding the onset of glucose intolerance. *Histopathology* 1985; **9**: 237.

28. Mauriac P. Hepatomegalie, nanisme, obesite dans le diabete infantile: pathogenie du syndrome. *Presse Med* 1946; **54**: 826.

29. Jacobs JE, Birnbaum BA, Shapiro MA, Langlotz CP *et al*. Diagnostic criteria for fatty infiltration of the liver on contrast-enhanced helical CT. *AJR* 1998; **171**: 659–64.

30. Grimm IS, Schindler W, Haluszka O. Steatohepatitis and fatal hepatic failure after biliopancreatic diversion. *Am J Gastroenterol* 1992; **87**: 775–9.

31. Faloon WM. Hepatobiliary effects of obesity and weight reducing surgery. *Semin Liver Dis* 1988; **8**: 218–28.

32. Nazim M, Stamp G, Hodgson HJF. Nonalcoholic steatohepatitis associated with small intestinal diverticulosis and bacterial overgrowth. *Hepatogastroenterology* 1989; **36**: 349–51.

33. Farrell GC. Steatohepatitis. In Farrell GC (ed.), *Drug-induced Liver Disease*. Churchill Livingstone: Edinburgh, 1995: 431–8.
34. Angulo P, Keach JC, Batts KP, Lindor KD. Independent predictors of liver fibrosis in patients with non-alcoholic steatohepatitis. *Hepatology* 1999; **30**: 1356–62.
35. James O, Day C. Non-alcoholic steatohepatitis: another disease of affluence. *Lancet* 1999; **353**: 1634–6.
36. Ferranini E. Insulin resistance, iron and the liver. *Lancet* 2000; **355**: 2181–2.
37. Knobler H, Schattner A, Zhornicki T *et al*. Fatty liver—an additional and treatable feature of the insulin resistance syndrome. *Quart. J Med* 1999; **92**: 73–9.
38. Marchesini G, Brizi M, Morselli-Labate AM, Bianchi G *et al*. Association of nonalcoholic fatty liver disease with insulin resistance. *Am J Med* 1999; **107**: 450–55.
39. Leclerq IA, Farrell GC, Field J, Bell DR *et al*. CYP2E1 and CYP4A as microsomal catalysts of lipid peroxides in urine non-alcoholic steatohepatitis. *J Clin Invest* 2000; **105**: 1067–75.
40. Kersten S, Seydoux J, Peters JM, Gonzalez FJ *et al*. Peroxisome proliferator-activated receptor alpha mediates the adaptive response to fasting. *J Clin Invest* 1999; **103**: 1489–98.
41. Tilg H, Diehl AM. Cytokines in alcoholic and non-alcoholic steatohepatitis. *N Engl J Med* 2000; **343**: 1467–76.
42. van Hoek B. Non-alcohol steatohepatitis: state-of-the-art. *Br Med J* 2001; **16** (suppl): 28(IX)–28(X).
43. Grove J, Daly AK, Bassendine MF, Gilvarry E, Day CP. Interleukin 10 promotor region polymorphisms and susceptibility to advanced alcoholic liver disease. *Gut* 2000; **46**: 540–45.
44. Letteron P, Fromenty B, Terris B *et al*. Acute and chronic hepatic steatosis lead to *in vivo* lipid peroxidation in mice. *J Hepatol* 1996; **24**: 200.
45. Braillon A, Capron JP, Herve MA, Degott C, Quenum C. Liver in obesity. *Gut* 1985; **26**: 133–9.
46. Krentz AJ, Baily CJ, Melander A. Thiazolidinediones for type 2 diabetes. *Br Med J* 2000; **321**: 252–3.
47. Fong DG, Nehra V, Lindor KD, Buchman AL. Metabolic and nutritional considerations in nonalcoholic fatty liver. *Hepatology* 2000; **32**: 3–10.
48. Klein CJ, Stanek GS, Wiles CE III. Overfeeding macronutrients to critically ill adults: metabolic complications. *J Am Diet Assoc* 1998; **98**: 795–806.
49. Shronts EP. Essential nature of choline with implications for total parenteral nutrition. *J Am Diet Assoc* 1997; **97**: 639–46.
50. Laurin J, Lindor KD, Crippin JS, Gossard A *et al*. Ursodeoxycholic acid or clofibrate in the treatment of non-alcohol-induced steatohepatitis. *Hepatology* 1996; **23**: 1464–7.
51. Lavine JE. Vitamin E treatment of nonalcoholic steatohepatitis in children: a pilot study. *J Pediat* 2000; **136**: 734–8.
52. Langtry HD, Balfour JA. Glimepiride. A review of its use in the management of type 2 diabetes mellitus. *Drugs* 1998; **55**: 563–84.
53. Yang CC, Chen CY, Lin XZ *et al*. Pyogenic liver abscess in Taiwan: emphasis on gasforming liver abscess in diabetics. *Am J Gastroenterol* 1993; **88**: 1911.
54. Milder MS, Cook JD, Sunday S *et al*. Idiopathic hemochromatosis. An interim report. *Medicine* 1980; **59**: 39.
55. Niederau C, Fischer R, Sonnenberg A *et al*. Survival and causes of death in cirrhotic and non-cirrhotic patients with primary hemochromatosis. *N Engl J Med* 1985; **313**: 1256.
56. Dymock IW, Cassar J, Pyke DA *et al*. Observations on the pathogenesis, complications and treatment of diabetes in 115 cases of haemochromatosis. *Diabetes* 1972; **52**: 203.

57. Ernst O, Sergent G, Bonvarlet P, Canva-Delcambre V *et al.* Hepatic iron overload: diagnosis and quantification with MR imaging. *AJR* 1997; **168**: 1205–8.

58. Lawrence SP, Caminer SJ, Yavorski RT, Borosky BD *et al.* Correlation of liver density by magnetic resonance imaging and hepatic iron levels. A non-invasive means to exclude homozygous hemochromatosis. *J Clin Gastroenterol* 1996; **23**: 113–17.

59. Cotler SJ, Bronner MP, Press RD, Carlson TH *et al.* End-stage liver disease without hemochromatosis associated with elevated hepatic iron index. *J Hepatol* 1998; **29**: 257–62.

60. Ramrakhiani S, Bacon BR. Hemochromatosis: advances in molecular genetics and clinical diagnosis. *J Clin Gastroenterol* 1998; **27**: 41–46.

61. Chalasani N, Gitlin N. Role of hepatic iron index in the management of iron overload syndromes in 1990s. *Am J Gastroenterol* 1998; **93**: 1385–6.

62. Press RD, Flora K, Gross C, Rabkin JM, Corless CL. Hepatic iron overload: direct HFE (HLA-H) mutation analysis vs. quantitative iron assays for the diagnosis of hereditary hemochromatosis. *Am J Clin Pathol* 1998; **109**: 577–84.

63. Adams PC, Bradley C, Henderson AR. Evaluation of the hepatic iron index as a diagnostic criterion for genetic hemochromatosis. *J Lab Clin Med* 1997; **130**: 509–14.

64. Bacon BR. Diagnosis and management of hemochromatosis. *Gastroenterology* 1997; **113**: 995–9.

65. Beutler E. The significance of the 187G (H63D) mutation in hemochromatosis. *Am J Human Genet* 1997; **61**: 762–4.

66. Moirand R, Mortaji AM, Loreal O *et al.* A new syndrome of liver iron overload with normal transferrin saturation. *Lancet* 1997; **349**: 95–7.

67. Griffiths JD, Dymock IW, Davies EWG *et al.* Occurrence and prevalence of diabetic retinopathy in hemochromatosis. *Diabetes* 1971; **20**: 766.

68. Hadziyannis S, Karamanos B. Diabetes mellitus and chronic hepatitis C virus infection. *Hepatology* 1999; **29**: 604–5.

69. Farbis P, Betterle C, Floreani A, Greggio NA *et al.* Development of type 1 diabetes mellitus during interferon alfa therapy for chronic HCV hepatitis. *Lancet* 1992; **340**: 548.

70. Fattovich G, Giustina G, Favarato S, Ruol A *et al.* A survey of adverse events in 11 241 patients with chronic viral hepatitis treated with α-interferon. *J Hepatol* 1996; **24**: 38–47.

71. Konrad T, Vicini P, Zeuzem S, Toffolo G *et al.* Interferon-α improves glucose tolerance in diabetic and non-diabetic patients with HCV-induced liver disease. *Exp Clin Endocrinol Diabetes* 1999; **107**: 343–9.

72. Mason AL, Lau JYN, Hoang N, Qian KP *et al.* Association of diabetes mellitus and chronic hepatitis C virus infection. *Hepatology* 1999; **29**: 328–33.

73. Strassburg CP, Obermayer-Straub P, Manns MP. Autoimmunity in hepatitis C and D virus infection. *J Viral Hepat* 1996; **3**: 49–59.

74. Honeyman MC, Stone NL, Harrison LC. T-cell epitopes in type I diabetes autoantigen tyrosine phosphatase IA-2: potential for mimicry with rotavirus and other environmental agents. *Mol Med* 1998; **4**: 231–9.

75. Choudhuri K, Gregorio GV, Mieli-Vergani G, Vergani D. Immunological cross-reactivity to multiple autoantigens in patients with liver kidney microsomal type 1 autoimmune hepatitis. *Hepatology* 1998; **28**: 1177–81.

76. Walton C, Walton S. Primary biliary cirrhosis in a diabetic male with dermatitis herpetiformis. *Clin Exp Dermatol* 1987; **12**: 46–7.

77. Prince MA, Vialettes B, Zevaco-Mattei C, Vague P. Clinical characteristics and etiological markers in insulin-dependent diabetes associated with an organ-specific autoimmune disease. *Acta Diabetol Lat* 1983; **20**: 221–9.

78. Csaszar A, Abel T. Receptor polymorphisms and diseases. *Eur J Pharmacol* 2001; **414**: 9–22.

79. Obermayer-Straub P, Manns MP. Autoimmune polyglandular syndromes. *Ballière's Clin Gastroenterol* 1998; **12**: 293–315.

80. Borgaonkar MR, Morgan DG. Primary biliary cirrhosis and type II autoimmune polyglandular syndrome. *Can J Gastroenterol* 1999; **13**: 767–70.

81. Ko GT, Szeto CC, Yeung VT, Chow CC *et al*. Autoimmune polyglandular syndrome and primary biliary cirrhosis. *Br J Clin Pract* 1996; **50**: 344–6.

82. Chapman BA, Wilson IR, Frampton CM *et al*. Prevalence of gallbladder disease in diabetes mellitus. *Dig Dis Sci* 1996; **41**: 2222–8.

83. De Santis A, Attili AF, Corradini SG *et al*. Gallstones and diabetes: a case control study in a free living population sample. *Hepatology* 1997; **25**: 787–90.

84. Hayes PC, Patrick A, Roulston JE *et al*. Gallstones in diabetes mellitus: prevalence and risk factors. *Eur J Gastroenterol Hepatol* 1992; **4**: 55–9.

85. Feldman M, Feldman M Jr. The incidence of cholelithiasis, cholesterolosis and liver disease in diabetes mellitus: an autopsy study. *Diabetes* 1954; **3**: 305–7.

86. Haffner SM, Diehl AK, Michell BD, Stern MP, Hazuda HP. Increased prevalence of clinical gallbladder disease in subjects with non-insulin-dependent diabetes mellitus. *Am J Epidemiol* 1990; **132**: 327–35.

87. Persson GE, Thulin AJG, Prevalence of gallstone disease in patients with diabetes mellitus. *Eur J Surg* 1991; **157**: 579–82.

88. Laakso M, Suhonen M, Julkunen R, Pyorola K. Plasma insulin, serum lipids and lipoproteins in gallstone disease in non-insulin dependent diabetic subjects: a case control study. *Gut* 1990; **31**: 344–7.

89. Ruhl CE, Everhart JE. Association of diabetes, serum insulin and C-peptide with gallbladder disease. *Hepatology* 2000; **31**: 299–303.

90. Hahm JS, Park JY, Park KG *et al*. Gallbladder motility in diabetes mellitus using real-time ultrasonography. *Am J Gastroenterol* 1996; **91**: 2391–4.

91. Chapman BA, Chapman TM, Frampton CM *et al*. Gallbladder volume. Comparison of diabetics and controls. *Dig Dis Sci* 1998; **43**: 344–8.

92. Jansen E, van Petersen AS, Lemkes HHPJ, Tjon A Tham R *et al*. Gallbladder motility in insulin-dependent diabetic patients with and without autonomic neuropathy. *Eur J Gastroenterol Hepatol* 1998; **10**: A83–4.

93. Fiorucci S, Bosso R, Scionti L *et al*. Neurohumoral control of gallbladder motility in healthy subjects and diabetic patients with or without autonomic neuropathy. *Dig Dis Sci* 1990; **35**: 1089–97.

94. Keshavarzian A, Dunne M, Iber FL. Gallbladder volume and emptying in insulin requiring male diabetics. *Dig Dis Sci* 1987; **32**: 824–8.

95. Rushakoff RA, Goldfine ID, Beccaria LJ, Mathur A *et al*. Reduced postprandial cholecystokinin (CCK) secretion in patients with non-insulin-dependent diabetes mellitus. *J Clin Endocrinol Metab* 1993; **76**: 489–93.

96. Stone B, Gavaler JS, Belle SM *et al*. Impairment of gallbladder emptying in diabetes mellitus. *Gastroenterology* 1988; **95**: 170–76.

97. Catnach SM, Ballinger AB, Stevens M *et al*. Erythromycin induces supranormal gallbladder contraction in diabetic autonomic neuropathy. *Gut* 1993; **34**: 1123–7.

98. Glasbrenner B, Dominquez-Munoz E, Riepl RL, Vetsi A, Malfertheiner P. Cholecystokinin and pancreatic polypeptide release in diabetic patients with and without autonomic neuropathy. *Dig Dis Sci* 1995; **40**: 406–11.

99. Mitsukawa T, Takemura J, Ohgo S *et al*. Gallbladder function and plasma cholecystokinin levels in diabetes mellitus. *Am J Gastroenterol* 1990; **85**: 981–5.

100. De Boer SY, Masclee AAM, Lam WF *et al.* Effect of hyperglycemia on gallbladder motility in type I diabetes mellitus. *Diabetologia* 1994; **37**: 75–81.

101. De Boer SY, Masclee AAM, Jebbink MCW *et al.* Effect of acute hyperglycemia on gallbladder contraction induced by cholecystokinin in humans. *Gut* 1993; **34**: 1128–32.

102. Del Favero G, Caroli A, Meggiato T *et al.* Natural history of gallstones in non-insulin dependent diabetes mellitus. A prospective 5-year follow-up. *Dig Dis Sci* 1994; **39**: 1704–7.

103. Landau O, Deutsch AA, Kott I, Rinlin E, Reiss R. The risk of cholecystectomy for acute cholecystitis in diabetic patients. *Hepatogastroenterology* 1992; **39**: 437–8.

104. Ikard RW. Gallstones, cholecystitis and diabetes. *Surg Gynecol Obstet* 1990; **171**: 528–32.

105. Aucott J, Cooper GS, Bloom AD, Aron DC. Management of gallstones in diabetic patients. *Arch Intern Med* 1993; **153**: 1053–8.

106. Lowell JA, Stratta RJ, Taylor RJ, Bynon JS *et al.* Cholelithiasis in pancreatic and kidney transplant recipients with diabetes. *Surgery* 1993; **114**: 858–64.

107. Barbineau TJ, Bothe A. General surgery considerations in the diabetic patient. *Infect Dis Clin North Am* 1995; **9**: 183–93.

108. Henderson JR, Daniel PM. A comparative study of the portal vessels connecting the endocrine and exocrine pancreas, with a discussion of some functional implications. *Q J Exp Physiol* 1979; **64**: 151–8.

109. Snook JT. Effect of diet, adrenalectomy, diabetes and actinomycin D on exocrine pancreas. *Am J Physiol* 1968; **215**: 1329–33.

110. Mössner J, Logsdon CD, Goldfine ID, Williams JA. Regulation of pancreatic acinar cell insulin receptors by insulin. *Am J Physiol* 1984; **247**: G155–60.

111. Lee KY, Zhou L, Ren XS, Chang TM, Chey WY. An important role of endogenous insulin on exocrine pancreatic secretion in rats. *Am J Physiol* 1990; **258**: G268–74.

112. Lam WF, Gielkens HAJ, Coenraad M, Lamers CBHW, Masclee AAM. Effect of insulin on basal and cholecystokinin stimulated exocrine pancreatic secretion in humans. *Pancreas* 1999; **18**: 252–8.

113. Gielkens HAJ, Lam WF, Coenraad M, Frölich M *et al.* Effect of insulin on basal and cholecystokinin stimulated gallbladder motility in humans. *J Hepatol* 1998; **28**: 595–602.

114. Chey WY, Shaw H, Shuman CR. External pancreatic secretion in diabetes mellitus. *Ann Int Med* 1963; **59**: 812–21.

115. Frier M, Saunders JHB, Wormsley KG, Bouchier AD. Exocrine pancreatic function in juvenile-onset diabetes mellitus. *Gut* 1976; **17**: 685–91.

116. Lankisch PG, Manthey G, Otto J *et al.* Exocrine pancreatic function in insulin dependent diabetes mellitus. *Digestion* 1982; **25**: 211–16.

117. Domschke W, Tympner F, Dorsche S, Derling L. Exocrine pancreatic function in juvenile diabetics. *Dig Dis Sci* 1975; **20**: 309–12.

118. El-Newihi H, Dooley CP, Saad C, Staples J *et al.* Impaired exocrine pancreatic function in diabetics with diarrhea and peripheral neuropathy. *Dig Dis Sci* 1988; **33**: 705–10.

119. Hardt PD, Krauss A, Bretz L *et al.* Pancreatic exocrine function in patients with type 1 and type 2 diabetes mellitus. *Acta Diabetol* 2000; **37**: 105–10.

120. Frier BM, Faber OK, Binder C, Elliot HL. The effect of residual insulin secretion on exocrine pancreatic function in juvenile-onset diabetes mellitus. *Diabetologia* 1978; **14**: 301–4.

121. Adler G, Beglinger C, Braun U *et al.* Interaction of the cholinergic system and cholecystokinin in the regulation of endogenous and exogenous stimulation of pancreatic secretion in humans. *Gastroenterology* 1991; **100**: 537–43.

122. Fraser RJ, Horowitz M, Maddox AF, Harding PF *et al.* Hyperglycemia slows gastric emptying in type 1 (insulin-dependent) diabetes mellitus. *Diabetologia* 1990; **33**: 675–80.

123. Salter JM, Davidson IWF, Best CH. The pathologic effect of large amounts of glucagon. *Diabetes* 1957; **6**: 248–52.

124. Dyck WP, Rudick J, Hoexter B, Janowitz HD. Influence of glucagon on pancreatic exocrine secretion in man. *Gastroenterology* 1970; **58**: 532–9.

125. Lonovics J, Guzman S, Devitt PG *et al.* Action of pancreatic polypeptide on exocrine pancreas and on release of cholecystokinin and secretin. *Endocrinology* 1981; **108**: 1925–30.

126. Floyd JC Jr, Fajans SS, Pek S, Chance RE. A newly recognized pancreatic polypeptide: plasma levels in health and disease. *Recent Prog Horm Res* 1977; **33**: 519–70.

127. Masclee AAM, Lamers CBHW. Effect of endoscopic sclerotherapy of esophageal varices on vagus nerve integrity. *J Hepatol* 1994; **21**: 724–9.

128. Gepts W. Pathologic anatomy of the pancreas in juvenile diabetes mellitus. *Diabetes* 1965; **14**: 619–33.

129. Silva MER, Vezorro DP, Ursich MJM *et al.* Ultrasonographic abnormalities of the pancreas in IDDM and NIDDM patients. *Diabetes Care* 1993; **16**: 1296–7.

130. Kobayachi T, Nakanishi K, Kajio H *et al.* Histopathological changes of the pancreas in islet cell antibodies (ICA)-positive subjects before and after the clinical onset of insulin-dependent diabetes. *Diabetes* 1988; **37**: 24A (abstr)

131. Kobayachi T, Nakanishi K, Kajio H *et al.* Pancreatic cytokeratin: an antigen of pancreatic exocrine cell autoantibodies in type 1 (insulin-dependent) diabetes mellitus. *Diabetologia* 1990; **33**: 363–70.

132. Rayfield EJ, Seto Y. Viruses and the pathogenesis of diabetes mellitus. *Diabetes* 1987; **11**: 1126–37.

133. Nakanishi K, Kobayashi T, Miyashita H *et al.* Exocrine pancreatic ductograms in insulin dependent diabetes mellitus. *Am J Gastroenterol* 1994; **89**: 762–6.

134. Larsen S, Hilsted J, Tronier B, Worning H. Metabolic control and B cell function in patients with insulin-dependent diabetes mellitus secondary to chronic pancreatitis. *Metabolism* 1987; **36**: 964–7.

135. Sjoberg RJ, Kidd GS. Pancreatic diabetes mellitus. *Diabetes Care* 1989; **12**: 715–24.

136. Wideroff L, Gridley G, Mellemkjaer L *et al.* Cancer incidence in a population-based cohort of patients hospitalized with diabetes mellitus in Denmark. *J Natl Cancer Inst* 1997; **89**: 1360–65.

137. Everhart J, Wright D. Diabetes mellitus as a risk factor for pancreatic cancer. *J Am Med Assoc* 1995; **273**: 24–31.

138. Silverman DT, Schiffman M, Everhart J *et al.* Diabetes mellitus, other medical conditions and familial history of cancer as risk factors for pancreatic cancer. *Br J Cancer* 1999; **80**: 1830–37.

139. Pemert J, Larsson J, Westermark GT *et al.* Islet amyloid polypeptide in patients with pancreatic cancer and diabetes. *N Engl J Med* 1994; **330**: 313–18.

140. Morris DV, Nabarro JD. Pancreatic cancer and diabetes mellitus. *Diabet Med* 1984; **1**: 119–21.

141. Thow J, Samad A, Alberti KGMM. Epidemiology and general aspects of diabetes secondary to pancreatopathy. In Tiengo A *et al.* (eds), *Diabetes Secondary to Pancreatopathy*. Excerpta Medica: Amsterdam, 1988; 7–20.

142. Gorelick FS. Diabetes mellitus and the exocrine pancreas. *Yale J Biol Med* 1983; **56**: 271–5.

143. Donowitz M, Hendler R, Spiro HM *et al.* Glucagon secretion in acute and chronic pancreatitis. *J Intern Med* 1975; **83**: 778–81.

144. Bank S, Marks IN, Vinik AL. Clinical and hormonal aspects of pancreatic diabetes. *Am J Gastroenterol* 1975; **64**: 13–22.
145. Fortson MR, Freedman SN, Webster PD. Clinical assessment of hyperlipedemic pancreatitis. *Am J Gastroenterol* 1995; **90**: 134–9.
146. Lam WF, Masclee AAM, Muller ESM, Lamers CBHW. Effect of hyperglycemia on gastric acid secretion during the gastric phase of digestion. *Am J Physiol* 1997; **272**: G1116–21.
147. Schwartz TW. Pancreatic polypeptide: a hormone under vagal control. *Gastroenterology* 1983; **85**: 1411–25.
148. Sutherland DER. The case for pancreas transplantation. *Diabetes Metab* 1996; **22**: 132–8.
149. Smets YFC, Westendorp RGJ, van der Pijl JW *et al*. Effect of simultaneous pancreas–kidney transplantation on mortality and end-stage renal failure. *Lancet* 1999; **353**: 1915–19.
150. Gaber AO, Oxley D, Karas J *et al*. Changes in gastric emptying in recipients of successful combined pancreas–kidney transplants. *Dig Dis Sci* 1991; **9**: 437–43.
151. Brayman K, Morel Ph, Chau C *et al*. Influence of rejection episodes on the relationship between exocrine and endocrine function in bladder-drained pancreas transplants. *Transplant Proc* 1992; **24**: 921–3.

8

Impact of Gastrointestinal Function on Glycaemic Control

Ian A. Macdonald, Michael A. Nauck
and Marie-France Kong

Introduction

The fate of nutrients subsequent to their entry into the gastrointestinal tract in many ways determines the changes in glycaemia that accompany a meal; this is particularly important in patients with diabetes, as glucose regulation is impaired and even more so if hypoglycaemia counterregulation is also impaired. The stomach does not contribute to absorption of glucose, so the rate at which nutrients leave the stomach into the small intestine is a major determinant of inflow into the circulation. Nutrients themselves and gastrointestinal hormones have a profound influence on the velocity of gastric emptying (Chapter 4). In the case of glucose metabolism, one major point of regulation is the liver, which produces glucose in the postabsorptive state, but has to reduce this glucose output in order to avoid uncontrolled postprandial glucose excursions, as occur in diabetes mellitus. Insulin and glucagon play a major role in regulating hepatic glucose metabolism, but their regulation is determined in turn by gut hormones, including the 'incretin' hormones, gastric inhibitory polypeptide (GIP)

Gastrointestinal Function in Diabetes Mellitus. Edited by Michael Horowitz and Melvin Samsom
© 2004 John Wiley & Sons, Ltd ISBN: 0-471-89916-X

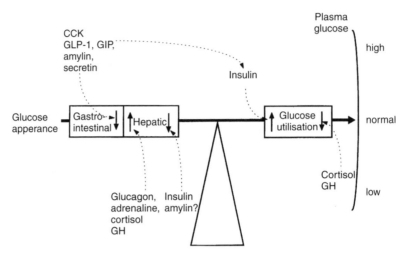

Figure 8.1   Schematic diagram of (gastrointestinal) factors affecting glucose concentrations in the fasting and postprandial states

and glucagon-like peptide 1 (GLP-1). The latter are responsible for approximately 50% of the amount of insulin secreted in response to a normal meal. Based on this knowledge, as illustrated in Figure 8.1, it is clear that abnormalities in any of these gastrointestinal functions will potentially have a major impact on glucose regulation.

The results of the DCCT [1] and the UKPDS studies [2] have shown conclusively that good glycaemic control reduces diabetic complications; treatment of type 1 and type 2 diabetes with insulin and oral hypoglycaemic agents and/or insulin, respectively, aims to reduce postprandial hyperglycaemic spikes, but this is only achieved in a minority of patients. Since the glycaemic response to oral carbohydrate and gastric emptying are related, modulation of the rate of gastric emptying, by dietary or pharmacological means, could be used to optimise glycaemic control. It has recently been shown that acute changes in the blood glucose concentration influence gastric and small intestinal function; thus, gastric emptying is slower during hyperglycaemia and faster during hypoglycaemia. This issue is discussed additionally in Chapters.

This chapter focuses on the role of gut hormones in the regulation of postprandial glucose concentration and the impact of pharmacological modulation of glycaemic control using gut hormones or their analogues. Within this chapter, the use of the term 'gastrointestinal function' is meant to include, where appropriate, contributions from the pancreas and liver as well.

Gut hormones and insulin secretion

Almost 100 years ago, Moore *et al.* described the blood-glucose-lowering activity of duodenal extracts [3], and in the late 1920s Zunz and LaBarre reported the release and action of a humoral substance from the gut mucosa, which decreased plasma glucose concentrations [4]. This lead to the *incretin concept*, which has received substantial attention in recent years, particularly because novel therapeutic strategies for type 2 diabetic patients can be derived from glucagon-like peptide 1 (GLP-1), one of the hormones involved [5,6].

The incretin effect

Incretin, in analogy to *excretin* (which stimulates exocrine pancreatic secretion), referred to the component of gut mucosal extracts that has the capacity to affect endocrine pancreatic secretion. Initially this was meant to be an increment in insulin secretion. The advent of insulin immunoassays in 1962 [7] made it possible to demonstrate the physiological importance of gut factors in the stimulation of insulin release: oral or intragastric/intraduodenal administration of glucose leads to a greater stimulation of insulin secretion than intravenous infusion of glucose [8,9]. This is the case, even though the rise in plasma glucose is greater in response to intravenous than to enteral glucose. The incretin effect refers to the phenomenon that oral glucose elicits a greater insulin secretory response than parenterally administered glucose (e.g. intravenous infusions) [10,11]. Incretin hormones are gut factors, released in response to nutrient ingestion, that stimulate pancreatic β-cells, especially when plasma glucose concentrations are elevated. The latter represents a safeguard against the release of high levels of incretin hormones by non-glucose nutrients (e.g. fat), which would otherwise potentially induce hypoglycaemia.

The above definitions represent modifications of those presented by Creutzfeldt in his 1978 Claude Bernard lecture [11]. One term that is often used is the *enteroinsular axis*, which was initially coined by Unger and Eisentraut [12] to refer to all connections between the gut and the islets of Langerhans i.e. substrates, nerves and (incretin) hormones. When used in this broader sense, not only effects on insulin, but also those on glucagon and pancreatic somatostatin etc. are subject to this definition. The incretin contribution can be estimated by the comparison of insulin secretory responses to glucose (e.g. 50 g) given by mouth and to an 'isoglycaemic' intravenous glucose infusion, administered on separate occasions. 'Isoglycaemic' means that the same plasma glucose profile that was determined after oral glucose is copied [13,14] in an experiment that is technically performed like a 'glucose clamp'; in this way the glycaemic stimulus to the β-cell is identical under both conditions. By comparing the insulin secretory responses, it became evident that the increases in insulin and C-peptide levels are substantially greater with oral than with intravenous glucose [13–15]. Several conclusions can be drawn from this type of experiment: (a) glucose is not the only stimulus for insulin secretion after oral glucose; (b) other factors (including gastrointestinal hormones with insulinotropic activity) are involved; (c) the quantitative importance of those additional factors approximates 50% of the insulin response; (d) the quantitative impact of the incretin effect is greater when insulin concentrations (i.e. comparing oral and isoglycaemic intravenous glucose loads) are evaluated—differences based on the measurement of C-peptide or the calculation of insulin secretion rates are substantially less [13,16]. It has become customary to quantify the incretin effect based on integrated incremental C-peptide (areas under the curve above baseline), according to the equation:

$$\text{Incretin effect}(\%) = (\text{AUC}_{CP}\ \text{oral} - \text{AUC}_{CP}\ i.v.)/\text{AUC}_{CP}\ oral \qquad (1)$$

Typical incretin contributions to insulin secretory responses after oral glucose range from approximately 25% for glucose loads of 25 g, to 60% for glucose loads of 100 g [13–16].

Gastric inhibitory polypeptide/glucose-dependent insulinotropic peptide (GIP)

GIP was originally named *gastric inhibitory polypeptide*, based on the biological function tested for in the bioassay used for its purification by Brown and co-workers: Gastric acid secretion was inhibited in vagally denervated (Heidenhain) gastric pouches [17,18]. Porcine gut mucosa was fractionated and further purified, until the amino acid sequence of proteolytic GIP fragments could be determined by the Edman technique. Purified GIP appeared to be a potent inhibitor of gastric acid and pepsin secretion in dogs [19]. Subsequent studies in humans with intact gastric innervation, however, have shed doubt as to whether GIP has a physiological role as a so-called 'enterogastrone' [20], a term used for a gut hormone that is released from the proximal small intestine after fat ingestion and inhibits gastric function. Soon after its discovery, purified GIP was shown to stimulate insulin secretion if administered to healthy human subjects together with glucose [21]. Based on this observation, research into the insulinotropic properties of GIP intensified and led to the concept of GIP being an incretin hormone. For this reason, the acronym GIP is now interpreted as *glucose-dependent insulinotropic peptide* [22]. Using immunohistochemistry, GIP-producing K cells have been detected in the mucosa of the upper small intestine of almost all species examined, including humans [23]. This was confirmed by electron microscopy [24]. Human K cells are characterised by secretory granules with small electron-dense cores surrounded by a concentric electron-lucent halo, but this differs between species. The human GIP gene is located on chromosome 17q and comprises six exons (Table 8.1) [25,26]. The appropriate messenger RNA is 800 base pairs (bp) long. GIP cDNA revealed a 459 bp open reading frame encoding the 153 amino acid peptide preproGIP. This sequence includes a signal peptide, most likely cleaved at amino acid glycine 21, as part of the 51 amino acid aminoterminal peptide. The carboxyterminal peptide

Table 8.1 Characterisation of the main incretin hormones, gastric inhibitory polypeptide (GIP) and glucagon-like peptide 1 (GLP-1), and their receptors (human data are mentioned whenever possible)

	GIP	GLP-1
Gene/precursor	ProGIP[26]	Proglucagon (intestinal)[264]
Chromosomal location	17 q, 10 kb	2 [265]
Number of exons	6	6
mRNA (bp)	800 bp	1101 bp [75]
cDNA (bp)	459 bp	537 bp [74]
Precursor (number of AA)	PreproGIP (153 AA)	Preproglucagon [264]
	ProGIP (132 AA)	Proglucagon (159 AA) [74]
Final product (number of AA)	GIP (42 AA)	GLP-1 (7–36 amide)/(7–37) (30/31 AA)
Other products	None	GLP-1, glicentin (enteroglucagon), oxyntomodulin, spacer peptides
Expression		
Gut	Duodenum, Jeunum [23,24]	small intestine (ileum) [79,80,88]
Other	Glandula submandibularis[28]	Brain, stomach [82]
Modulation of expression by		
Transcription	Glucose [28]	cAMP [266] Fasting (reduction) [99]
Translation	Not known	Not known
Receptor	[28,57,59]	[64,112]
Chromosomal location	19q13.2/13.3 [60]	6p21 [267]
Number of exons	14	7 [116]0
mRNA (bp)	> 2.15 kbp plus poly A tail	2.7 and 3.6 kbp (including poly A tails of different length [112]
cDNA (bp)	1389 bp	3066 bp [112]
Product (number of AA)	466	463 [112]

AA, amino acids; bp, base pairs.

is 60 amino acids in length [25,26] and is similar, but not identical, in the rat [27]. Within the family of secretin, glucagon, vasoactive intestinal peptide (VIP) etc., sequence homology between GIP and the other members is restricted to the biologically active part of precursor molecules, with greater variation in other domains.

Expression of the human GIP gene is controlled by a promoter containing a TATA box (TATAAGG), 28 bp upstream of the putative transcriptional start site. In addition, there is an 'enhancer core element' (at position −138) and there are two CAAT boxes (CCAAT at position −156 and CAAAT at position −169). The GIP promoter contains consensus sequences for an AP-1 and cAMP response elements (CREs; [28]). The expression of the GIP gene may be regulated by nutrients; GIP mRNA increases with oral glucose and fat loads in rats [29].

GIP release occurs after nutrient stimulation, primarily oral carbohydrate and fat [30,31]. Among carbohydrates, glucose, galactose and sucrose stimulate GIP secretion, whereas fructose, mannose and lactose have no effect, even after intestinal perfusion [32]. The increment in plasma GIP occurs within 15 min after starting to ingest nutrients and is more sustained after fat than sugars [30–33,34]. The release of GIP may be particularly dependent on the early phase of gastric emptying [35], but this needs to be studied in more detail. It is the fatty acid component of triglycerides that promotes the release of GIP—only long chain fatty acids (not medium or short chain fatty acids) have an effect [36]. It is also possible to stimulate GIP release with rather high doses and a special mixture of amino acids [37,38]. However, in response to physiological protein loads, GIP release is minimal [31,39,40]. Duodenal acidification also stimulates GIP release [41].

The secretion of GIP from upper intestinal K cells is closely associated with nutrient absorption. This is clearly the case for carbohydrates, since GIP release can be prevented by phlorizin [42] and for fat, because in exocrine pancreatic insufficiency the GIP response to fat is attenuated in the absence, but not the presence, of adequate enzyme supplementation [43]. In the latter case, the reduction in GIP response may account, at least in part, for the diminished insulin response; this can be improved with pancreatic enzyme replacement [43].

Several radioimmunoasays for the measurement of plasma GIP have been published and are available [39,41,44,45]. Most laboratories agree that basal GIP plasma levels are <100 pmol/l and that GIP concentrations can increase to >300 pmol/l after physiological nutrient stimulation. GIP, like other peptide hormones, is subject to proteolytic inactivation by the ubiquitous protease DPP IV (dipeptidyl peptidase IV)[46,47]. DPP IV produces des Tyr-Ala GIP or GIP 3–42, which is biologically inactive [48]. This process occurs in the circulation and is rapid, thereby limiting the half-life of biologically active GIP to about 2 min in experimental animals [49] and 7 min in humans [47]. Based on non-specific assays, which cannot differentiate GIP (1–42) from GIP (3–42), the half-life of GIP has been estimated to be around 20 min in human subjects [50–53]. The bulk elimination of GIP occurs via the kidney [54], with little or no contribution by the liver [55,56].

GIP receptors and intracellular signal transduction

The GIP receptor belongs to the family of G protein-coupled receptors with seven transmembrane domains [57–59]. It is similar to receptors for other peptides belonging to the glucagon–secretin family of peptide hormones [e.g. glucagon, glucagon-like peptides, secretin, vasoactive intestinal peptide (VIP), parathyroid hormone and growth hormone releasing factor]. The human GIP receptor gene is located on chromosome 19q [60]. The gene spans 13.8 kb and consists of 14 exons [59,61]. Mature messenger RNA contains a 1389 bp open reading frame coding for a 466 amino acid protein. The GIP receptor in other animal species is similar. Splice variants with unknown biological significance may exist. In the rat GIP receptors are expressed in pancreas, stomach, adipose tissue and the heart [57]. In addition, several brain loci (pituitary gland, cerebral cortex, hippocampus and olfactory bulb) and the adrenal cortex express GIP receptors [57]. The latter observation may be related to the rare food-induced Cushing's syndrome [62].

GIP receptors bind GIP [1–42] or the GIP fragment [1–30] with high affinity [58,61]. It is not clear, whether exendin-4 [1–39], a GLP-1 agonist (derived from the venom of *Heloderma suspectum*, the 'Gila monster') or exendin [9–39], a GLP-1 antagonist [63,64] also have the capacity to bind the GIP receptor [58,65]. If this were the case, the use of exendin [9–39] as an antagonist for GLP-1 in *in vivo* experiments would not be specific enough to discriminate between the actions of GIP and GLP-1. After binding of GIP to its receptor, the generation of cAMP is stimulated through the activation of adenylate cyclase via stimulatory G proteins [66]. The activation of protein kinase A also affects closure of ATP-dependent K^+ channels, opening of voltage-gated Ca^{2+} channels, the release of Ca^{2+} from intracellular stores, and the direct stimulation of exocytosis of insulin secretory granules from pancreatic β-cells, in a fashion similar to the signal transduction cascade induced by GLP-1 (Figure 8.2) [5,67].

Biological actions and physiological functions of GIP

The main function of GIP in humans is a glucose-dependent stimulation of insulin secretion. At basal plasma glucose concentrations very little happens, whereas at the levels of glycaemia associated with the postprandial period, GIP potently augments insulin secretion [21,52,68,69]. The effect of physiological doses of exogenous GIP during physiological increments of glucose concentrations is of comparable magnitude to the total incretin effect, assigning a major contribution to GIP [52,68]. In rats, GIP also stimulates glucagon secretion [70], but in normal and type 2 diabetic human subjects this is not the case [53,68]. In humans, stimulation of glucagon by exogenous GIP has only been observed in patients with cirrhosis who are known to have elevated preprandial glucagon levels [71]. In contrast to GLP-1, GIP has little, if any, effect on gastric emptying [72] and causes only minimal suppression of gastric acid secretion [20,73].

Glucagon-like peptide 1 (GLP-1)

GLP-1 was detected originally during analysis of the proglucagon gene sequence [74,75]. Two glucagon-like sequences, named glucagon-like peptides 1 and 2, with a high degree of sequence homology, were detected within the same

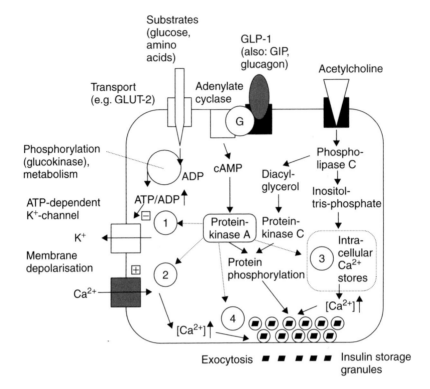

Figure 8.2 Schematic diagram of a pancreatic β-cell. The steps leading to insulin secretion are depicted: glucose transport via GLUT-2; metabolism of glucose raising the ATP:ADP ratio; closure of an ATP-dependent K$^+$ channel, causing depolarisation of the cell membrane; calcium influx through voltage-dependent L-type Ca^{2+} channels; GLP-1 can interact by binding to its receptor, promotion of cAMP synthesis and stimulation of protein kinase A. Largely by promoting phosphorylation of proteins, protein kinase A is able to interact with: (1) ATP-dependent K$^+$ channels; (2) L-type Ca^{2+} channels; (3) mobilisation of Ca^{2+} from intracellular stores; and (4) augmentation of storage granule exocytosis. For details, see text

precursor molecule ('proglucagon'). At that time, neither a corresponding peptide product nor their biological function were known. The suggested GLP-1 sequence was in part erroneous, because proteolytic processing was assumed to occur exclusively at dibasic amino acid recognition sites, leading to the sequence proglucagon 72–108 [GLP-1 (1–36 amide) or (1–37), sometimes referred to as 'full-length GLP-1']. Subsequently, it was found that the N-terminally 'truncated' GLP-1 [GLP-1 (7–36 amide) or (7–37)] was the predominant form synthesised *in vivo* and secreted into the circulation [76,77]. Holst has suggested that the term 'GLP-1' should only be used to refer to proglucagon (78–106 amide) [GLP-1 (7–36 amide)] [78]. According to this terminology, the non-amidated form, proglucagon [78–107] [GLP-1 (7–37)], would be called 'glycin-extended GLP-1'.

GLP-1 is a product of the proglucagon gene [74,75,79,80]. Proglucagon is expressed in the pancreas (α-cells in the islets of Langerhans). In the pancreatic α-cell, posttranslational processing by limited proteolysis leads mainly to glucagon synthesis, and both the GLP-1 and GLP-2 sequences, together with an 'intervening' sequence, remain part of a single product with hitherto unknown biological activity, the 'major proglucagon fragment' (MPGF) [81]. In the L-cells of the lower gastrointestinal tract (ileum, colon and rectum), proglucagon processing leads to the synthesis of enteroglucagon (glicentin) and the glucagon-like peptides 1 and 2 [79,80]. The products of posttranslational processing in the brain are similar to those of the gut [82]. Endocrine cells expressing the proglucagon gene and the prohormone convertase 3 (PC3, also called PC1) produce the intestinal (L-cell) pattern of products (i.e. mainly glicentin and GLP-1/GLP-2) [83–85], whereas PC2 seems to be the main processing enzyme for pancreatic (α-cell) products (glucagon and the 'major proglucagon fragment') [84,85]. Additional enzymes are probably needed.

GLP-1 is secreted from L-cells in the lower gut (ileum, colon and rectum [77,80,86–88]) after meals containing carbohydrate and fat [89–94]. Fructose, like glucose, stimulates GLP-1 release, although to a lesser degree [95].

In relation to the secretion of GLP-1 and other L-cell products, a paradox has been noted: GLP-1 secretion is initiated rapidly (within 5–10 min) after nutrient ingestion [52,53,92] although, as discussed, L-cells occur primarily in the lower gastrointestinal tract [86,88]. Here, they should not come into rapid contact with meal components, which have to be emptied from the stomach and pass through the upper parts of the small intestine (i.e. duodenum and jejunum). Basically, two explanations have been suggested: (a) there is an 'upper gut signal' (hormonal or neural) that is activated by the presence of nutrients in the proximal small intestine, which is then transferred to the L-cells; and (b) although relatively few L-cells are present in the proximal small intestine (at least when compared to the vast numbers present distally), the quantity is sufficient to allow GLP-1 secretion in the quantities that have been observed *in vivo*. This debate has not been resolved conclusively. However, it is recognised that surgical removal of parts of the ileum or the colon does modify the GLP-1 response to oral glucose [96] and that a larger nutrient load must enter the small intestine to stimulate GLP-1 when compared to GIP secretion [97]. As discussed, GIP-producing K cells are located mainly in the duodenum. Taken together, these findings argue in favour of GLP-1 release via direct contact of nutrients with the sparse L-cells in the jejunum and upper ileum. Quantitative considerations relating the GLP-1 content of the small intestinal mucosa to the amount of GLP-1 secreted in response to a typical nutrient stimulus also support this view: only approximately 1.5% of the amount of GLP-1 present in the total small intestine (and approximately 10–15% of the amount present in the upper jejunum) is secreted in response to a single oral stimulus with sucrose [5,96]. On the other hand, observations that neurotransmitters that are present in the enteric nervous system (i.e. bethanechol, a cholinergic agonist; bombesin; the ß-adrenergic agonist isoproterenol; and CGRP) have the capacity to stimulate GLP-1 release from the perfused ileum [93,98], are consistent with the concept of neural signalling via the intrinsic enteric nervous system from the upper to the lower small intestine. GIP, which is a potent stimulus to GLP-1 secretion in rodents [93], does not lead to elevations in plasma GLP-1 levels when infused into healthy or type 2 diabetic human subjects, i.e. GIP does not display GLP-1-releasing activity in humans [40,53]. L-cell density and GLP-1 'stores' are modified in response to experimental gut resections or dietary manipulations [99], such as a change in dietary fibre content [100].

There is evidence that obese subjects may secrete less GLP-1 after an oral carbohydrate load when compared to normal-weight subjects, while with fat as the nutritional stimulus, no difference was apparent [101]. This observation is of interest, given the effect of GLP-1 on feeding behaviour [102,103].

Measurement of the biologically active forms of GLP-1 in plasma (e.g. 'truncated' GLP-1 (7–36 amide) or (7–37), 'glycin-extended' GLP-1) [77,104] is possible but has proved difficult because, among other reasons, of *in vivo* N-terminal degradation by dipeptidyl peptidase IV [46,49,105,106], which leads to biologically inactive or even antagonistic GLP-1 (9–36 amide) or (9–37) [107], and the simultaneous presence of other molecules containing the GLP-1 sequence (e.g. the 'major proglucagon fragment' and GLP-1 (1–36 amide) or (1–37) as pancreatic products of processing). A sandwich ELISA that measures only GLP-1 with both intact N- and C-termini has now been introduced [108]. This assay has helped to characterise *in vitro* and *in vivo* degradation of GLP-1 [105,106,109]. Future sandwich assays, employing highly specific and high-affinity monoclonal antibodies, will hopefully resolve the discrepancies in GLP-1 concentrations reported by different laboratories. Basal (fasting) plasma GLP-1 concentrations between 2 and 15 pmol/l and stimulated (postprandial) concentrations of 20–50 pmol/l may be regarded as physiological. Disorders associated with rapid gastric emptying are accompanied by excessive plasma GLP-1 concentrations [110,111].

GLP-1 receptors and intracellular signal transduction

The GLP-1 receptor was first cloned from an insulinoma cell line [64,112]. It belongs to the '7 transmembrane domain' group of receptors and is expressed in β-cells of the pancreatic islets of Langerhans, in the lung, and in certain areas of the brain (see below). The presence of GLP-1 receptors on pancreatic endocrine α-cells is questionable [113–115]. Recent tissue surveys in rats [116], mice [117] and humans [118,119] have confirmed that mRNA coding for this pancreatic (β-cell) type GLP-1 receptor does not exist in liver, muscle and adipose tissue. GLP-1 receptors of the same deduced amino acid sequence are found in all tissues that have been examined [118].

Scrocchi *et al.* [120–122] recently described GLP-1 receptor 'knock-out' mice. The phenotype of these mice includes glucose intolerance and reduced insulin secretion, evident after intraperitoneal glucose administration, but no difference in body weight, although the acute, suppressive, effects of intracerebroventricular GLP-1 on food intake were seen in control, but not in receptor-negative, animals. Interestingly, these mice are characterised by an enhanced response to GIP, which might compensate for some of the consequences of 'knocked-out' GLP-1.

In pancreatic β-cells or similar insulinoma cell lines, cAMP has been described originally as the classical second messenger [123]. Recent studies, however, have established that an increment in cytoplasmic Ca^{++} is another important signalling pathway [124–127]. The rise in Ca^{++} is secondary to cAMP formation and is dependent on Na^+ inflow [128].

GLP-1 has traditionally been viewed as an *incretin* hormone, i.e. a gut factor that is released into the circulation after nutrient ingestion, which contributes to meal-induced insulin secretion as a result of its glucose-dependent insulinotropic properties [52,68,129,130]. In addition, GLP-1 suppresses glucagon secretion [53,131,132]. At the cellular level, GLP-1 has been shown to promote (pro)insulin biosynthesis and affect the production of other islet hormones [133] as well as β-cell replication and differentiation in general [134–139].

Insulin secretion and glucose-dependence of insulinotropic effects

A prominent feature of the insulinotropic effect of GLP-1 is its glucose-dependence [52,68,140–142]. Based on the work of Holz *et al.* [126,127] and Gromada *et al.* [67,143–146] the cell biology underlying the insulinotropic actions of GLP-1 has been elucidated in sufficient detail so that the phenomenon of its strict glucose dependence is understandable (see the excellent review by Gromada *et al.* [67]). Basically, there are four intracellular steps in the insulin secretory cascade that may be influenced by GLP-1 and other cAMP-increasing agents: (a) via protein kinase A there is a small, direct effect on the ATP-dependent potassium channel (closure) [126,145,146], which by itself, however, is insufficient to cause membrane depolarisation (which can only be achieved with high glucose concentrations or by the combination of GLP-1 and slightly elevated glucose levels); (b) there is a direct stimulation of L-type Ca^{2+}-channels causing augmented influx of calcium from extracellular sources [146,147]; (c) GLP-1 promotes release of calcium ions from intracellular Ca^{2+} stores [127]; (d) there is direct stimulation of exocytosis, which is quantitatively the most important contribution, probably by promoting a transition of storage granules into a readily releasable form [67,145,146]. Steps b–d, however, are dependent on closure of the ATP-dependent potassium channel to a degree that is sufficient to cause membrane depolarisation [145]. Therefore, overall insulinotropic activity strictly depends on 'elevated' glucose concentrations, the threshold being around 110 mg/dl (6 mmol/l). Clinically, this is demonstrated by the fact that high-dose intravenous administration of GLP-1 does not cause hypoglycaemia in healthy volunteers [141], and that a prolonged administration of GLP-1 in type 2 diabetic patients leads to a normalisation of glycaemia, which in turn causes insulin concentrations to fall into the basal range despite ongoing infusion of GLP-1 [148,149]. In comparison to the sulphonylurea glyburide, the insulinotropic effects of GLP-1 are more glucose-dependent [150], because sulphonylureas alone are able to depolarise β-cells. ß-Adrenergic counterregulation does not contribute to the maintenance of euglycaemia during exogenous administration of GLP-1 [151].

GLP-1 suppresses glucagon secretion in the isolated perfused pancreas [131,152]. It is not entirely clear whether or not there are GLP-1 receptors on pancreatic α-cells [113,118,119]. It is possible that the effects of GLP-1 on glucagon secretion are partly mediated by augmented insulin and/or somatostatin secretion [113]. The suppression of glucagon by exogenous GLP-1 probably makes a substantial contribution to the normalisation of fasting hyperglycaemia in type 2 diabetic patients [148,149]. Even in type 1 diabetic patients, a clear inhibition of glucagon secretion was observed, accompanied by a significant fall in plasma glucose [153]. The stimulation of glucagon secretion during hypoglycaemia is not affected by GLP-1 in healthy subjects [154], establishing that glucagonostatic effects of GLP-1 are glucose-dependent, as are the insulinotropic effects; similar results have been obtained in type 2-diabetic patients (Nauck MA, unpublished data).

Gastric effects

Gastric emptying is slowed by exogenous administration of GLP-1 (Figure 8.3) [155–158], with the consequence that dependent functions (such as 'intestinal phase' pancreatic exocrine secretion) are also reduced. Gastric acid secretion

Figure 8.3   Gastric emptying (upper panels), plasma glucose concentrations (second row of panels), plasma insulin (third row of panels) and plasma glucagon (bottom panels) in response to a mixed liquid meal (containing amino acids and sucrose) in young healthy subjects (left; redrawn from [158]) and in type 2 diabetic patients (right; redrawn from [157]) under the influence of a pharmacological infusion of GLP-1 (7–36 amide) (1.2 pmol/kg^{-1}/min^{-1}) or placebo. The bar on top indicates the duration of the infusion (30–240 min) and the arrow shows the time point of meal administration (through a nasogastric tube). In healthy subjects, GLP-1 retards gastric emptying, prevents a postprandial rise in glycaemia, stimulates preprandial and reduces postprandial insulin secretion (secondary to impaired substrate availability due to the retardation of gastric emptying), and suppresses glucagon. In type 2 diabetic patients, gastric emptying is similarly retarded, but glucose levels fall and insulin secretion is stimulated despite the absence of a rise in glycaemia (due to the glucose-dependence of GLP-1's insulinotropic actions). Glucagon rises more after the meal with placebo than in healthy subjects, but this increment is completely prevented by GLP-1; this is also evident type 2 diabetic patients

has been found to be suppressed by GLP-1 in some [159,160] but not in all [20] studies.

Other 'extrapancreatic effects'

The controversy as to whether GLP-1 can interact with liver, muscle, and adipose tissue directly is based on descriptions of GLP-1 effects on glucose transport and glycogen metabolism in such tissues at GLP-1 concentrations exceeding 1 nmol/l (1000 pmol/l) [161–166]. There are also contradictory

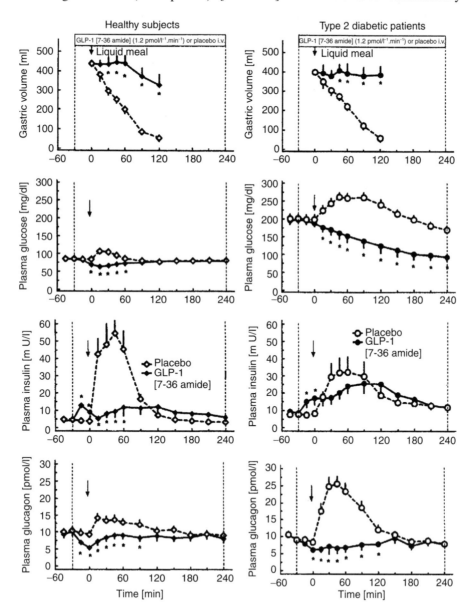

reports [167,168]. Specific binding sites for labelled GLP-1 have been described by some but not all groups [169–173]. These binding sites do not seem to be identical to the pancreatic (β-cell) GLP-1 receptor as characterised by molecular genetic methods, because there appears to be no β-cell type GLP-1 receptor mRNA in these tissues [64,112,118,119]. Therefore, if one postulates that GLP-1 has direct effects on 'peripheral tissues', independent from GLP-1-induced changes in the concentrations of insulin and glucagon, one has to hypothesise additional receptor species that have not hitherto been characterised at the molecular level.

At least in humans, the influence of circulating GLP-1 on processes involved in the regulation of carbohydrate homeostasis is dependent on the changes in insulin and glucagon secretion described above [174]; a direct effect on insulin sensitivity originally described in type 1 diabetic patients [175] could not be confirmed in healthy subjects [176] or in type 2 diabetic patients [177].

Additional GLP-1 targets

GLP-1 stimulates the transcription of genes coding for β-cell components involved in the process of glucose sensing and insulin synthesis and secretion (insulin, GLUT-1 and hexokinase) [178]. GLP-1 also stimulates phosphorylation of GLUT-2, the liver β-cell-specific glucose transporter [179]. GLP-1 stimulates TSH secretion from pituitary cells, although only at high concentrations [180], enhances secretion of luteinising hormone (LH)-releasing hormone in a hypothalamic cell line [181] and stimulates cAMP production and calcitonin release in a murine C cell line [182]. Another group of potential functions relates to the presence of GLP-1 [183,184] and its receptor [112,118,185] in the brain: GLP-1 injected into the cerobrospinal fluid in μg amounts reduces food intake, especially in satiated rats [102,186,187]. Water intake is also affected [186,187]. It is probable that GLP-1 is synthesised in the brain [82] and functions as a neurotransmitter to affect food and water intake. An alternative possibility is that GLP-1 present in the bloodstream may bind to receptors present in the subfornical organ and area postrema [82]. This is of particular interest, since the effects of plasma GLP-1 on gastric functions (acid secretion and possibly gastric emptying) are dependent on an intact vagus nerve [156], and because exogenous GLP-1 (and perhaps endogenously secreted GLP-1 from the gut) may also regulate food intake in humans [103,188]. It is not clear, to what extent retarded gastric emptying contributes to reduced appetite, increased satiety and an overall reduction in nutrient intake.

Relative importance of GIP, GLP-1 and/or additional incretin hormones

Exendin (9–39) is a specific peptide GLP-1 receptor antagonist and its use has made it possible to examine the net effect of endogenously secreted GLP-1 in experimental animals. Administration of exendin (9–39) reduced insulin secretory responses after enteral stimulation with nutrients [129,130]. At the same time the plasma glucose responses were greater, suggesting a more 'diabetic' state. The fact that a specific peptide antagonist for the GIP receptor [GIP fragment (7–30)] [189] also leads to a major reduction in meal-induced insulin secretion in rats can be accounted for by either a similarly important incretin role for GIP or to the fact that, in rodents, GIP is a GLP-1 secretagogue [93,190]. As discussed, this mediation of GLP-1 release via GIP certainly is not active in humans [40,53]. The question arises as to which hormone is the more potent incretin. After meals, GLP-1 concentrations peak at approximately 15–40 pmol/l, substantially lower levels than are typical for GIP (100–500 pmol/l) [52,53]. Therefore, exogenous GLP-1, administered in a dose that mimics physiological increments in plasma GLP-1 concentrations, only slightly augments insulin secretion in response to a physiological glycaemic increment, contributing some 25% to the incretin effect [52] or less than 15% to total postprandial insulin secretion. Furthermore, the insulin-stimulatory role of GLP-1 is counteracted by the slowing of gastric emptying, which reduces substrate-stimulated insulin secretion and the permissive increment in glycaemia. Since exendin (9–39) has been used as a GLP-1 receptor antagonist in humans [191], it can be expected that the physiological importance of insulinotropic effects of GLP-1 will be clarified in the near future. When exendin (9–39) was infused into healthy volunteers, the glycaemic profile after oral glucose was steeper and insulin responses tended to be higher [192].

Other hormones have been examined as potential incretin hormones, but clearly do not fulfil the criteria outlined by Creutzfeldt [11], e.g. CCK [69,193]. Another interesting aspect is the possibility of gut hormones that suppress, rather than augment, postprandial insulin secretion. One hormone with this potential is somatostatin, which occurs ubiquitously, but may be secreted from the gut mucosa after nutrient intake. Exogenous administration of somatostatin 28, resulting in plasma concentrations that are typically reached in a postprandial situation, lowered insulin responses [194,195]. Although the interaction of such a 'decretin' with insulin stimulatory hormones and the quantitative impact are poorly defined, these findings raise the likelihood that the postprandial regulation of insulin secretion by gastrointestinal hormones is even more complicated than currently known. Pancreatic innervation does not appear to be a prerequisite, as evidenced by a normal incretin effect in pancreas-transplanted patients whose pancreas is denervated [196,197].

Gut hormones in type 2 diabetes

Since type 2 diabetes is characterised by defective insulin secretion [198], especially in response to meals, possible disturbances of the enteroinsular axis in type 2 diabetic patients have received considerable attention. The broad hypothesis is that disorders of the secretion, or insulinotropic activity, of physiologically important incretin hormones contribute to the delay in insulin secretory activity that is typically seen during the 'early phase' of the postprandial insulin response.

The incretin effect has been quantified in type 2 diabetic patients and found to be reduced in magnitude [14]; in some patients, a complete lack of a measurable incretin effect was noted. The incretin response appeared to be independent of patient characteristics such as age, degree of obesity and treatment. These observations indicate that type 2 diabetes is associated with abnormalities in either the secretion of incretin hormones or their insulinotropic activity.

Secretion of GIP and GLP-1 in type 2 diabetic patients

It is clear from a number of studies that there is no obvious undersecretion of GIP in response to typical nutrient stimuli (glucose, fat or mixed meals) in patients with type 2 diabetes in comparison to non-diabetic subjects of comparable age and degree of obesity [199–201]. Rather, there is evidence that a small, but significant, enhancement of GIP responses is characteristic of type 2 diabetic patients [202,203]. These old observations do not, however, take into account the fact that GIP is degraded by dipeptidyl peptidase IV [46,204], to a product which by itself is biologically inactive, but was probably detected by the immunoassays used. Therefore, at present it can not be excluded that the concentration of biologically active, intact GIP (1–42) differs between healthy and type 2 diabetic patients. Given the substantial interest in the possible therapeutic role of GLP-1 in type 2 diabetic patients, data on the secretion of GLP-1 in type 2 diabetic vs. metabolically healthy subjects are relatively scarce. Initial studies with small numbers of subjects were contradictory [53,205]: one study described an enhanced GLP-1 secretion after a 100 g oral glucose in type 2 diabetic patients [205]; another found the contrary after a 50 g oral glucose [53]. Recently, data have been presented to support the concept of a reduced GLP-1 secretory response in type 2 diabetic patients [206]. The discrepancies between different studies, in some cases even from the same laboratory, may reflect the quality of the assay methods used, especially in the late 1980s and early 1990s. On the other hand, both patient characteristics and their glucose concentrations could have had a direct influence on the release of incretin hormones, although such effects have not been clearly established.

Actions of GIP and GLP-1 in type 2 diabetic patients

A considerable number of reports are available that have examined the insulinotropic activity of exogenous GIP in type 2 diabetic patients. Typical infusion rates that gave rise to postprandial-like plasma concentrations were 0.8–1.5 pmol/kg^{-1}/min. In all studies the insulinotropic activity of exogenous GIP in type 2 diabetic patients was negligible [207–209]. When this was compared to healthy subjects, insulin responses in type 2 diabetic patients were reduced [210]. Whereas earlier studies used synthetic GIP of the porcine amino acid sequence, the same result has been reproduced using synthetic human GIP [53,211]. Therefore, there is little doubt that GIP has almost no insulinotropic activity in type 2 diabetic patients. It is not clear whether this is due to: (a) the general inability of diabetic β-cells to respond to any insulin secretory stimulus; (b) a loss of 'glucose-potentiation', because GIP is a glucose-dependent insulinotropic stimulus and may have a diminished effect simply because glucose no longer initiates the processes that are required for GIP to exert its insulinotropic effect; or (c) a specific 'GIP blindness' of type 2 diabetic β-cells. The latter is suggested by the potent insulinotropic effect of GIP's partner incretin hormone, GLP-1, in the same patients (see below).

As a whole, the effects mediated by GLP-1 counteract many of the peculiarities of the type 2 diabetic phenotype, namely: (a) disturbed glucose-induced insulin secretion [198]; (b) hyperglucagonaemia [212]; (c) abnormally rapid gastric emptying (which may occur in a subgroup of 'early type 2-diabetic patients' [213]); (d) a slight reduction in β-cell mass and pancreatic insulin content [214,215]; (e) hyperphagia/obesity [216]; and (f) insulin resistance [198]. Regarding the first five characteristics, there is general agreement that GLP-1 has the potential to be antidiabetogenic, but the effects of GLP-1 on insulin sensitivity remain contentious [174,176,177]; *in vivo* examinations describe at most minor influences of GLP-1 on insulin action, even at very high plasma concentrations [175].

Animal experiments had suggested a comparable reduction in insulinotropic activity of GIP and GLP-1 in streptozotocin-diabetic rats [217]. Surprisingly, however, pharmacological concentrations of GLP-1, in contrast to those of GIP, triggered an almost normal, rapid release of insulin in, 'mild', diet-treated type 2 diabetic patients, who were compared to control subjects under identical hyperglycaemic clamp conditions (8.75 mmol/l) [53,211]. Similar observations were made by Elahi *et al.* [218]. The other facets of GLP-1 bioactivity are also preserved in type 2 diabetic patients: glucagon concentrations are lowered [53,148,149] and gastric emptying is slowed [157], as in control subjects. A prominent direct effect of GLP-1 on insulin sensitivity or insulin resistance seems unlikely [177].

Gut hormones in type 1 diabetes

The secretion and action of GIP and GLP-1 have also studied in patients with type 1 diabetes. Since their main target is insulin secretion, and because islet β-cells are more or less destroyed in type 1 diabetes, their impact on islet function is smaller in this clinical situation. The secretion of GIP has been assessed in type 1 diabetic patients [44] and found to be reduced early after the diagnosis was made. During clinical remission ('honeymoon phase'), GIP secretion reverted to normal. This subject has been reviewed by Krarup [45].

Obviously, the insulinotropic response to the exogenous administration of GIP is smaller in type 1 diabetic patients than in type 2 diabetic patients and healthy volunteers [210].

Although the secretion of GLP-1 in patients with type 1 diabetes has not been studied, the effects of exogenous GLP-1 have been reported. When infused intravenously into fasting, insulinopenic, hyperglycaemic patients, glucagon is lowered by approximately 50% and plasma glucose reduced by 61 mg/dl (3.4 mmol/l) [153]. If administered before meals, the meal-related increment in glycaemia is reduced [219,220]. It is not clear whether this offers a useful adjunct to insulin treatment.

Pharmacological influences

Since it is recognised that gastric emptying has an impact on glycaemic control (discussed in Chapter 4), strategies to modify gastric emptying could potentially be used to optimise diabetic control. It can be postulated that pharmacological improvement of delayed gastric emptying, or slowing gastric emptying in patients with rapid emptying, would result in better glycaemic control. Potentially, even in patients with a normal velocity of gastric emptying, its retardation and the resulting slower entry of nutrients into the circulation could be improved by the altered metabolic capacity in patients with both type 1 and type 2 diabetes. In principle, this can be done using dietary manipulations or pharmacological approaches.

Gastric emptying

A number of studies have evaluated the effect of slowing of gastric emptying on glycaemic control in both type 1 and type 2 diabetes [5,221–224]. Thus, some food components, such as guar gum [225], soluble fibre [224] and low glycaemic index foods, have been shown to reduce postprandial hyperglycaemia in type 2 diabetes, presumably by retarding gastric emptying, as well as by slowing intestinal carbohydrate absorption. Pramlintide [223] and GLP-1 [5,220] reduce postprandial hyperglycaemia in patients with uncomplicated type 1 diabetes by slowing gastric emptying [226,227].

Native human amylin is relatively insoluble and has an inherent tendency to self-aggregate and adhere to various surfaces upon contact (discussed in Chapter 2). Pramlintide is a trisubstituted human amylin analogue, which has been shown to have biological activities comparable to that of human amylin [228]. In patients with uncomplicated type 1 diabetes, acute administration of pramlintide reduces postprandial hyperglycaemia [223,229,230], presumably as a result of slower gastric emptying [226,227]. Kong et al. [227] showed that an intravenous infusion of pramlintide markedly slowed emptying of both solid and liquid components of a meal. Since the dose of pramlintide used was clearly 'supraphysiological' and intravenous infusion of pramlintide would be impractical clinically, the dose–response effect of subcutaneous injections of pramlintide on gastric emptying was then examined. It was also determined whether administration of the drug before one meal had an impact on gastric emptying of a subsequent meal [226]. The three doses of pramlintide that were used all delayed emptying of the solid component of the first meal without any significant difference between them (Figure 8.4). Pramlintide had no effect on gastric emptying of the second meal (Figure 8.4).

In patients with type 2 diabetes, slowing of gastric emptying, whether induced by dietary modifications [224,231], administration of cholecystokinin [232], GLP-1 [5,157,220] or pramlintide [223], reduces postprandial glucose levels. In the subset of type 1 patients who have normal (or occasionally rapid) gastric emptying, pramlintide has the potential to be a useful adjunct to insulin treatment by slowing gastric emptying and optimising the coordination between absorption of ingested nutrients and insulin delivery. The beneficial effects of pramlintide may potentially be more marked in type 2 diabetic patients, since type 2 diabetes is characteristically associated with delayed insulin release and, occasionally, with accelerated gastric emptying [233–236]. This concept is supported by a study by Thompson et al. [223], who reported that an intravenous infusion of pramlintide reduced postprandial plasma glucose concentrations in type 2 diabetic patients. However, the beneficial effect of pramlintide was seen in insulin-treated patients and in patients treated with diet and/or oral hypoglycaemic agents (sulphonylureas) who had suboptimal glycaemic control (glycated haemoglobin > 8%). These patients presumably had more advanced ß-cell failure and lower amylin concentrations and it remains to be seen whether 'replacement' of amylin in this subset of patients will prove to be a new approach to the management of type 2 diabetes. Clinical trials to evaluate the long-term effects of modulation of gastric emptying on glycaemic control in both type 1 and type 2 diabetes are now required.

Intestinal function

Acarbose has been the first antidiabetic medication designed to act through an influence on intestinal functions. Basically, it is a carbohydrate-mimetic, acting as a competitive inhibitor of brush border enzymes known as α-glucosidases. Starch and certain oligo-, tri- and disaccharides are substrates that are digested more slowly in the presence of acarbose. This reduces the inflow of glucose into the circulation and moves chyme into lower parts of the gastrointestinal tract. As a consequence, acarbose primarily reduces postprandial glycaemic increments, but also lowers fasting glucose concentrations in the longer term. The accentuation of 'physiological malassimilation' (i.e. undigested carbohydrate reaching the large intestine) causes bacterial decomposition of remaining carbohydrates, leading to meteorism and flatulence in some patients. This can often be prevented

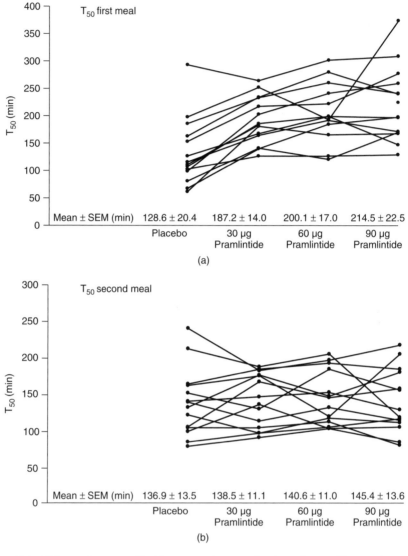

Figure 8.4 Effects of s.c. pramlintide on gastric emptying in patients with type 1 diabetes. (A) Half-emptying timer (T_{50}) of the solid component of the first meal after placebo, 30 μg, 60 μg and 90 μg pramlintide injections. (B) Half-emptying timer (T_{50}) of the solid component of the second meal after placebo, 30 μg, 60 μg and 90 μg pramlintide injections. All three doses of pramlintide delayed emptying of the solid component of the first meal to the same extent. There was no effect of any dose on gastric emptying of the second meal. From Kong *et al.* [226] with permission from Springer-Verlag © 1998

by starting treatment at a low dose (once daily, 25–50 mg) and increasing it over weeks (up to 50–100 mg three times daily); 5–10% of patients, certainly <15%, will have to stop treatment because of gastrointestinal side effects. While these side effects might be unpleasant, they are not dangerous. Acarbose is not absorbed from the gut to any substantial degree, so that it is free of serious side effects and may be used safely in patients with renal failure, for whom most other oral antidiabetic treatments are contraindicated. The overall effect on gly-caemia is equivalent to 0.5% reduction in glycated haemoglobin in the largest trial performed. This is somewhat less than that observed in response to sulpho-nylureas and metformin. Other α-glucosidase inhibitors have been used with similar success, e.g. miglitol. It has been demonstrated in healthy subjects that α-glucosidase inhibition augments endogenous, meal-induced GLP-1 secretion [237–239]. This might provide a novel and alternative approach to elevate GLP-1 plasma concentrations into the 'therapeutic' range, because clinically effective plasma levels are only three to four fold higher than concentrations measured after stimulating endogenous release by nutrient ingestion [53,240,241]. How-ever, the stimulation of GLP-1 secretion by α-galactosidase inhibition cannot be demonstrated in type 2 diabetic patients eating regular meals (Bergmann, Ritzel and Nauck, unpublished).

A similar approach has been taken to the treatment of obesity (including obese patients with type 2 diabetes), using a drug to inhibit the activity of pancreatic lipase. Thus, tetrahydrolipostatin (orlistat) reduces the digestion of dietary fat and is of value as part of a weight-reducing diet in the treatment of obesity [242].

GLP-1

Exogenous GLP-1 of the amino acid sequence (7–37) or (7–36 amide) typically leads to a true normalisation of plasma glucose concentrations into the physi-ological basal range: 60–100 mg/dl (3.3–5.6 mmol/l) within 3–4 h in fasting type 2 diabetic patients [148,149,240,241] (Figure 8.5). Continued administra-tion of GLP-1 does not lead to hypoglycaemia, because the insulinotropic actions [52,68,140,141] and the glucagonostatic effect [148,149,154] are strictly glucose-dependent and little or no insulin is secreted at glucose concentrations below 90 mg/dl (5 mmol/l), even with large doses of GLP-1. However, the glucose-lowering effect wanes after stopping the infusion [241,243]. Continued administration, on the other hand, leads to a reduction of postprandial glucose concentrations by GLP-1 [157,241]. In long-term experiments, the efficacy of intravenous GLP-1 in type 2 diabetic patients has been maintained for 7 days without loss of activity (tachyphylaxis) [244]. In animal experiments, there was no loss of activity over 5 days [142]. With repeated injections of GLP-1 in type 2 diabetic patients, stable effects were observed over a period up to 6 weeks [245,246,247]. The suppression of plasma glucagon concentrations by GLP-1 is also observed in type 1 diabetic patients [153]. As suggested by a delayed incre-ment in glucose, insulin, C-peptide, glucagon, and pancreatic polypeptide after meals after administration of GLP-1 in type 1-diabetic patients [175,219,220], the retarding effect on gastric emptying appears to be preserved in this group as well. The long-term intravenous infusion of peptide hormones such as GLP-1

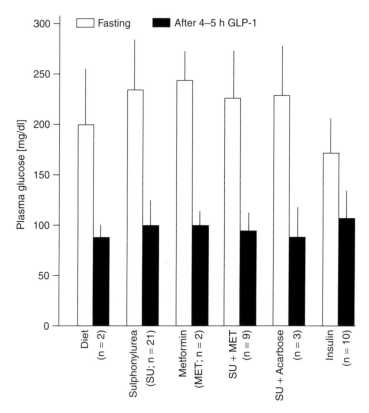

Figure 8.5 Comparison of GLP-1 effects in type 2 diabetic patients who had previously been treated with different approaches from diet to insulin (thus representing different stages of type 2 diabetes); 47 patients previously analysed and published [6,148,149,243,250] are shown. In each group, fasting glycaemia is shown as white columns (mean ±SD) and glucose concentrations measured 4–5 h after starting GLP-1 administrations (either intravenous infusions or two subcutaneous injections, 1.5 nmol/kg, given at 0 and 120 min) are shown. GLP-1 was equally effective in all groups of type 2 diabetic patients tested

is not a feasible approach to treat type 2 diabetic patients. Subcutaneous injections of GLP-1 produce large peaks in plasma concentrations which, however, are maintained for only a short duration [106,248–250]. Therefore, there are attempts to administer GLP-1 as a slow-release preparation. This can be achieved by, 'microencapsulation' [251] or by using biologically erodable microspheres [252]. A second approach is the development of GLP-1 analogues, which should ideally maintain all of the pharmacodynamic activities, while having a better pharmacokinetic profile (longer duration of action of up to 24 h [253]). Such GLP-1 derivatives or analogues are being developed for clinical studies [254]. In the long term, GLP-1 receptor agonists should preferably be short peptides (such as has been recently described for erythropoietin [255]) or even inorganic compounds that can be administered orally. A tablet has recently been described that is designed to adhere to the buccal mucosa and release its content (GLP-1) through direct absorption from the oral cavity [256]. At present, the resulting plasma profile resembles that observed after subcutaneous injection.

Exendin-4

Exendin-4 is a 39 amino acid peptide derived from the salivary secretions of *Heloderma suspectum* (the 'Gila monster'). It displays more than 50% sequence homology to GLP-1, and binds to the GLP-1 receptor with an affinity equal to, or even greater than, that of GLP-1 [257,258]. According to recent studies, exendin-4 shares many of the therapeutic activities of GLP-1, but is characterised by a considerably longer duration of action. Accordingly, a single subcutaneous injection of exendin-4 can maintain a lower average plasma glucose concentration in animal models of type 2 diabetes for 24 h [259]. There is no significant acute toxicity associated with exendin-4 administration to humans [260], so that clinical trials in patients with diabetes are being performed.

Dipeptidyl peptidase IV inhibition

The fact that 'therapeutic' concentrations of GLP-1 are three to four-fold higher [5,157,158] than normal postprandial concentrations [77,157] has led to the idea that activating or stimulating endogenous GLP-1 could represent a means of reducing plasma glucose in type 2 diabetic patients. Since the action of a ubiquitous exopeptidase, dipeptidyl peptidase IV (DPP IV) [46,105,106], rapidly inactivates GLP-1 by forming GLP-1 (9–36 amide/9–37), this enzyme has become a target for enhancing the biological activity of endogenous or exogenous GLP-1. First, GLP-1 analogues resistant to the action of DPP IV are being evaluated as longer-acting drugs [253]. Second, inhibitors of the enzyme are in early clinical trial phases, which are thought to provide evidence for an augmented incretin stimulation of insulin secretion (i.e. via halting degradation and inactivation of both GIP and GLP-1). In animal experiments, enhanced biological activity of GLP-1 has already been demonstrated [47,261,262]. The potency of these drugs will probably be limited by the fact that the DPP IV degradation product itself [GLP-1 (9–36 amide)] has a short half-life, so that complete inhibition of DPP IV alone can only be expected to triple the intact GLP-1 concentrations, without having a major effect on the duration of the postprandial elevation. Nevertheless, this approach makes sense, especially since the majority of GLP-1 already leaves the gut in its degraded, i.e. inactive, form. Initial clinical trials have demonstrated a beneficial effect on glucose concentrations and glycated haemoglobin levels in type 2 diabetic patients [263]. This is therefore a typical example of therapeutic interventions aiming at normoglycaemia by altering gastrointestinal function, in this case by modifying the gut's endocrine activity.

Outlook

The developments outlined above make the relation between gastrointestinal function and glycaemic control a matter that is not only of interest with regard to physiological processes, but is also of relevance to problems encountered in diabetes. Thus, the role of gastrointestinal factors in the pathophysiology of diabetes can be better understood by recent insights into the interplay of motility, nutrient absorption, hormone secretion and action, and metabolic adaptation. This field is expanding more and more into the area of pharmacology, with the development of several novel therapeutic strategies, e.g. amylin analogues (pramlintide), GLP-1 derivatives or analogues and specific inhibitors of peptide digestion/absorption. The successful development of these agents promises to expand therapeutic options for the treatment of diabetes mellitus.

References

1. Diabetes Control and Complications Trial Group, The effect of intensive treatment of diabetes on the development of long-term complications in insulin-dependent diabetes mellitus. *N Engl J Med* 1993; **329**: 977–86.
2. United Kingdom Prospective Diabetes Study Group, Intensive blood glucose control with sulphonylureas or insulin compared with conventional treatment and risk of complications in patients with type 2 diabetes (UKPDS 33). *Lancet* 1998; **352**: 837–53.
3. Moore B, Edie ES, Abram JH. On the treatment of diabetes mellitus by acid extract of duodenal mucous membrane. *Biochem J* 1906; **1**: 28–38.
4. Zunz E, and La Barre J. Contributions a l'étude des variations physiologiques de la sérétion interne du pancréas: relations entre les sérétions externe et interne di pancréas. *Arch Int Physiol* 1929; **31**: 20–44.
5. Nauck MA *et al*. Glucagon-like peptide-1 (GLP-1) as a new therapeutic approach for Type 2 diabetes. *Exp Clin Endocrinol Diabetes* 1997; **105**: 187–95.
6. Nauck MA, Holst JJ, Willms B. Glucagon-like peptide 1 and its potential in the treatment of non-insulin-dependent diabetes mellitus. *Horm Metab Res* 1997; **29**: 411–6.
7. Berson SA, Yalow RS. Immunoassay of plasma insulin. *Ciba Coll Endocrinol* 1962; **41**: 182–201.
8. Elrick H *et al*. Plasma insulin response to oral and intravenous glucose administration. *J Clin Endocrinol Metab* 1964; **24**: 1076–82.
9. McIntyre N, Holdsworth CD, Turner DS. Intestinal factors in the control of insulin secretion. *J Clin Endocrinol* 1965; **25**: 1317–24.
10. Perley MJ, Kipnis DM. Plasma insulin responses to oral and intravenous glucose: studies in normal and diabetic subjects. *J Clin Invest* 1967; **46**: 1954–62.
11. Creutzfeldt W. The incretin concept today. *Diabetologia* 1979; **16**: 75–85.
12. Unger RH, Eisentraut AM. Entero-insular axis. *Arch Int Med* 1969; **123**: 261–6.
13. Nauck MA *et al*. Incretin effects of increasing glucose loads in man calculated from venous insulin and C-peptide responses. *J Clin Endocrinol Metab* 1986; **63**: 492–8.
14. Nauck M *et al*. Reduced incretin effect in type 2 (non-insulin-dependent) diabetes. *Diabetologia* 1986; **29**: 46–54.
15. Tillil H *et al*. Dose-dependent effects of oral and intravenous glucose on insulin secretion and clearance in normal humans. *Am J Physiol* 1988; **254**: E349–57.

16. Shuster LT *et al.* Incretin effect due to increased secretion and decreased clearance of insulin in normal humans. *Diabetes* 1988; **37**: 200–203.

17. Brown JC *et al.* Preparation of highly active enterogastrone. *Can J Physiol Pharmacol* 1969; **47**: 113–14.

18. Brown JC, Mutt V, Pederson RA. Further purification of a polypeptide demonstrating enterogastrone activity. *J Physiol* 1970; **209**: 57–64.

19. Pederson RA, Brown JC. Inhibition of histamine-, pentagastrin- and insulin-stimulated canine gastric secretion by pure 'gastric inhibitory polypeptide'. *Gastroenterology* 1972; **62**: 393–400.

20. Nauck MA *et al.* Lack of effect of synthetic human gastric inhibitory polypeptide and glucagon-like peptide 1 (7–36 amide) infused at near-physiological concentrations on pentagastrin-stimulated gastric acid secretion in normal human subjects. *Digestion* 1992; **52**: 214–21.

21. Dupré J *et al.* Stimulation of insulin secretion by gastric inhibitory polypeptide in man. *J Clin Endocrinol Metab* 1973; **37**: 826–8.

22. Brown JC, Pederson RA. GI hormones and insulin secretion. In *Endocrinology. Proceedings of the Vth International Congress Endocrinology* 1976; vol 2, 568–70.

23. Buffa B *et al.* Identification of the intestinal cell storing gastric inhibitory polypeptide. *Histochemistry* 1975; **43**: 249–55.

24. Buchan AMJ *et al.* Electron immunocytochemical evidence of the K cell localisation of gastric inhibitory polypeptide (GIP) in man. *Histochemistry* 1978; **56**: 37–44.

25. Takeda J *et al.* Sequence of an intestinal cDNA encoding human gastric inhibitory polypeptide precursor. *Proc Natl Acad Sci USA* 1987; **84**: 7005–8.

26. Inagaki N *et al.* Gastric inhibitory polypeptide: structure and chromosomal location of the human gene. *Mol Endocrinol* 1989; **3**: 1014–21.

27. Tseng CC *et al.* Glucose-dependent insulinotropic peptide: structure of the precursor and tissue-specific expression in rat. *Proc Natl Acad Sci USA* 1993; **90**: 1992–6.

28. Wolfe M *et al.* Glucose-dependent insulinotropic polypeptide (GIP). In Greeley GHJ (ed.). *Gastrointestinal Endocrinology*. Humana: Totowa, NJ, 1999; 439–66.

29. Tseng CC, Jarboe LA, Wolfe MM. Regulation of glucose-dependent insulinotropic peptide gene expression by a glucose meal. *Am J Physiol* 1994; **266**: G887–91.

30. Pederson RA, Schubert HE, Brown JC. Gastric inhibitory polypeptide. Its physiologic release and insulinotropic action in the dog. *Diabetes* 1975; **24**: 1050–56.

31. Cleator IG, Gourlay RH. Release of immunoreactive gastric inhibitory polypeptide (IR-GIP) by oral ingestion of food substances. *Am J Surg* 1975; **130**: 128–35.

32. Sykes S *et al.* Evidence for preferential stimulation of gastric inhibitory polypeptide secretion by the rat by actively transported carbohydrates and their analogues. *J Endocrinol* 1980; **5**: 210–17.

33. Sirinek KR *et al.* Release of gastric inhibitory polypeptide: comparison of glucose and fat as stimuli. *Surg Forum* 1974; **25**: 361–3.

34. Krarup T, Holst JJ, Larsen KL. Responses and heterogeneity of IR-GIP after intraduodenal glucose and fat. *Am J Physiol* 1985; **249**: E195–E200.

35. Horowitz M *et al.* The effect of short-term dietary supplementation with glucose on gastric emptying of glucose and fructose and oral glucose tolerance in normal subjects. *Diabetologia* 1996; **39**: 481–6.

36. O'Dorisio TM, Cataland S. Effect of diet on GIP release. In *Gut hormones*. Bloom SR, Polak JM. (eds), Churchill Livingstone: Edinburgh, 1981; 269–72.

37. Thomas FB *et al.* Stimulation of secretion of gastric inhibitory polypeptide and insulin by intraduodenal amino acid perfusion. *Gastroenterology* 1976; **70**: 523–7.

38. Thomas FB *et al.* Selective release of gastric inhibitory polypeptide release by intraduodenal amino acid perfusion in man. *Gastroenterology* 1978; **74**: 1261–5.

39. Sarson DL, Bryant MG, Bloom SR. A radioimmunoassay of gastric inhibitory polypeptide in human plasma. *J Endocrinol* 1980; **85**: 487–96.

40. Fieseler P, *et al*. Physiological augmentation of amino acid-induced insulin secretion by GIP and GLP-I but not by CCK-8. *Am J Physiol* 1995; **268**: E949–55.

41. Ebert R, Illmer K, Creutzfeldt W. Release of gastric inhibitory polypeptide (GIP) by intraduodenal acidification in rats and humans and abolition of the incretin effect of acid by GIP-antiserum in rats. *Gastroenterology* 1979; **76**: 515–23.

42. Ebert R, Creutzfeldt W. Decreased GIP secretion through impairment of absorption. In Wimersma Greidanus TB (ed.), *Frontiers in Hormone Research*. Karger: Basel, 1980; 192–201.

43. Ebert R, Creutzfeldt W. Reversal of impaired GIP and insulin secretion in patients with pancreatogenic steatorrhea following enzyme substitution. *Diabetologia* 1980; **19**: 198–204.

44. Krarup T *et al*. Diminished immuno-reactive gastric inhibitory polypeptide response to a meal in newly diagnosed type I diabetics. *J Clin Endocrinol Metab* 1983; **56**: 1306–12.

45. Krarup T. Immunoreactive gastric inhibitory polypeptide. *Endocrinol Rev* 1988; **9**: 122–33.

46. Mentlein R, Gallwitz B, Schmidt WE. Dipeptidyl-peptidase IV hydrolyses gastric inhibitory polypeptide, glucagon-like peptide-1(7–36)amide, peptide histidine methionine and is responsible for their degradation in human serum. *Eur J Biochem* 1993; **214**: 829–35.

47. Deacon CF *et al*. Dipeptidyl peptidase IV inhibition reduces the degradation and clearance of GIP and potentiates its insulinotropic and antihyperglycemic effects in anesthetized pigs. *Diabetes* 2001; **50**: 1588–97.

48. Schmidt WE *et al*. Commercially available preparations of porcine glucose-dependent insulinotropic polypeptide (GIP) contain a biologically inactive GIP-fragment and cholecystokinin-33–39. *Endocrinology* 1987; **120**: 835–7.

49. Kieffer TJ, McIntosh CH, Pederson RA. Degradation of glucose-dependent insulinotropic polypeptide and truncated glucagon-like peptide 1 *in vitro* and *in vivo* by dipeptidyl peptidase IV. *Endocrinology* 1995; **136**: 3585–96.

50. Elahi D *et al*. Pancreatic α- and β-cell responses to GIP infusion in normal man. *Am J Physiol* 1979; **237**: E185–91.

51. Sarson DL, Hayter RC, Bloom SR. The pharmacokinetics of porcine glucose-dependent insulinotropic polypeptide (GIP) in man. *Eur J Clin Invest* 1982; **12**: 457–61.

52. Nauck MA *et al*. Additive insulinotropic effects of exogenous synthetic human gastric inhibitory polypeptide and glucagon-like peptide-1-(7–36) amide infused at near-physiological insulinotropic hormone and glucose concentrations. *J Clin Endocrinol Metab* 1993; **76**: 912–17.

53. Nauck MA *et al*. Preserved incretin activity of glucagon-like peptide 1 (7–36 amide) but not of synthetic human gastric inhibitory polypeptide in patients with type 2 diabetes mellitus. *J Clin Invest* 1993; **91**: 301–7.

54. O'Dorisio TM *et al*. Renal effects on serum gastric inhibitory polypeptide (GIP). *Metabolism* 1977; **26**: 651–6.

55. Chap Z *et al*. Absence of hepatic extraction of gastric inhibitory polypeptide in conscious dogs. *Dig Dis Sci* 1987; **32**: 280–84.

56. Hanks JB *et al*. The hepatic extraction of gastric inhibitory polypeptide and insulin. *Endocrinology* 1984; **115**: 1011–18.

57. Usdin TB *et al*. Gastric inhibitory polypeptide receptor, a member of the secretin-vasoactive intestinal peptide receptor family, is widely distributed in peripheral organs and the brain. *Endocrinology* 1993; **133**: 2861–70.

58. Gremlich S *et al*. Cloning, functional expression, and chromosomal localization of the human pancreatic islet glucose-dependent insulinotropic polypeptide receptor. *Diabetes* 1995; **44**: 1202–8.

59. Yamada Y *et al*. Human gastric inhibitory polypeptide receptor: cloning of the gene (GIPR) and cDNA. *Genomics* 1995; **29**: 773–6.

60. Stoffel M *et al*. Assignment of the gastric inhibitory polypeptide receptor gene (GIPR) to chromosome band 19q13.2–q13.3 by fluorescence *in situ* hybridization. *Genomics* 1995; **28**: 607–9.

61. Volz A *et al*. Molecular cloning, functional expression, and signal transduction of the GIP-receptor cloned from a human insulinoma. *FEBS Lett* 1995; **373**: 23–9.

62. Lacroix A *et al*. Gastric inhibitory polypeptide-dependent cortisol hypersecretion—a new cause of Cushing's syndrome. *N Engl J Med* 1992; **327**: 974–80.

63. Göke R *et al*. Exendin-4 is a high potency agonist and truncated exendin-(9–39)-amide an antagonist at the glucagon-like peptide 1-(7–36)-amide receptor of insulin-secreting β-cells. *J Biol Chem* 1993; **268**: 19650–5.

64. Thorens B *et al*. Cloning and functional expression of the human islet GLP-1 receptor. Demonstration that exendin-4 is an agonist and exendin-(9–39) an antagonist of the receptor. *Diabetes* 1993; **42**: 1678–82.

65. Wheeler MB *et al*. Functional expression of the rat pancreatic islet glucose-dependent insulinotropic polypeptide receptor: ligand binding and intracellular signaling properties. *Endocrinology* 1995; **136**: 4629–39.

66. Siegel EG *et al*. Comparison of the effect of GIP and GLP-1 (7–36 amide) on insulin release from rat pancreatic islets. *Eur J Clin Invest* 1992; **22**: 154–7.

67. Gromada J, Holst JJ, Rorsman P. Cellular regulation of islet hormone secretion by the incretin hormone glucagon-like peptide 1. *Pflügers Arch Eur J Physiol* 1998; **435**: 583–94.

68. Kreymann B *et al*. Glucagon-like peptide-1 7–36: a physiological incretin in man. *Lancet* 1987; **2**: 1300–304.

69. Nauck MA *et al*. Insulinotropic properties of synthetic gastric inhibitory peptide in man: interactions with glucose, phenylalanine, and cholecystokinin-8. *J Clin Endocrinol Metab* 1989; **69**: 654–62.

70. Pederson RA, Brown JC. The insulinotropic action of gastric inhibitory polypeptide in the perfused rat pancreas. *Endocrinology* 1976; **99**: 780–85.

71. Dupré J *et al*. Stimulation of glucagon secretion by gastric inhibitory polypeptide in patients with hepatic cirrhosis and hyperglucagonemia. *J Clin Endocrinol Metab* 1991; **72**: 125–9.

72. Ebert R, Aschenbeck J, Creutzfeldt W. Wirkung von humanem Gastric Inhibitory Polypeptide (GIP) auf die Magenentleerung (abstr). *Z Gastroenterol* 1989; **27**: 516.

73. Maxwell V *et al*. Effect of gastric inhibitory polypeptide on pentagastrin-stimulated acid secretion in man. *Dig Dis Sci* 1980; **24**: 113–16.

74. Bell GI *et al*. Exon duplication and divergence in the human preproglucagon gene. *Nature* 1983; **304**: 368–71.

75. Lopez LC *et al*. Mammalian pancreatic proglucagon contains three glucagon-related peptides. *Proc Natl Acad Sci USA* 1983; **80**: 5485–9.

76. Ørskov C *et al*. Complete sequences of glucagon-like peptide-1 from human and pig small intestine. *J Biol Chem* 1989; **264**: 12826–9.

77. Ørskov C *et al*. Tissue and plasma concentrations of amidated and glycine-extended glucagon-like peptide 1 in humans. *Diabetes* 1994; **43**: 535–9.

78. Holst JJ. Glucagon-like peptide 1: a newly discovered gastrointestinal hormone. *Gastroenterology* 1994; **107**: 1848–55.

79. Mojsov S, Weir GC, Habener JF. Insulinotropin: glucagon-like peptide I (7–37) co-encoded in the glucagon gene is a potent stimulator of insulin release in the perfused rat pancreas. *J Clin Invest* 1987; **79**: 616–19.

80. Ørskov C *et al*. Pancreatic and intestinal processing of proglucagon in man. *Diabetologia* 1987; **30**: 874–81.

81. Patzelt C, Schiltz E. Conversion of proproglucagon in pancreatic α-cells: the major endproducts are glucagon and a single peptide, the major proglucagon fragment, that contains two glucagon-like peptides. *Proc Natl Acad Sci USA* 1984; **81**: 5007–11.

82. Ørskov C *et al*. Glucagon-like peptide 1 receptors in the subfornical organ and the area postrema are accessible to circulating glucagon-like peptide 1. *Diabetes* 1996; **45**: 832–5.

83. Rouillé Y *et al*. Proglucagon is processed to glucagon by prohormone convertase PC2 in α TC1-6 cells. *Proc Natl Acad Sci USA* 1994; **91**: 3242–6.

84. Rouillé Y, Martin S, Steiner DF. Differential processing of proglucagon by the sub-tilisin-like prohormone convertase PC2 and PC3 to generate either glucagon or glucagon-like peptide. *J Biol Chem* 1995; **270**: 26488–96.

85. Dhanvantari S, Seidah NG, Brubaker PL. Role of prohormone convertases in the tissue-specific processing of proglucagon. *Mol Endocrinol* 1996; **10**: 342–55.

86. Varndell IM *et al*. Localization of glucagon-like peptide (GLP) immunoreactants in human gut and pancreas using light and electron microscopic immunocytochemistry. *J Histochem Cytochem* 1985; **33**: 1080–86.

87. Ørskov C. Glucagon-like peptide-1, a new hormone of the entero-insular axis. *Diabetologia* 1992; **35**: 701–11.

88. Eissele R *et al*. Glucagon-like peptide-1 cells in the gastrointestinal tract and pancreas of rat, pig and man. *Eur J Clin Invest* 1992; **22**: 283–91.

89. Ørskov C *et al*. Glucagon-like peptides GLP-1 and GLP-2, predicted products of the glucagon gene, are secreted separately from pig small intestine but not pancreas. *Endocrinology* 1986; **119**: 1467–75.

90. Shima K *et al*. Release of glucagon-like peptide 1 immunoreactivity from the perfused rat pancreas. *Acta Endocrinol Copenh* 1987; **114**: 531–6.

91. Sasaki H *et al*. GLP-1 secretion coupled with Na/glucose transporter from the isolated perfused canine ileum. *Digestion* 1993; **54**: 365–7.

92. Herrmann C *et al*. Glucagon-like peptide-1 and glucose-dependent insulin-releasing polypeptide plasma levels in response to nutrients. *Digestion* 1995; **56**: 117–26.

93. Herrmann-Rinke C *et al*. Regulation of glucagon-like peptide-1 secretion from rat ileum by neurotransmitters and peptides. *J Endocrinol* 1995; **147**: 25–31.

94. Rocca AS, Brubaker PL. Stereospecific effects of fatty acids on proglucagon-derived peptide secretion in fetal rat intestinal cultures. *Endocrinology* 1995; **136**: 5593–9.

95. Kong MF *et al*. Effects of oral fructose and glucose on plasma GLP-1 and appetite in normal subjects. *Peptides* 1999; **20**: 545–51.

96. Nauck MA *et al*. Release of glucagon-like peptide 1 [GLP-1 (7–36 amide)], gastric inhibitory polypeptide (GIP) and insulin in response to oral glucose after upper and lower intestinal resections. *Z Gastroenterol* 1996; **34**: 159–66.

97. Schirra J *et al*. Gastric emptying and release of incretin hormones after glucose ingestion in humans. *J Clin Invest* 1996; **97**: 92–103.

98. Dumoulin V *et al*. Regulation of glucagon-like peptide-1-(7–36) amide, peptide YY, and neurotensin secretion by neurotransmitters and gut hormones in the isolated vascularly perfused rat ileum. *Endocrinology* 1995; **136**: 5182–8.

99. Hoyt EC *et al*. Effects of fasting, refeeding, and intraluminal triglyceride on proglucagon expression in jejunum and ileum. *Diabetes* 1996; **45**: 434–9.

100. Reimer RA, McBurney MI. Dietary fiber modulates intestinal proglucagon messenger ribonucleic acid and postprandial secretion of glucagon-like peptide-1 and insulin in rats. *Endocrinology* 1996; **137**: 3948–56.

101. Ranganath LR *et al*. Attenuated GLP-1 secretion in obesity: cause or consequence? *Gut* 1996; **38**: 916–19.

102. Turton MD *et al*. A role for glucagon-like peptide-1 in the central regulation of feeding. *Nature* 1996; **379**: 69–72.

103. Flint A *et al*. Glucagon-like peptide-1 promotes satiety and suppresses energy intake in humans. *J Clin Invest* 1998; **101**: 515–20.

104. Ørskov C, Holst JJ. Radio-immunoassays for glucagon-like peptides 1 and 2 (GLP-1 and GLP-2). *Scand J Clin Lab Invest* 1987; **47**: 165–74.

105. Deacon CF, Johnsen AH, Holst JJ. Degradation of glucagon-like peptide-1 by human plasma *in vitro* yields an N-terminally truncated peptide that is a major endogenous metabolite *in vivo*. *J Clin Endocrinol Metab* 1995; **80**: 952–7.

106. Deacon CF *et al*. Both subcutaneously and intravenously administered glucagon-like peptide 1 are rapidly degraded from the NH_2-terminus in type 2 diabetic patients and in healthy subjects. *Diabetes* 1995; **44**: 1126–31.

107. Grandt D *et al*. Is GLP-1 (9–36)amide an endogenous antagonist at GLP-1 receptors? (abstr). *Digestion* 1994; **55**: 302.

108. Pridal L *et al*. Comparison of sandwich enzyme-linked immunoadsorbent assay and radioimmunoassay for determination of exogenous glucagon-like peptide-1(7–36)amide in plasma. *J Pharm Biomed Anal* 1995; **13**: 841–50.

109. Deacon CF *et al*. Glucagon-like peptide 1 undergoes differential tissue-specific metabolism in the anesthetized pig. *Am J Physiol Endocrinol Metab* 1996; **271**: E458–64.

110. Miholic J *et al*. Emptying of the gastric substitute, glucagon-like peptide-1 (GLP-1), and reactive hypoglycemia after total gastrectomy. *Dig Dis Sci* 1991; **36**: 1361–70.

111. Miholic J *et al*. Postprandial release of glucagon-like peptide-1, pancreatic glucagon, and insulin after esophageal resection. *Digestion* 1993; **54**: 73–8.

112. Thorens B. Expression cloning of the pancreatic beta cell receptor for the gluco-incretin hormone glucagon-like peptide 1. *Proc Natl Acad Sci USA* 1992; **89**: 8641–5.

113. Heller RS, Aponte GW. Intra-islet regulation of hormone secretion by glucagon-like peptide-1-(7–36) amide. *Am J Physiol* 1995; **269**: G852–60.

114. Moens K *et al*. Expression and functional activity of glucagon, glucagon-like peptide 1, and glucose-dependent insulinotropic peptide receptors in rat pancreatic islet cells. *Diabetes* 1996; **45**: 257–61.

115. Kofod H, Kirk O, Adelhorst K. β-Cell receptors for glucagon/GLP-1? Properties of exendin(9–39) in mouse islets. *Acta Physiol Scand* 1996; **157**: 347.

116. Bullock BP, Heller RS, Habener JF. Tissue distribution of messenger ribonucleic acid encoding the rat glucagon-like peptide-1 receptor. *Endocrinology* 1996; **137**: 2968–78.

117. Campos RV, Lee YC, Drucker DJ. Divergent tissue-specific and developmental expression of receptors for glucagon and glucagon-like peptide-1 in the mouse. *Endocrinology* 1994; **134**: 2156–64.

118. Wei Y, Mojsov S. Tissue-specific expression of the human receptor for glucagon-like peptide-1: brain, heart and pancreatic forms have the same deduced amino acid sequences. *FEBS Lett* 1995; **358**: 219–24.

119. Wei Y, Mojsov S. Distribution of GLP-1 and PACAP receptors in human tissues. *Acta Physiol Scand* 1996; **157**: 355–7.

120. Scrocchi LA *et al*. Glucose intolerance but normal satiety in mice with a null mutation in the glucagon-like peptide 1 receptor gene. *Nature Med* 1996; **2**: 1254–8.

121. Scrocchi LA *et al*. Identification of glucagon-like peptide 1 (GLP-1) actions essential for glucose homeostasis in mice with disruption of GLP-1 receptor signaling. *Diabetes* 1998; **47**(4): 632–9.

122. Scrocchi LA *et al*. Elimination of glucagon-like peptide 1R signaling does not modify weight gain and islet adaptation in mice with combined disruption of leptin and GLP-1 action. *Diabetes* 2000; **49**: 1552–60.

123. Göke R *et al*. Signal transmission after GLP-1(7–36)amide binding in RINm5F cells. *Am J Physiol* 1989; **257**: G397–401.

124. Yada T, Itoh K, Nakata M. Glucagon-like peptide-1-(7–36)amide and a rise in cyclic adenosine $3',5'$-monophosphate increase cytosolic free Ca^{2+} in rat pancreatic β-cells by enhancing Ca^{2+} channel activity. *Endocrinology* 1993; **133**: 1685–92.

125. Britsch S *et al*. Glucagon-like peptide-1 modulates Ca^{2+} current but not K^+ ATP current in intact mouse pancreatic β-cells. *Biochem Biophys Res Commun* 1995; **207**: 33–9.

126. Holz GG, Kuhtreiber WM, Habener JF. Pancreatic β-cells are rendered glucose-competent by the insulinotropic hormone glucagon-like peptide-1(7–37). *Nature* 1993; **361**: 362–5.

127. Holz GG, Leech CA, Habener JF. Activation of a cAMP-regulated Ca^{2+}-signaling pathway in pancreatic β-cells by the insulinotropic hormone glucagon-like peptide-1. *J Biol Chem* 1995; **270**: 17749–57.

128. Kato M, Ma HT, Tatemoto K. GLP-1 depolarizes the rat pancreatic β-cell in a Na^+-dependent manner. *Regul Pept* 1996; **62**: 23–7.

129. Kolligs F *et al*. Reduction of the incretin effect in rats by the glucagon-like peptide 1 receptor antagonist exendin (9–39) amide. *Diabetes* 1995; **44**: 16–19.

130. Wang Z *et al*. Glucagon-like peptide-1 is a physiological incretin in rat. *J Clin Invest* 1995; **95**: 417–21.

131. Ørskov C, Holst JJ, Nielsen OV. Effect of truncated glucagon-like peptide-1 [proglucagon-(78–107) amide] on endocrine secretion from pig pancreas, antrum, and non-antral stomach. *Endocrinology* 1988; **123**: 2009–13.

132. Kawai K *et al*. Comparison of the effects of glucagon-like peptide-1-(1–37) and -(7–37) and glucagon on islet hormone release from isolated perfused canine and rat pancreases. *Endocrinology* 1989; **124**: 1768–73.

133. Fehmann HC, Göke R, Göke B. Cell and molecular biology of the incretin hormones glucagon-like peptide-1 and glucose-dependent insulin releasing polypeptide. *Endocr Rev* 1995; **16**: 390–410.

134. Buteau J *et al*. Glucagon-like peptide-1 promotes DNA synthesis, activates phosphatidylinositol 3-kinase and increases transcription factor pancreatic and duodenal homeobox gene 1 (PDX-1) DNA binding activity in β(INS-1)-cells. *Diabetologia* 1999; **42**: 856–64.

135. Buteau J *et al*. Glucagon-like peptide 1 induces pancreatic β-cell proliferation via transactivation of the epidermal growth factor receptor. *Diabetes* 2003; **52**: 124–32.

136. Perfetti R *et al*. Glucagon-like peptide-1 induces cell proliferation and pancreatic-duodenum homeobox-1 expression and increases endocrine cell mass in the pancreas of old, glucose-intolerant rats. *Endocrinology* 2000; **141**: 4600–605.

137. Hui H, Wright C, Perfetti R. Glucagon-like peptide 1 induces differentiation of islet duodenal homeobox-1-positive pancreatic ductal cells into insulin-secreting cells. *Diabetes* 2001; **50**: 785–96.

138. Farilla L *et al*. Glucagon-like peptide-1 promotes islet cell growth and inhibits apoptosis in Zucker diabetic rats. *Endocrinology* 2002; **143**: 4397–408.

139. Bulotta A *et al*. Cultured pancreatic ductal cells undergo cell cycle re-distribution and β-cell-like differentiation in response to glucagon-like peptide-1. *J Mol Endocrinol* 2002; **29**: 347–60.

140. Göke R *et al.* Glucose-dependency of the insulin stimulatory effect of glucagon-like peptide-1 (7–36) amide on the rat pancreas. *Res Exp Med Berl* 1993; **193**: 97–103.

141. Qualmann C *et al.* Insulinotropic actions of intravenous glucagon-like peptide-1 (GLP-1) (7–36 amide) in the fasting state in healthy subjects. *Acta Diabetol* 1995; **32**: 13–16.

142. Hargrove DM *et al.* Glucose-dependent action of glucagon-like peptide-1 (7–37) *in vivo* during short- or long-term administration. *Metabolism* 1995; **44**: 1231–7.

143. Gromada J *et al.* Stimulation of cloned human glucagon-like peptide 1 receptor expressed in HEK 293 cells induces cAMP-dependent activation of calcium-induced calcium release. *FEBS Lett* 1995; **373**: 182–6.

144. Gromada J *et al.* Glucagon-like peptide I increases cytoplasmic calcium in insulin-secreting βTC3-cells by enhancement of intracellular calcium mobilization. *Diabetes* 1995; **44**: 767–74.

145. Gromada J *et al.* Multisite regulation of insulin secretion by cAMP-increasing agonists: evidence that glucagon-like peptide 1 and glucagon act via distinct receptors. *Pflüger's Arch* 1997; **434**: 515–24.

146. Gromada J *et al.* Glucagon-like peptide 1 (7–36) amide stimulates exocytosis in human pancreatic β-cells by both proximal and distal regulatory steps in stimulus-secretion coupling. *Diabetes* 1998; **47**: 57–65.

147. Suga S *et al.* GLP-1 (7–36) amide activates L-type Ca^{2+} channels of pancreatic β-cells through cAMP signaling. *Jpn J Physiol* 1997; **47**(suppl 1): S13–14.

148. Nauck MA *et al.* Normalization of fasting hyperglycaemia by exogenous glucagon-like peptide 1 (7–36 amide) in type 2 (non-insulin-dependent) diabetic patients. *Diabetologia* 1993; **36**: 741–4.

149. Nauck MA *et al.* Normalization of fasting glycaemia by intravenous GLP-1 [(7–36 amide) or (7–37)] in type 2-diabetic patients. *Diabetic Med* 1998; **15**: 937–45.

150. Hargrove DM *et al.* Comparison of the glucose dependency of glucagon-like peptide-1 (7–37) and glyburide *in vitro* and *in vivo*. *Metabolism* 1996; **45**: 404–9.

151. Toft-Nielsen M *et al.* No effect of β-adrenergic blockade on hypoglycaemic effect of glucagon-like peptide-1 (GLP-1) in normal subjects. *Diabet Med* 1996; **13**: 544–8.

152. Komatsu R *et al.* Glucagonostatic and insulinotropic action of glucagonlike peptide I-(7–36)-amide. *Diabetes* 1989; **38**: 902–5.

153. Creutzfeldt WO *et al.* Glucagonostatic actions and reduction of fasting hyperglycemia by exogenous glucagon-like peptide I(7–36) amide in type 1 diabetic patients. *Diabetes Care* 1996; **19**: 580–86.

154. Nauck MA *et al.* Effects of glucagon-like peptide 1 on counterregulatory hormone responses, cognitive functions, and insulin secretion during hyperinsulinemic, stepped hypoglycemic clamp experiments in healthy volunteers. *J Clin Endocrinol Metab* 2002; **87**: 1239–46.

155. Wettergren A *et al.* Truncated GLP-1 (proglucagon 78–107 amide) inhibits gastric and pancreatic functions in man. *Dig Dis Sci* 1993; **38**: 665–73.

156. Wettergren A *et al.* Glucagon-like peptide-1 7–36 amide and peptide YY from the L-cell of the ileal mucosa are potent inhibitors of vagally induced gastric acid secretion in man. *Scand J Gastroenterol* 1994; **29**: 501–5.

157. Willms B *et al.* Gastric emptying, glucose responses, and insulin secretion after a liquid test meal: effects of exogenous glucagon-like peptide-1 (GLP-1)-(7–36) amide in type 2 (non-insulin-dependent) diabetic patients. *J Clin Endocrinol Metab* 1996; **81**: 327–32.

158. Nauck MA *et al.* Glucagon-like peptide 1 inhibition of gastric emptying outweighs its insulinotropic effects in healthy humans. *Am J Physiol* 1997; **273**: E981–8.

159. Schjoldager BT *et al.* GLP-1 (glucagon-like peptide 1) and truncated GLP-1, fragments of human proglucagon, inhibit gastric acid secretion in humans. *Dig Dis Sci* 1989; **34**: 703–8.

160. O' Halloran DJ *et al*. Glucagon-like peptide-1 (7–36)-NH$_2$: a physiological inhibitor of gastric acid secretion in man. *J Endocrinol* 1990; **126**: 169–73.
161. Ruiz Grande C *et al*. Lipolytic action of glucagon-like peptides in isolated rat adipocytes. *Peptides* 1992; **13**: 13–16.
162. Villanueva Penacarrillo ML *et al*. Potent glycogenic effect of GLP-1(7–36)amide in rat skeletal muscle. *Diabetologia* 1994; **37**: 1163–6.
163. Egan JM *et al*. Glucagon-like peptide-1(7–36) amide (GLP-1) enhances insulin-stimulated glucose metabolism in 3T3-L1 adipocytes: one of several potential extrapancreatic sites of GLP-1 action. *Endocrinology* 1994; **135**: 2070–75.
164. Valverde I *et al*. Glucagon-like peptide 1: a potent glycogenic hormone. *FEBS Lett* 1994; **349**: 313–16.
165. Valverde I, VillanuevaPenacarrillo ML. *In vitro* insulinomimetic effects of GLP-1 in liver, muscle and fat. *Acta Physiol Scand* 1996; **157**: 359–60.
166. Miki H *et al*. Glucagon-like peptide-1(7–36)amide enhances insulin-stimulated glucose uptake and decreases intracellular cAMP content in isolated rat adipocytes. *Biochim Biophys Acta* 1996; **1312**: 132–6.
167. Fürnsinn C, Ebner K, Waldhäusl W. Failure of GLP-1(7–36)amide to affect glycogenesis in rat skeletal muscle. *Diabetologia* 1995; **38**: 864–7.
168. Nakagawa Y *et al*. Glucagon-like peptide-1 (7–36) amide and glycogen synthesis in the liver. *Diabetologia* 1997; **40**: 1241–2.
169. Merida E *et al*. Presence of glucagon and glucagon-like peptide-1-(7–36)amide receptors in solubilized membranes of human adipose tissue. *J Clin Endocrinol Metab* 1993; **77**: 1654–7.
170. Valverde E *et al*. Immunocytochemical and ultrastructural characterization of endocrine cells and nerves in the intestine of *Rana temporaria*. *Tissue Cell* 1993; **25**: 505–16.
171. Valverde I *et al*. Presence and characterization of glucagon-like peptide-1(7–36) amide receptors in solubilized membranes of rat adipose tissue. *Endocrinology* 1993; **132**: 75–9.
172. Villanueva Penacarrillo ML *et al*. Glucagon-like peptide-1 binding to rat hepatic membranes. *J Endocrinol* 1995; **146**: 183–9.
173. Delgado E *et al*. Glucagon-like peptide-1 binding to rat skeletal muscle. *Peptides* 1995; **16**: 225–9.
174. Toft-Nielsen M-B, Madsbad S, Holst JJ. The effect of glucagon-like peptide I (GLP-1) on glucose elimination in healthy subjects depends on the pancreatic glucoregulatory hormones. *Diabetes* 1996; **45**: 552–6.
175. Gutniak MK *et al*. Antidiabetogenic effect of glucagon-like peptide-1 (7–36)amide in normal subjects and patients with diabetes mellitus. *N Engl J Med* 1992; **326**: 1316–22.
176. Ørskov L *et al*. GLP-1 does not acutely affect insulin sensitivity in healthy man. *Diabetologia* 1996; **39**: 552–6.
177. Åhren B, Larsson H, Holst JJ. Effects of glucagon-like peptide-1 on islet function and insulin sensitivity in non-insulin-dependent diabetes mellitus. *J Clin Endocrinol Metab* 1997; **82**: 473–78.
178. Wang Y *et al*. Glucagon-like peptide-1 affects gene transcription and messenger ribonucleic acid stability of components of the insulin secretory system in RIN 1046-38 cells. *Endocrinology* 1995; **136**: 4910–17.
179. Thorens B *et al*. Protein kinase A-dependent phosphorylation of GLUT 2 in pancreatic β-cells. *J Biol Chem* 1996; **271**: 8075–81.
180. Beak SA *et al*. Glucagon-like peptide-1 (GLP-1) releases thyrotropin (TSH): characterization of binding sites for GLP-1 on α-TSH cells. *Endocrinology* 1996; **137**: 4130–38.

181. Beak SA *et al*. Glucagon-like peptide-1 stimulates luteinizing hormone-releasing hormone secretion in a rodent hypothalamic neuronal cell line. *J Clin Invest* 1998; **101**: 1334–41.

182. Lamari Y *et al*. Expression of glucagon-like peptide 1 receptor in a murine C cell line: regulation of calcitonin gene by glucagon-like peptide 1. *FEBS Lett* 1996; **393**: 248–52.

183. Shimizu I *et al*. Identification and localization of glucagon-like peptide-1 and its receptor in rat brain. *Endocrinology* 1987; **121**: 1076–82.

184. Kauth T, Metz J. Immunohistochemical localization of glucagon-like peptide 1. Use of poly- and monoclonal antibodies. *Histochemistry* 1987; **86**: 509–15.

185. Kanse SM *et al*. Identification and characterization of glucagon-like peptide-1 7–36 amide-binding sites in the rat brain and lung. *FEBS Lett* 1988; **241**: 209–12.

186. Tang Christensen M *et al*. Central administration of GLP-1-(7–36) amide inhibits food and water intake in rats. *Am J Physiol* 1996; **271**: R848–56.

187. Navarro M *et al*. Colocalization of glucagon-like peptide-1 (GLP-1) receptors, glucose transporter GLUT-2, and glucokinase mRNAs in rat hypothalamic cells: evidence for a role of GLP-1 receptor agonists as an inhibitory signal for food and water intake. *J Neurochem* 1996; **67**: 1982–91.

188. Gutzwiller JP *et al*. Glucagon-like peptide-1 is a physiologic regulator of food intake in humans. *Gastroenterology* 1997; **112**(suppl): A1153.

189. Tseng C-C *et al*. Postprandial stimulation of insulin release by glucose-dependent insulinotropic peptide (GIP). Effect of a specific glucose-dependent insulinotropic polypeptide receptor antagonist in the rat. *J Clin Invest* 1996; **98**: 2440–45.

190. Roberge JN and Brubaker PL. Regulation of intestinal proglucagon-derived peptide secretion by glucose-dependent insulinotropic peptide in a novel enteroendocrine loop. *Endocrinology* 1993; **133**: 233–40.

191. Schirra J *et al*. Exendin (9–39) amide is an antagonist of glucagon-like peptide-1 (7–36) amide in humans. *J Clin Invest* 1998; **101**: 1421–30.

192. Edwards CMB *et al*. GLP-1 has a physiological role in the control of postprandial glucose in man. Studies with the antagonist exendin 9–39. *Diabetes* 1999; **48**: 86–93.

193. Baum F *et al*. Role of endogenously released cholecystokinin in determining postprandial insulin levels in man: effects of loxiglumide, a specific cholecystokinin receptor antagonist. *Digestion* 1992; **53**: 189–99.

194. Ensinck JW *et al*. Effect of ingested carbohydrate, fat, and protein on the release of somatostatin-28 in humans. *Gastroenterology* 1990; **98**: 633–8.

195. Ensinck JW *et al*. Endogenous somatostatin-28 modulates postprandial insulin secretion. Immunoneutralization studies in baboons. *J Clin Invest* 1997; **100**: 2295–302.

196. Clark JDA *et al*., Studies of the entero-insular axis following pancreas transplantation in man: neural or hormonal control? *Diabet Med*, 1989; **6**: 813–17.

197. Nauck MA *et al*. Preserved incretin effect in type 1 diabetic patients with end-stage nephropathy treated by combined heterotopic pancreas and kidney transplantation. *Acta Diabetol* 1993; **30**: 39–45.

198. DeFronzo RA. The triumvirate: ß-cell, muscle and liver. A collusion responsible for NIDDM. *Diabetes* 1988; **37**: 667–87.

199. Crockett SE, Mazzaferri EL, Cataland S. Gastric inhibitory peptide (GIP) in maturity-onset diabetes mellitus. *Diabetes* 1976; **25**: 931–5.

200. Ross SA, Brown JC, J Dupré. Hypersecretion of gastric inhibitory polypeptide following oral glucose in diabetes mellitus. *Diabetes* 1977; **26**: 525–9.

201. May JM, Williams RH. The effect of endogenous gastric inhibitory polypeptide on glucose-induced insulin secretion in mild diabetes. *Diabetes* 1978; **27**: 849–55.

202. Jones IR *et al*. The glucose-dependent insulinotropic polypeptide response to oral glu-cose and mixed meals is increased in patients with type 2 (non-insulin-dependent) diabetes mellitus. *Diabetologia* 1989; **32**: 668–77.

203. Creutzfeldt W, Nauck M. Gut hormones and diabetes mellitus. *Diabet Metab Rev* 1992; **8**: 149–77.

204. Deacon CF, Nauck MA, Meier J, Hucking K, *et al*. Degradation of endogenous and exogenous gastric inhibitory polypeptide in healthy and in type 2 diabetic subjects as revealed using a new assay for the intact peptide *J Clin Endocrinol Metab* 2000; **85**: 3575–81.

205. Ørskov C *et al*. Proglucagon products in plasma of non-insulin-dependent diabetics and nondiabetic controls in the fasting state and after oral glucose and intravenous arginine. *J Clin Invest* 1991; **87**: 415–23.

206. Vilsbøll T *et al*. Reduced postprandial concentrations of intact biologically active glucagon-like peptide 1 in type 2 diabetic patients. *Diabetes* 2001; **50**: 609–13.

207. Amland PF *et al*. Effects of intravenously infused porcine GIP on serum insulin, plasma C-peptide, and pancreatic polypeptide in non-insulin-dependent diabetes in the fasting state. *Scand J Gastroenterol* 1985; **20**: 315–20.

208. Jorde R, Burhol PG. The insulinotropic effect of gastric inhibitory polypeptide in non-insulin-dependent diabetes. *Ital J Gastroenterol* 1987; **19**: 76–8.

209. Jones IR *et al*. The effects of glucose-dependent insulinotropic polypeptide infused at physiological concentrations in normal subjects and type 2 (non-insulin-dependent) dia-betic patients on glucose tolerance and β-cell secretion. *Diabetologia* 1987; **30**: 707–12.

210. Krarup T *et al*. Effect of porcine gastric inhibitory polypeptide on ß-cell function in type 1 and type 2 diabetes mellitus. *Metabolism* 1988; **36**: 677–82.

211. Meier JJ *et al*. Reduced insulinotropic effect of gastric inhibitory polypeptide in first-degree relatives of patients with type 2 diabetes. *Diabetes* 2001; **50**: 2497–504.

212. Gerich JE, Abnormal glucagon secretion in type 2 (non-insulin-dependent) diabetes mellitus: causes and consequences. In Creutzfeldt W, Lefèbvre P (eds), *Diabetes Mel-litus: Pathophysiology and Therapy*. Springer Verlag: Berlin, Heidelberg, 1989; 127–33.

213. Frank JW *et al*. Mechanism of accelerated gastric emptying and hyperglycemia in patients with type 2 diabetes mellitus. *Gastroenterology* 1995; **109**: 755–65.

214. Rahier J, Goebbels RM, and Henquin JC Cellular composition of the human diabetic pancreas. *Diabetologia* 1983; **24**: 366–71.

215. Rahier JRD, Ibrahim M Channaoui K. Islet cell populations in obese subjects and type 2 (non-insulin-dependent) diabetic patients (abstr). *Diabetologia* 1989; **32**(suppl 1): 532A.

216. Ohlson L-O *et al*. The influence of body fat distribution on the incidence of diabetes mellitus. *Diabetes* 1985; **34**: 1055–8.

217. Suzuki S *et al*. Reduced insulinotropic effects of glucagonlike peptide 1-(7–36)-amide and gastric inhibitory polypeptide in isolated perfused diabetic rat pancreas. *Diabetes* 1990; **39**: 1320–25.

218. Elahi D *et al*. The insulinotropic actions of glucose-dependent insulinotropic polypep-tide (GIP) and glucagon-like peptide-1 (7–37) in normal and diabetic subjects. *Regul Pept* 1994; **51**: 63–74.

219. Dupré J *et al*. Glucagon-like peptide 1 reduces postprandial glycemic excursions in IDDM. *Diabetes* 1995; **44**: 626–30.

220. Dupré J *et al*. Subcutaneous glucagon-like peptide 1 combined with insulin normalizes postcibal glycemic excursions in IDDM. *Diabetes Care* 1997; **20**: 381–4.

221. Schwartz JG *et al*. Treatment with an oral proteinase inhibitor slows gastric emptying and acutely reduces glucose and insulin levels after a liquid meal in type II diabetic patients. *Diabetes Care* 1994; **17**: 255–62.

222. Thompson RG *et al.* Pramlintide: a human amylin analogue reduced postprandial plasma glucose, insulin, and C-peptide concentrations in patients with type 2 diabetes. *Diabet Med* 1997; **14**: 547–55.

223. Thompson RG *et al.* Effects of pramlintide, an analog of human amylin, on plasma glucose profiles in patients with IDDM: results of a multicenter trial. *Diabetes* 1997; **46**: 632–6.

224. Torsdottir I *et al.* A small dose of soluble alginate-fiber affects postprandial glycaemia and gastric emptying in humans with diabetes. *J Nutr* 1991; **121**: 795–9.

225. French SJ, Read NW. Effect of guar gum on hunger and satiety after meals of different fat content: relationship with gastric emptying. *Am J Clin Nutr* 1994; **59**: 87–91.

226. Kong M-F *et al.* The effect of single doses of pramlintide on gastric emptying of two meals in IDDM. *Diabetologia* 1998; **41**: 577–83.

227. Kong M-F *et al.* Infusion of pramlintide, a human amylin analogue, delays gastric emptying in men with IDDM. *Diabetologia* 1997; **40**: 82–8.

228. Janes S *et al.* The selection of pramlintide for clinical evaluation. *Diabetes* 1996; **45**(suppl 2): 235A (abstr).

229. Kolterman OG *et al.* Reduction of postprandial hyperglycaemia in subjects with IDDM by intravenous infusion of AC137, a human amylin analogue. *Diabetes Care* 1995; **18**: 1179–82.

230. Thompson RG, Gottlieb AB, Peterson J. The human amylin analogue AC137 reduces mean 24 hour glucose in type 1 diabetes. *Diabetologia* 1995; **38**(suppl 1): A44 (abstr).

231. Schwartz JG *et al.* Treatment with an oral proteinase inhibitor slows gastric emptying and acutely reduces glucose and insulin levels after a liquid meal in type 2 diabetic patients. *Diabetes Care* 1994; **17**: 255–62.

232. Phillips WT, Schwartz JG, McMahan CA. Reduced postprandial blood glucose levels in recently diagnosed non-insulin-dependent diabetics secondary to pharmacologically induced delayed gastric emptying. *Dig Dis Sci* 1993; **38**: 51–8.

233. Phillips WT, Schwartz JG, McMahan CA. Rapid gastric emptying of an oral glucose solution in type 2 diabetic patients. *J Nucl Med* 1992; **33**: 1496–500.

234. Frank JW *et al.* Mechanism of accelerated gastric emptying of liquids and hyperglycaemia in patients with type 2 diabetes mellitus. *Gastroenterology* 1995; **109**: 755–65.

235. Schwartz JG *et al.* Rapid gastric emptying of a solid pancake meal in type 2 diabetic patients. *Diabetes Care* 1996; **19**: 468–71.

236. Kong M-F *et al.* Euglycaemic hyperinsulinaemia does not affect gastric emptying in type 1 and type 2 diabetes mellitus. *Diabetologia* 1999; **42**: 365–72.

237. Qualmann C *et al.* Glucagon-like peptide 1 (7–36 amide) secretion in response to luminal sucrose from the upper and lower gut. A study using α-glucosidase inhibition (acarbose). *Scand J Gastroenterol* 1995; **30**: 892–6.

238. Göke B *et al.* Voglibose (AO-128) is an efficient α-glucosidase inhibitor and mobilizes the endogenous GLP-1 reserve. *Digestion* 1995; **56**: 493–501.

239. Ranganath L *et al.* Delayed gastric emptying occurs following acarbose administration and is a further mechanism for its antihyperglycaemic effect. *Diabet Med* 1998; **15**: 120–24.

240. Rachman J *et al.* Normalization of insulin responses to glucose by overnight infusion of glucagon-like peptide 1 (7–36) amide in patients with NIDDM. *Diabetes* 1996; **45**: 1524–30.

241. Rachman J *et al.* Near-normalization of diurnal glucose concentrations by continuous administration of glucagon-like peptide 1 (GLP-1) in subjects with NIDDM. *Diabetologia* 1997; **40**: 205–211.

242. Drent ML *et al*. Orlistat (RO-18-0647), a lipase inhibitor, in the treatment of human obesity: a multiple dose study. *Int J Obesity* 1995; **19**: 221–6.

243. Willms B *et al*. Overnight GLP-1 normalizes fasting but not daytime plasma glucose values in NIDDM patients. *Exp Clin Endocrinol Diabetes* 1998; **106**: 103–7.

244. Larsen J *et al*. Glucagon-like peptide-1 infusion must be maintained for 24 h/day to obtain acceptable glycemia in type 2 diabetic patients who are poorly controlled on sulphonylurea treatment. *Diabetes Care* 2001; **24**: 1416–21.

245. Juntti-Berggren L *et al*. The antidiabetogenic effect of GLP-1 is maintained during a 7-day treatment period and improves diabetic dislipoproteinemia in NIDDM patients. *Diabetes Care* 1996; **19**: 1200–206.

246. Todd JJ *et al*. Glucagon-like peptide 1: a trial of treatment of non-insulin dependent diabetes mellitus. *Eur J Clin Invest* 1997; **27**: 533–6.

247. Zander M *et al*. Effect of a 6-week course of glucagon-like peptide 1 on glycaemic control, insulin sensitivity, and β-cell function in type 2 diabetes: a parallel group study. *Lancet* 2002; **359**: 824–30.

248. Gutniak MK *et al*. Subcutaneous injection of the incretin hormone glucagon-like peptide 1 abolishes postprandial glycemia in NIDDM. *Diabetes Care* 1994; **17**: 1039–44.

249. Ritzel R *et al*. Pharmacokinetic, insulinotropic, and glucagonostatic properties of GLP-1 (7–36 amide) after subcutaneous injection in healthy volunteers. Dose–response relationships. *Diabetologia* 1995; **38**: 720–25.

250. Nauck MA *et al*. Effects of subcutaneous glucagon-like peptide 1 [GLP-1 (7–36 amide)] in patients with NIDDM. *Diabetologia* 1996; **39**: 1546–53.

251. Johnson OFL *et al*. A month-long effect from a single injection of microencapsulated human growth hormone. *Nature Med* 1996; **2**: 795–9.

252. Mathiowitz E *et al*. Biologically erodable microspheres as potential oral drug delivery systems. *Nature* 1997; **386**: 410–14.

253. Deacon CF *et al*. Dipeptidyl peptidase IV resistant analogues of glucagon-like peptide-1 which have extended metabolic stability and improved biological activity. *Diabetologia* 1998; **41**: 271–8.

254. Juhl CB *et al*. Bedtime administration of NN2211, a long-acting GLP-1 derivative, substantially reduces fasting and postprandial glycemia in type 2 diabetes. *Diabetes* 2002; **51**: 424–9.

255. Wrighton NC *et al*. Small peptide as potent mimetics of the protein hormone erythropoietin. *Science* 1996; **273**: 458–63.

256. Gutniak MK *et al*. Potential therapeutic levels of glucagon-like peptide 1 achieved in humans by a buccal tablet. *Diabetes Care* 1996; **19**: 843–8.

257. Raufman JP *et al*. Truncated glucagon-like peptide-1 interacts with exendin receptors on dispersed acini from guinea pig pancreas. Identification of a mammalian analogue of the reptilian peptide exendin-4. *J Biol Chem* 1992; **267**: 21432–7.

258. Eng J *et al*. Isolation and characterization of exendin-4, an exendin-3 analogue, from *Heloderma suspectum* venom. Further evidence for an exendin receptor on dispersed acini from guinea pig pancreas. *J Biol Chem* 1992; **267**: 7402–5.

259. Young AA, Gedulin BR, Rink TJ Dose–responses for the slowing of gastric emptying in a rodent model by glucagon-like peptide (7–36) NH_2, amylin, cholecystokinin, and other possible regulators of nutrient uptake. *Metabolism* 1996; **45**: 1–3.

260. Edwards CMB *et al*. Exendin-4 reduces fasting and postprandial glucose and decreases energy intake in healthy volunteers. *Am J Physiol* 2001; **281**: E155–61.

261. Deacon CF, Highes TE, Holst JJ. Dipeptidyl peptidase IV inhibition potentiates the insulinotropic effect of glucagon-like peptide 1 in the anesthetized pig. *Diabetes* 1998; **47**: 764–9.

262. Balkan B *et al.* Sustained improvement of glucose tolerance by DPP-IV inhibition after chronic treatment with NVP-DPP728 (abstr). *Diabetologia* 1999; **42**(suppl 1): A41.

263. Åhren B *et al.* Inhibition of dipeptidyl peptidase IV improves metabolic control over a 4-week study period in type 2 diabetes. *Diabetes Care* 2002; **25**: 869–75.

264. Bell GI. The glucagon superfamily: precursor structure and gene organization. *Peptides* 1986; **7**(suppl 1): 27–36.

265. Irwin DM. Ancient duplications of the human proglucagon gene. *Genomics* 2002; **79**: 741–6.

266. Drucker DJ, Brubaker PL. Proglucagon gene expression is regulated by a cyclic AMP-dependent pathway in rat intestine. *Proc Natl Acad Sci USA* 1989; **86**: 3953–7.

267. Stoffel M *et al.* Human glucagon-like peptide-1 receptor gene. Localization to chromosome band 6p21 by fluorescence *in situ* hybridization and linkage of a highly polymorphic simple tandem repeat DNA polymorphism to other markers on chromosome 6. *Diabetes* 1993; **42**: 1215–18.

9

Evaluation of Gastrointestinal Autonomic Function

Miriam Thumshirn and Michael Camilleri

Introduction

The autonomic nervous system is involved in the modulation of normal gastrointestinal function. It consists of an extrinsic control, exerted by the parasympathetic and sympathetic nervous system, and an intrinsic control imposed by the enteric plexuses (the 'little brain' in the digestive tract) (Figure 9.1). Sympathetic input to the enteric nervous system (ENS) facilitates contraction (α-fibres) or relaxation (β-fibres) of sphincteric muscles and inhibits non-sphincteric muscles. In addition, norepinephrine (noradrenaline) released from sympathetic nerve fibres inhibits submucosal secretomotor neurons directly. Activation of parasympathetic efferent nerves results in excitation of non-sphincteric smooth muscles and has a stimulatory effect on secretion in the gastrointestinal tract. The ENS, an integrated neural network within the walls of the digestive tract, is semi-autonomous and possesses specific programmes for motor responses (such as peristaltic reflexes) and a regional rate of contractions. The latter is generated by a self-excitable electrical syncytium consisting of the interstitial cells of

Gastrointestinal Function in Diabetes Mellitus. Edited by Michael Horowitz and Melvin Samsom
© 2004 John Wiley & Sons, Ltd   ISBN: 0-471-89916-X

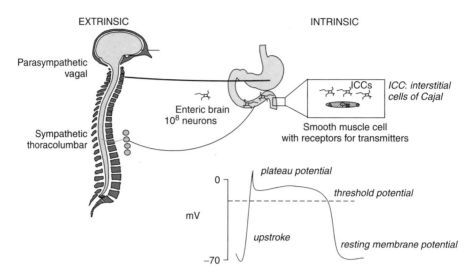

Figure 9.1   Control of gastrointestinal motility. Note the extrinsic or autonomic nervous system modulates the function of the enteric nervous system, which controls smooth muscle cells through transmitters. Adapted from Camilleri and Phillips [35] with permission

Cajal, which function as a pacemaker system. Current evidence indicates that the extrinsic nervous system has a predominantly modulatory role, with primary control through the ENS [1]. The integration of the central nervous system, parasympathetic and sympathetic nerves and the ENS results in integrated activity in different regions of the gut and coordination of digestive tract activity with that of other organs. Thus, derangements of the extrinsic nerves at any level may result in disordered gastrointestinal motility and secretion [2].

As discussed in other chapters, the aetiology of gastrointestinal dysfunction in diabetes mellitus appears to be multifactorial. Potential causes include vagal nerve dysfunction (autovagotomy), sympathetic and enteric nerve damage, and the direct effects of hyperglycaemia on the autonomic nervous system.

Vagal dysfunction (both 'reversible' and 'irreversible') is probably critical in the pathophysiology of diabetic gastroenteropathy. This is supported by the observation that the vagally-mediated acid secretion that occurs in response to sham feeding is frequently attenuated in diabetes [3]. The rapid small bowel transit, evident in some patients, may be due to vagotomy or loss of the sympathetically mediated 'brake' of the small intestine. Whereas parasympathetic denervation is likely to be important in the aetiology of constipation, sympathetic dysfunction may contribute to stool incontinence by reducing resting anal tone. The majority of studies have found that disordered gut motor function occurs more frequently in those patients with evidence of autonomic nerve function (usually assessed by cardiovascular reflex tests); however, the association is certainly not strong. This may, potentially, be because gastrointestinal autonomic function was not evaluated in most cases. As discussed in Chapter 4, acute changes in the blood glucose concentration have reversible effects on both gut motility and autonomic nerve function. For example, acute hyperglycaemia slows gastric emptying in patients with type 1 diabetes mellitus [4] and retards small intestinal transit [5]. In the colon, acute hyperglycaemia inhibits the colonic reflex response to gastric distension [6].

As discussed in Chapter 2, animal models of diabetes have revealed a number of morphological changes in the autonomic nerve supply to the gut. In contrast, the human studies which are more limited have yielded inconsistent observations. While histopathological studies have in some cases revealed substantial changes in vagal nerve morphology in diabetes mellitus, including a reduction in the density of unmyelinated axons and a smaller calibre of surviving axons [7], other studies have provided little evidence of a fixed pathologic process in neural tissue [8]. Abnormalities in the sympathetic nervous system have been reported in patients with diabetes-related diarrhoea and postural hypotension with giant sympathetic neurons, dendritic swelling of postganglionic neurons in prevertebral and paravertebral ganglia, and reduced fibre density in the splanchnic nerves [9]. A recent case report of a patient with long-standing type 1 diabetes demonstrated a marked decrease in interstitial cell of Cajal (ICC) volume and absence of the ICC network within the circular smooth muscle layer of the small intestine. A defect at the level of ICCs would be expected to have substantial effects on gastrointestinal motility by resulting in decreased inhibitory, and increased excitatory, innervation [10].

As well as morphological changes, disturbances in neurotransmitter expression within the ENS may play a critical role in diabetes-related gastrointestinal dysmotility. As discussed in Chapter 2, animal studies have provided evidence of reductions in neuronal nitric oxide synthesis (nNOS) expression and nitric oxide (NO)-mediated relaxation of gastric muscle strips in diabetes [11,12]. The defects in nNOS expression were apparently confined to the gastrointestinal tract, and the decreased expression of nNOS, as well as the decreased gastric emptying observed, were both corrected by administration of the phosphodiesterase type 5 inhibitor, sildenafil, which acts as a NO donor [13]. The concept of a role for NO mechanisms in disease is also supported by limited human data [10].

Evaluation of autonomic function

In the evaluation of patients with diabetes who have gastrointestinal symptoms, it is rarely necessary to test autonomic function formally, since the information is unlikely to lead to substantial alterations in either investigation or therapy. In particular, the outcome of such tests should not be used as a surrogate for formal investigation of gastrointestinal function. It also remains to be established whether the outcome of tests for autonomic function has predictive value for either prognosis of symptoms (e.g. chronicity or risk of recurrence) or the response to pharmacological therapy (e.g. prokinetic drugs), although there are data to suggest that this may be the case [13].

While autonomic function tests can identify disturbances in the extrinsic neurologic control of the viscera [14], there are, regrettably, very few tests that specifically assess the autonomic innervation to the gastrointestinal tract. The suggestion that in conditions such as diabetes mellitus, which are associated with length-dependent neuropathy, abnormal cardiovascular reflexes are an excellent predictor of dysfunction of the abdominal vagus and provide a good evaluation of the overall function of the autonomic supply to the abdominal viscera [3] requires additional confirmation.

The clinical evaluation of patients for autonomic dysfunction should start with a careful review of symptoms. Several symptoms, including postural dizziness, lack of sweating, failure of erection or ejaculation, difficulty with bladder emptying or recurrent urinary tract infections, and dryness of the eyes, mouth or vagina, may be indicative of autonomic dysfunction (Table 9.1). An infrequently sought symptom in patients with diabetes is gustatory sweating of the face, which reflects parasympathetic denervation [15]. Postprandial hypotension, which is distinct from orthostatic hypotension, occurs frequently in patients with diabetic autonomic neuropathy and may result in syncope and falls.

Laboratory tests

The aims of laboratory evaluation of sympathetic and parasympathetic function are to detect autonomic failure, determine its distribution, quantitate its severity, and identify the autonomic system involved (e.g. sudomotor, adrenergic, cardiovagal). The tests of autonomic function can be subdivided into three categories: (a) sympathetic adrenergic tests; (b) sympathetic cholinergic tests; and (c) vagal tests.

Table 9.2 shows a list of the autonomic function tests that are commonly performed in autonomic reflex laboratories. There are a number of pitfalls in

Table 9.1 Symptoms and signs suggestive of autonomic dysfunction

Sympathetic	Parasympathetic
Failure of pupils to dilate in the dark	Fixed dilated pupils
Fainting, orthostatic dizziness	Lack of pupillary accommodation
Constant heart rate with orthostatic hypotension	Sweating during mastication of certain foods
Absent piloerection	Decreased gut motility
Absent sweating	Dry eyes and mouth
Impaired ejaculation	Dry vagina
Paralysis of dartos muscle	Impaired erection
	Difficulty with emptying urinary bladder; recurrent urinary tract infections

Adapted from Camilleri [2].

Table 9.2 Commonly performed autonomic nervous function tests

Test	Physiological functions tested	Rationale	Comments/ PITFALLS
Sympathetic function			
Thermoregulatory sweat test (% surface area of anhydrosis)	Preganglionic and postganglionic cholinergic	Stimulation of hypothalamic temperature control centres	Cumbersome, whole body test
Quantitative sudomotor axon reflex test (sweat output, latency)	Postganglionic cholinergic	Antidromic stimulation of peripheral fibre by axonal flex	Needs specialized facilities
Heart rate and blood pressure responses			
Orthostatic tilt test	Adrenergic	Baroreceptor reflex	Impaired responses if intravascular volume is reduced
Postural adjustment ratio	Adrenergic	Baroreceptor reflex	Impaired responses if intravascular volume is reduced
Cold pressor test	Adrenergic	Baroreceptor reflex	Impaired responses if intravascular volume is reduced
Sustained hand grip	Adrenergic	Baroreceptor reflex	Impaired responses if intravascular volume is reduced
Plasma norepinephrine response to:			
Postural changes	Postganglionic adrenergic	Baroreceptor stimulation	Moderate sensitivity, impaired response if intravascular volume is reduced
Intravenous edrophonium	Postganglionic adrenergic	Anticholinesterase 'stimulates' postganglionic fibre at prevertebral ganglia	False negatives caused by contributions to plasma norepinephrine from many organs
Parasympathetic function			
Heart rate (RR) variation with deep breathing	Parasympathetic	Vagal afferents stimulated by lung stretch	Best cardiovagal test available, but not a test of abdominal vagus
Supine/erect heart rate	Parasympathetic	Vagal stimulation by change in central blood volume	Cardiovagal test
Valsalva ratio (heart rate, maximum/ minimum)	Parasympathetic	Vagal stimulation by change in central blood volume	Cardiovagal test

(*continued overleaf*)

Table 9.2   (*continued*)

Test	Physiological functions tested	Rationale	Comments/ PITFALLS
Gastric acid secretory or plasma pancreatic polypeptide response to modified sham feeding or hypoglycaemia	Parasympathetic	Stimulation of vagal nuclei by sham feeding or hypoglycaemia	Abdominal vagal test, critically dependent on avoidance of swallowing food during test
Nocturnal penile tumescence	Pelvic parasympathetic	Integrity of S_{2-4}	Plethysmographic technique requiring special facilities
Cystometrographic response to bethanechol	Pelvic parasympathetic	Increase in intravesical pressure suggests postganglionic denervation supersensitivity	Tests parasympathetic supply to bladder, not bowel

From Camilleri and Ford [14] with permission.

the application and interpretation of autonomic function tests, e.g. tests of sympathetic adrenergic function are critically dependent on the state of hydration of the patient, which may be particularly important in patients with diabetes. Thus, patients must be adequately hydrated before testing sympathetic adrenergic function. Attention should also be paid to the potential interference with autonomic function tests of medical therapy given for other conditions—medications including benzodiazepines (used as sedatives or anxiolytics), β-adrenergic antagonists and α_2-agonists (for treatment of hypertension) or α_1-antagonists (for treatment of bladder outlet obstruction), and 'over-the-counter' cough and cold medications should be stopped several days prior to testing (for a duration of at least five times the half-life of the specific medication).

Sympathetic adrenergic tests

Cardiovascular tests [14]

Orthostatic hypotension   In response to a head-up tilt at 80° to the horizontal, a decline in systolic or diastolic blood pressure without a compensatory increase in pulse rate is indicative of sympathetic adrenergic dysfunction. Upright tilt normally results in a transient reduction in systolic, mean and diastolic blood pressure, followed by recovery of normal blood pressure within 1 min. The blood pressure response to tilt is entirely dependent upon sympathetic adrenergic function; the fall should normally be less than 25 mmHg in systolic and 15 mmHg in diastolic blood pressure. Adrenergic sympathetic dysfunction is characterised by a marked reduction in blood pressure on upright tilt and absence of recovery. A similar measurement is the postural adjustment ratio, in which arterial blood pressure is measured with the arm in different positions relative to the level of the heart.

Valsalva manoeuvre   Heart rate and blood pressure responses are evaluated during forced expiration against a closed glottis. For the Valsalva manoeuvre, the patient is in a rested and recumbent position and is asked to blow into the tubing of a sphygmomanometer to maintain the column of mercury at 40–50 mmHg for 15–20 s. The Valsalva manoeuvre has several components, including a sympathetic adrenergic component that maintains the blood pressure response. The change in pulse rate during phase IV (after cessation of forced expiration) in the Valsalva manoeuvre is a vagally-mediated parasympathetic response (see below). Thus, the Valsalva manoeuvre cannot be regarded as a pure sympathetic test; it evaluates predominantly sympathetic adrenergic function, but is also dependent on intact vagal innervation. In phase II, forced expiration against a closed glottis results in reduction in venous return to the central circulation, thereby decreasing blood pressure and cardiac output. A sympathetically mediated, compensatory tachycardia normally serves to maintain cardiac output and this can be detected accurately as a shortening of the interval between successive QRS complexes on the electrocardiogram. During phase IV of the manoeuvre (i.e. following cessation of forced expiration) the glottis is open and venous return and cardiac output are restored, resulting in an overshoot of the blood pressure and compensatory bradycardia. The 'Valsalva ratio' refers to the comparison of parameters during phases II and IV. In autonomic dysfunction, the phase IV responses of blood pressure overshoot and the compensatory bradycardia is typically lost.

Measurement of plasma norepinephrine   Sympathetic adrenergic function can be assessed by measurement of plasma norepinephrine (noradrenaline) in the supine and standing postures, or in response to intravenous (i.v.) edrophonium [16]. When the patient is supine, a low plasma norepinephrine concentration suggests a postganglionic sympathetic adrenergic lesion. Failure of the plasma norepinephrine level to increase when the patient stands up is suggestive of either a preganglionic or postganglionic sympathetic disturbance.

Another test of the sympathetic postganglionic adrenergic fibre is the plasma norepinephrine response to i.v. edrophonium. Administration of the short-acting anticholinesterase, edrophonium induces a transient increase of endogenous cholinergic activity in the prevertebral sympathetic ganglia by rapid and short-lived inhibition of acetylcholinesterase. This results in a rapid release of norepinephrine from the postganglionic sympathetic fibres into the plasma, which can be detected in blood samples taken every 1 or 2 min over a period of 10 min. However, the plasma norepinephrine response is not a sensitive measure of sympathetic abdominal innervation because there is a significant contribution to plasma norepinephrine levels from other vascular beds, particularly the pulmonary circulation and kidneys [17].

Superior mesenteric arterial (SMA) blood flow   The SMA blood flow is under baroreflex control. Measurement of SMA blood flow by duplex ultrasonography is a non-invasive and reproducible test of abdominal sympathetic function [18,19]. These are technically demanding studies that are operator-dependent and not routinely available. In our laboratory, changes in SMA blood flow are assessed during the following perturbations: autonomic stress with the cold pressor test, upright tilt, and the combination of upright tilt and meal ingestion. Impaired regulation of splanchnic–mesenteric vascular resistance and blood pooling are probably important in the development of orthostatic and postprandial hypotension in patients with autonomic failure. In a group of patients with neurogenic orthostatic hypotension predominantly associated with diabetic autonomic neuropathy, we reported that different patterns of SMA blood flow and resistance can be assessed by performing a tilt test in the postprandial period [19] (Figure 9.2). Normally, systemic arterial pressure is maintained despite the marked (2–3.5-fold) increase in SMA blood flow postprandially, as a result of compensatory contraction of the peripheral vasculature. Autonomic failure is characterized by a negative correlation between the rise of postprandial SMA blood flow and the fall of postprandial blood pressure (Figure 9.3). Thus, during the postprandial period, the increase in SMA blood flow is less in some patients in whom there is not a decrease in systemic pressure. On the

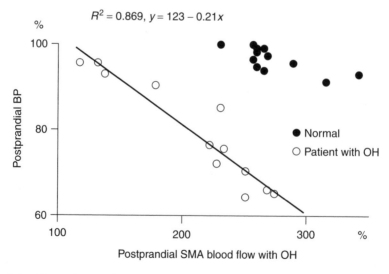

Figure 9.2   Change in superior mesenteric artery blood flow after meal and tilt. OH, orthostatic hypotension. From Fujimura *et al.* [19], with permission

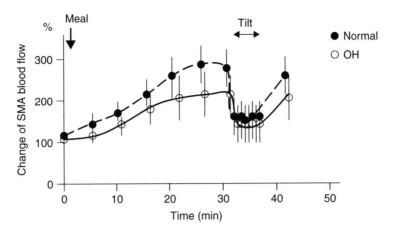

Figure 9.3   Correlation between the rise in postprandial superior mesenteric artery blood flow and the fall in postprandial blood pressure. Note that, in healthy subjects, systemic arterial pressure is maintained postprandially despite the marked increase in SMA blood flow during the digestive phase. OH, orthostatic hypotension. From Fujimura *et al.* [19], with permission

other hand, those with a more normal increase in SMA blood flow develop severe systemic hypotension postprandially, since they are unable to constrict their vascular beds. It appears, therefore, that monitoring systemic arterial pressure during postprandial SMA blood flow studies enhances interpretation of the observations. The sensitivity and specificity of this test relative to other evidence of sympathetic adrenergic dysfunction requires further elucidation.

Rectal mucosal blood flow

Emmanuel and Kamm have reported that measurement of rectal mucosal blood flow is highly reproducible (coefficient of variation 0.05–0.06) and responsive to physiological perturbations, such as eating and ovulatory status, and to autonomically active drugs and nerve stimulation [20]. The procedure involves placement of a laser Doppler flow meter probe into the rectum via a rigid sigmoidoscope. This probe measures the frequency shift in light reflected from a moving object which, in tissue, predominantly arises from red blood cells. The principle is similar to measurements of skin vasomotor reflex using skin Doppler [21]. Tissue measurements of blood flow by Doppler, including transcranial Doppler sonography [22], are currently used to measure general autonomic control in conditions such as orthostatic hypotension. The application of rectal mucosal blood flow measurements in disease has also been proposed [23]. Baseline rectal mucosal blood is less in patients with slow transit than those with normal transit constipation. Moreover, the magnitude of the reduction in flow induced by inhalation of the muscarinic antagonist, ipratropium, is less in slow transit constipation than in normal transit constipation [23]. These data suggest that cholinergic neural input to the colon may be reduced in slow transit constipation; in contrast, sympathetic β_2 stimulation had no effect, either in health or in patients with constipation. The role of rectal mucosal blood flow testing in disease states, including diabetes, requires further study.

Sympathetic cholinergic tests

Sweat tests

Thermoregulatory sweat test [14]   This test identifies the area of the body with anhydrosis after the whole body is covered with alizarin red powder and the patient exposed to an environment of 44–50°C and 40–50% relative humidity for up to 30 min. Normally, < 5% body surface area should be anhydrotic. An increase in core body temperature of 1°C is required. An abnormal increase in the area of anhydrosis is indicative of a lesion at any site from the hypothalamic temperature control centre to the sweat gland in the skin. Thus, abnormal sweating may result from either preganglionic or postganglionic sympathetic dysfunction, or from a disease of sweat glands.

Quantitative sudomotor axon reflex test (QSART)   The quantitative evaluation of the latency, output and duration of sweating following iontophoresis of acetylcholine into the skin evaluates the integrity of postganglionic cholinergic sympathetic function [24]. In most autonomic function laboratories, responses are recorded from the forearm and three lower extremity sites (the lateral proximal aspect of the leg, the medial distal aspect of the leg, and the proximal portion of the foot over the extensor digitorum brevis muscle). This is also a sensitive test of peripheral nerve function. The response to iontophoresis of acetylcholine into the skin is recorded in a compartment of a multicompartmental sweat cell that is physically separated from the stimulus compartment, where the small electrical current is applied to transfer the charged molecules of acetylcholine into the skin. This test stimulates an axon reflex; if the postganglionic cholinergic sympathetic neuron is intact (Figure 9.4), the impulse from iontophoresed acetylcholine stimulates the peripheral axon antidromically; this subsequently stimulates the axon of the neighbouring skin so that sweat glands are stimulated to produce sweat, which is measured for latency and output. The QSART is a sensitive and reproducible test of peripheral autonomic dysfunction in patients with diabetic neuropathy [24].

Vagal tests

Two types of test are commonly performed to assess vagal function [14].

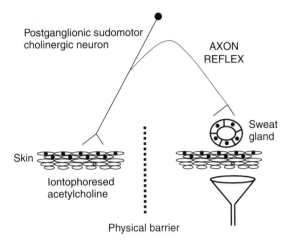

Figure 9.4 Quantitative sudomotor axon reflex test. Iontophoresed acetylcholine stimulates the postganglionic nerve antidromically to set up a reflex stimulation of physically separated sweat glands

Cardiovagal tests

Heart rate (R wave to R wave) response to deep breathing and Valsalva ratio

Inflation and deflation of the lungs stimulate vagal afferents that change the pulse rate reflexly through vagal efferents. Thus, reductions in pulse rate occur with inspiration, and increases accompany expiration. During deep breathing (6 breaths/min), the interval between successive R waves on the electrocardiogram (RR interval) and the induction of vagovagal reflex bradycardia are determined. Impairment of pulse rate variations (oscillations) is indicative of vagal dysfunction. It should be recognised that the magnitude of these oscillations is related to both the position and age of the patient, as well as the rate of breathing, and caution is needed in interpreting this test if the testing protocol is not standardized and the age-related normal values are not provided. A variant measurement to the absolute change in heart rate is the '30:15 ratio', in which the heart rate response to standing is evaluated by comparing RR intervals around the 30th and 15th beats after standing [25,26].

As discussed, the Valsalva ratio is derived from the longest (usually in phase IV) and the shortest (usually in phase II) RR interval on the electrocardiogram during the Valsalva manoeuvre. A reduced index indicates parasympathetic dysfunction.

The spectrum of pulse interval variations can be analysed by power spectral methods. Thus, the more sophisticated power spectral analysis of the respiratory-related and non-respiratory-related peaks provides information about the autonomic nervous system. As expected, the respiratory peak (> 0.1 Hz) reflects vagal function; the non-respiratory peak provides information about sympathetic function, but is also dependent on vagal tone [27,28]. This adaptation is used mostly as a research tool [29]; however, it is important to emphasise that the more sophisticated spectral analysis studies do not permit an unequivocal assessment of vagal vs. sympathetic function. Moreover, the heart rate spectral components may be less than ideal surrogates for *abdominal* sympathetic and parasympathetic tone, since central control of vasomotor and gastrointestinal functions may be independently regulated [30].

Test of abdominal vagal function

Plasma pancreatic polypeptide response to sham feeding (Figure 9.5)

The plasma pancreatic polypeptide response during 30 min of modified sham feeding, i.e. chewing and spitting a sandwich, measures abdominal vagal function. Blood samples for pancreatic polypeptide are collected into chilled ethylenediamine tetra-acetic acid (EDTA) tubes, once at baseline before sham feeding, and then at regular intervals over 30 min during the sham feeding. Plasma concentrations of pancreatic polypeptide are determined by radioimmunoassay [31]. An increase from baseline of > 25 pg/ml is considered normal [32,33]; failure of plasma pancreatic polypeptide levels to increase by > 25 pg/ml after modified sham feeding suggests abdominal vagal dysfunction. Other laboratories

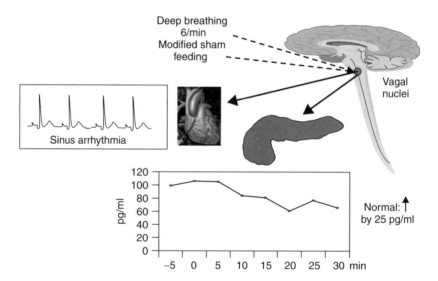

Figure 9.5   Abdominal vagal function test. Modified sham feeding stimulates the vagal nuclei which, in turn, stimulate pancreatic acinar D cells to secrete pancreatic polypeptide. This is reflected by a change in circulating levels of the hormone (normally, a change of > 25 pg/ml)

assess the pancreatic polypeptide response to insulin-induced hypoglycaemia, which stimulates the vagal nuclei directly.

The composite autonomic scoring scale

In the autonomic reflex laboratory at the Mayo Clinic, we frequently use a quantitative composite score [34] to describe the severity of autonomic failure and to follow the progression of disease and the response to therapy. The composite autonomic scoring scale spans a 10-point scale from 0 = normal to 10 = autonomic failure, and is based on the autonomic reflex screen, which includes evaluation of the sympathetic cholinergic function (the quantitative sudomotor axon reflex), cardiovagal function (the heart rate response to deep breathing and the Valsalva ratio), and sympathetic adrenergic function (the beat-to-beat blood pressure measurements in response to tilt and the Valsalva manoeuvre). The severity scale of the autonomic test is semiquantitative and equates to 0 = normal, 1 = mild, 2 = moderate and 3 = severe for cardiovagal and sympathetic cholinergic function. Adrenergic dysfunction is scored maximally at 4.

Conclusion

Autonomic function tests are usually applied in clinical practice at centres where the Neurology Department has interest in these tests; they serve to some extent as surrogates for visceral extrinsic neural dysfunctions if gastrointestinal motility tests are not available. However, the recent development of non-invasive and accurate motility tests, scintigraphy, breath tests and ultrasonography has reduced this need. The careful assessment of symptoms referable to autonomic dysfunction is essential. While there are several sophisticated and detailed autonomic tests available, the heart period response to deep breathing or standing, and blood pressure response to tilt, are the easiest tests to perform and are generally available in most centres. It remains to be established whether the outcome of these tests provides information that is of prognostic value in patients with gastrointestinal dysmotilities, including diabetes.

References

1. Wood JD. Enteric neurophysiology. *Am J Physiol* 1984; **247**: 6585–98.
2. Camilleri M. Disorders of gastrointestinal motility in neurologic disease. *Mayo Clin Proc* 1990; **65**: 825–46.
3. Buysschaert M, Donckier J, Dive A, Ketelslegers J-M, Lambert AE. Gastric acid and pancreatic polypeptide responses to sham feeding are impaired in diabetic subjects with autonomic neuropathy. *Diabetes* 1985; **34**: 1181–5.

4. Fraser RJ, Horowitz M, Maddox AF, Harding PE *et al*. Hyperglycaemia slows gastric emptying in type 1 (insulin-dependent) diabetes mellitus. *Diabetologia* 1990; **33**: 675–80.

5. Russo A, Fraser R, Horowitz M. The effect of acute hyperglycaemia on small intestinal motility in normal subjects. *Diabetologia* 1996; **39**: 984–989.

6. Sims MA, Hasler WL, Chey WD, Kim MS, Owyang C. Hyperglycemia inhibits mechanoreceptor-mediated gastrocolonic responses and colonic peristaltic reflexes in healthy humans. *Gastroenterology* 1995; **108**: 350–59.

7. Guy RJ, Dawson JL, Garrett JR, Laws JW *et al*. Diabetic gastroparesis from autonomic neuropathy: surgical considerations and changes invagus nerve morphology. *J Neurol Neurosurg Psychiat* 1984; **47**: 686–91.

8. Yoshida MM, Shuffler MD, Sumi MS. There are no morphological abnormalities of the gastric wall or abdominal vagus in patients with gastroparesis. *Gastroenterology* 1988; **94**: 907–14.

9. Low PA, Walsh JC, Huang CY, Mcleod JG. The sympathetic nervous system in diabetic neuropathy: a clinical and pathological study. *Brain* 1975; **98**: 341–56.

10. He CL, Soffer EE, Ferris CD, Walsh RM *et al*. Loss of interstitial cells of Cajal and inhibitory innervation in insulin-dependent diabetes. *Gastroenterology* 2001; **121**: 427–34.

11. Wrzos HF, Cruz A, Polavarapu R, Shearer D, Ouyang A. Nitric oxide synthase (NOS) expression in the myenteric plexus of streptozotocin-diabetic rats. *Dig Dis Sci* 1997; **42**: 2106–10.

12. Watkins CC, Sawa A, Jaffrey S, Blackshaw S *et al*. Insulin restores neuronal nitric oxide synthase expression and function that is lost in diabetic gastropathy. *J Clin Invest* 2000; **106**: 373–84.

13. Camilleri M, Balm RK, Zinsmeister AR. Determinants of response to a prokinetic agent in neuropathic chronic intestinal motility disorder. *Gastroenterology* 1994; **106**: 916–23.

14. Camilleri M, Ford MJ. Functional gastrointestinal disease and the autonomic nervous system: a way ahead? *Gastroenterology* 1994; **106**: 1114–18.

15. Shaw JE, Parker R, Hollis S, Gokal R, Boulton AJ. Gustatory sweating in diabetes mellitus. *Diabet Med* 1996; **13**: 1033–7.

16. Leveston SA, Shah SD, Cryer PE. Cholinergic stimulation of norepinephrine release in man. *J Clin Invest* 1979; **64**: 374–80.

17. Esler M, Jennings G, Lambert G, Meredith I *et al*. Overflow of catecholamine neurotransmitter to the circulation: source, fate and functions. *Physiol Rev* 1990; **70**: 963–85.

18. Chaudhuri KR, Thomaides T, Mathias CJ. Abnormality of superior mesenteric artery blood flow responses in human sympathetic failure. *J Physiol (Lond)* 1992; **457**: 477–89.

19. Fujimura J, Camilleri M, Low PA, Novak V *et al*. Effect of perturbations and a meal on superior mesenteric artery flow in patients with orthostatic hypotension. *J Auton Nerv Syst* 1997; **67**: 15–23.

20. Emmanuel AV, Kamm MA. Laser Doppler measurement of rectal mucosal blood flow. *Gut* 1999; **45**: 64–9.

21. Low PA, Neumann C, Dyck PJ, Fealey RD, Tuck RR. Evaluation of skin vasomotor reflexes by using laser Doppler velocimetry. *Mayo Clin Proc* 1983; **58**: 583–92.

22. Novak V, Novak P, Spies JM, Low PA. Autoregulation of cerebral blood flow in orthostatic hypotension. *Stroke* 1998; **29**: 104–11.

23. Emmanuel AV, Kamm MA. Laser Doppler flowmetry as a measure of extrinsic colonic innervation in functional bowel disease. *Gut* 2000; **46**: 212–17.

24. Low PA, Zimmerman BR, Dyck PJ. Comparison of distal sympathetic with vagal function in diabetic neuropathy. *Muscle Nerve* 1986; **9**: 592–6.

25. Ewing DJ, Campbell IW, Murray A, Neilson JM, Clarke BF. Immediate heart-rate response to standing: simple test for autonomic neuropathy in diabetes. *Br Med J* 1978; **1**: 145–7.

26. Ewing DJ, Clarke BF. Diagnosis and management of diabetic autonomic neuropathy. *Br Med J Clin Res Ed* 1982; **285**: 916–18.

27. Novak P, Novak V. Time-frequency mapping of the heart rate, blood pressure and respiratory signals. *Med Biol Eng Comput* 1993; **31**: 103–10.

28. Novak V, Novak P, De Champlain J, Le Blanc AR *et al.* Influence of respiration on heart rate and blood pressure fluctuations. *J Appl Physiol* 1993; **74**: 617–26.

29. Bharucha AE, Novak V, Camilleri M, Zinsmeister AR *et al.* α_2-Adrenergic modulation of colonic tone during hyperventilation. *Am J Physiol* 1997; **273**: G1135–40.

30. Janig W, McLachlan EM. Specialized functional pathways are the building blocks of the autonomic nervous system. *J Auton Nerv Syst* 1992; **41**: 3–13.

31. Koch MB, Go VLW, DiMagno EP. Can plasma human pancreatic polypeptide be used to detect disease of the exocrine pancreas? *Mayo Clin Proc* 1985; **60**: 259–65.

32. Taylor I, Feldman M, Richardson C, Walsh J. Gastric and cephalic stimulation of human pancreatic polypeptide release. *Gastroenterology* 1978; **75**: 432–7.

33. Camilleri M, Balm RK, Low PA. Autonomic dysfunction in patients with chronic intestinal pseudo-obstruction. *Clin Auton Res* 1993; **3**: 95–100.

34. Low PA. Composite autonomic scoring scale for laboratory quantification of generalized autonomic failure. *Mayo Clin Proc* 1993; **68**: 748–52.

35. Camilleri M, Phillips SF. Disorders of small intestinal motility. In Ouyang A (ed.), *Motility Disorders*. Gastroenterology Clinics of North America, Vol. 18. W. B. Saunders: Philadelphia, PA, 1989; 405–24.

INDEX

Gastrointestinal Function in Diabetes Mellitus.   Edited by Michael Horowitz and Melvin Samsom
© 2004 John Wiley & Sons, Ltd   ISBN: 0-471-89916-X